Handbook of Urology

Handbook of Urology

Edited by

J. Kellogg Parsons, MD, MHS, FACS
Associate Professor of Urology
Moores Comprehensive Cancer Center
UC San Diego Health System
La Jolla, CA, USA

John B. Eifler, MD
Resident, Urological Surgery
The James Buchanan Brady Urological Institute and Department of Urology
The Johns Hopkins School of Medicine
Baltimore, MD, USA

Misop Han, MD, MS
Associate Professor of Urology and Oncology
The James Buchanan Brady Urological Institute and Department of Urology
The Johns Hopkins School of Medicine
Baltimore, MD, USA

WILEY Blackwell

Wiley-Blackwell is an imprint of John Wiley & Sons, formed by the merger of Wiley's global Scientific, Technical and Medical business with Blackwell Publishing.

Registered office: John Wiley & Sons, Ltd, The Atrium, Southern Gate, Chichester, West Sussex, PO19 8SQ, UK

Editorial offices: 9600 Garsington Road, Oxford, OX4 2DQ, UK
The Atrium, Southern Gate, Chichester, West Sussex, PO19 8SQ, UK
111 River Street, Hoboken, NJ 07030-5774, USA

For details of our global editorial offices, for customer services and for information about how to apply for permission to reuse the copyright material in this book please see our website at www.wiley.com/wiley-blackwell

Library of Congress Cataloging-in-Publication Data
Handbook of urology / edited by J. Kellogg Parsons, John B. Eifler, Misop Han.
p. ; cm.
Includes bibliographical references and index.
ISBN 978-0-470-67256-3 (softback : alk. paper) – ISBN 978-1-118-71373-0 (Pub) –
ISBN 978-1-118-71374-7 (PDF) – ISBN 978-1-118-71375-4 (Mobi) – ISBN 978-1-118-71376-1
I. Parsons, J. Kellogg. II. Eifler, John B. III. Han, Misop.
[DNLM: 1. Urologic Diseases–Handbooks. 2. Female Urogenital Diseases–Handbooks.
3. Male Urogenital Diseases–Handbooks. WJ 39]
RC871
616.6–dc23

2013013055

A catalogue record for this book is available from the British Library.

Wiley also publishes its books in a variety of electronic formats. Some content that appears in print may not be available in electronic books.

Cover image: © James Benet istockphoto.com
Cover design by Andrew Magee Design Ltd

01 2014

Contents

Contributors

Ifeanyichukwu Anusionwu, MD
Resident, Urological Surgery
The James Buchanan Brady Urological Institute and Department of Urology
The Johns Hopkins School of Medicine
Baltimore, MD, USA

Mark W. Ball, MD
Resident, Urological Surgery
The James Buchanan Brady Urological Institute and Department of Urology
The Johns Hopkins School of Medicine
Baltimore, MD, USA

Trinity J. Bivalacqua MD, PhD
Associate Professor of Urology and Oncology
The James Buchanan Brady Urological Institute and Department of Urology
The Johns Hopkins School of Medicine
Baltimore, MD, USA

Arthur L. Burnett, MD, MBA
Patrick C. Walsh Professor of Urology
The James Buchanan Brady Urological Institute and Department of Urology
The Johns Hopkins School of Medicine
Baltimore, MD, USA

John B Eifler, MD
Resident, Urological Surgery
The James Buchanan Brady Urological Institute and Department of Urology
The Johns Hopkins School of Medicine
Baltimore, MD, USA

Nicholas C. Field, MD, MBA
Southern Alberta Institute of Urology
University of Calgary
Calgary, AB, Canada

Bishoy A. Gayed, MD
Chief Resident
University of Pittsburgh Medical Center
Pittsburgh, PA, USA

Angela D. Gupta, MD
Resident, Urological Surgery
The James Buchanan Brady Urological Institute and Department of Urology
The Johns Hopkins School of Medicine
Baltimore, MD, USA

Elias Hyams, MD
Instructor and Fellow
The James Buchanan Brady Urological Institute and Department of Urology
The Johns Hopkins School of Medicine
Baltimore, MD, USA

Matthew Eric Hyndman MD, PhD
Attending Physician
Rockyview General Hospital
Calgary, AB, Canada

Adam Kern, MD
Resident, Urological Surgery
The James Buchanan Brady Urological Institute and Department of Urology
The Johns Hopkins School of Medicine
Baltimore, MD, USA

Stacy Loeb, MD
Assistant Professor of Urology and Population Health
Department of Urology
New York University School of Medicine and Manhattan Veterans Affairs Medical Center
New York, NY, USA

Ahmed Magheli, MD, PhD
Attending Physician and Assistant Professor
Department of Urology
Charité Universitätsmedizin Berlin
Berlin, Germany

Markus Margreiter, MD, FEBU
Assistant Professor of Urology
Department of Urology
Medical University Vienna
Vienna, Austria

Eric Z Massanyi, MD
Pediatric Urology
The James Buchanan Brady Urological Institute and Department of Urology
The Johns Hopkins School of Medicine
Baltimore, MD, USA

Brian Matlaga, MD MPH
Associate Professor
The James Buchanan Brady Urological Institute and Department of Urology
The Johns Hopkins School of Medicine
Baltimore, MD, USA

Jeffrey K. Mullins, MD
Resident, Urological Surgery
The James Buchanan Brady Urological Institute and Department of Urology
The Johns Hopkins School of Medicine
Baltimore, MD, USA

Phillip M. Pierorazio, MD
Chief Resident, Urological Surgery
The James Buchanan Brady Urological Institute and Department of Urology
The Johns Hopkins School of Medicine
Baltimore, MD, USA

Ashley E Ross, MD, PhD
Assistant Professor Urology, Oncology and Pathology
The James Buchanan Brady Urological Institute and Department of Urology
The Johns Hopkins School of Medicine
Baltimore, MD, USA

Michelle Jo Semins, MD
Assistant Professor in Urology
University of Pittsburgh Medical Center
Pittsburgh, PA, USA

Varun Sharma MS, MCh (Urology)
Assistant Professor
Institute of Kidney Diseases and Research Centre
Institute of Transplantation Sciences (IKDRC - ITS)
Ahmedabad, Gujarat, India

Debasish Sundi MD
Resident
The James Buchanan Brady Urological Institute and Department of Urology
The Johns Hopkins School of Medicine
Baltimore, MD, USA

Kristina D. Suson, MD
Attending Physician, Pediatric Urology
Children's Hospital of Michigan
Detroit, MI, USA

Kenneth S Tseng, MD, MPH
Resident
The James Buchanan Brady Urological Institute and Department of Urology
The Johns Hopkins School of Medicine
Baltimore, MD, USA

Robert M. Turner II, MD
Resident
Department of Urology
University of Pittsburgh
Pittsburgh, PA, USA

Preface to the First Edition

Urology residency is challenging, both for the prodigious knowledge required to be a competent urologist and for the paucity of time available to acquire it. Our intention in writing the *Handbook of Urology* is to distill pertinent topics to the bare essentials that can be easily digested in one night of reading. Urology trainees selected the content of each chapter, drawing upon their experiences during training.

Each chapter is preceded by an abstract, a bulleted summary of key points, multiple choice questions and detailed answers, as well as key pitfalls and clinical vignettes. Important results from seminal clinical studies are included and should guide a more thorough review of the topic. As a result, I feel this book is an ideal reference for residents in urology and will also augment the in-service study material currently available.

I am indebted to the exceptional residents and fellows of the The James Buchanan Brady Urological Institute and Department of Urology of the The Johns Hopkins School of Medicine, whose insightfulness and industry were critical to the preparation of this resource.

Finally, I am grateful for the mentorship and expertise of my co-editors, J. Kellogg Parsons, MD, and Misop Han, MD, without whom this book would not be possible.

John B. Eifler, M.D.
Department of Urologic Surgery
Vanderbilt University Medical Center
Nashville, TN
USA

Section 1 Infections

1 Infections of the urinary tract

Mark W. Ball

The James Buchanan Brady Urological Institute and Department of Urology, The Johns Hopkins School of Medicine, Baltimore, MD, USA

KEY POINTS

- Urinary tract infections (UTIs) are commonly diagnosed maladies and account for a significant number of healthcare visits and dollars.
- Infections of the bladder include uncomplicated cystitis, complicated cystitis, pyocystis, and emphysematous cystitis.
- Infections of the kidney include pyelonephritis, emphysematous pyelonephritis, xanthogranulomatous pyelonephritis, infected hydronephrosis, renal abscess and perinephric abscess.
- Infections of the genitalia and reproductive organs include orchitis, epididymitis, prostatitis, and Fournier gangrene.

CASE STUDY

A previously healthy 27-year-old woman presents to the Emergency Department with fever to 39°C, tachycardia to 150 bpm, respirations of 25 breaths per minute, and a leukocytosis to 13,000 WBC. Urinalysis is significant for large leukocyte esterase, positive nitrite, and bacteria are too numerous to count. CT of the abdomen and pelvis reveals a 6-mm left mid-ureteral stone with ipsilateral hydronephrosis and perinephric fat stranding.

The patient is taken emergently to the operating room for left-sided ureteral stent placement. Upon cannulating the ureter, purulent urine drains from the ureteral orifice. Postoperatively, the patient has a profound systemic inflammatory response syndrome (SIRS), requiring several days of mechanical ventilation, vasoactive infusions, and broad-spectrum antibiotics. She eventually makes a full recovery.

Nomenclature

Urinary tract infection (UTI) refers to bacterial invasion of the urothelium causing an inflammatory response. When the site of infection is known, it is more informative to name the site of infection; in other words, cystitis should be used for bladder infection and pyelonephritis for kidney injection, rather than using the generic UTI. Bacteriuria, on the other hand, refers to the presence of bacteria in the urine, which may be either asymptomatic or associated with infection. Pyuria refers to the presence of white blood cells (WBCs) in the urine, which can occur in the setting of either infection or other inflammatory states (nephrolithiasis, malignancy, or foreign body).

Epidemiology

UTI is the most common bacterial infection, responsible for at least 7 million office visits and 100,000 hospitalizations per year. Most infections are diagnosed

Handbook of Urology, First edition. J. Kellogg Parsons, John B. Eifler and Misop Han.
Published 2014 by John Wiley & Sons, Ltd.

based on clinical symptoms and a suggestive urinalysis (UA). This algorithm, however, misses 20% of patients who will have positive urine cultures and causes unnecessary treatment of 50% of patients who will not go on to have a positive urine culture. The bacteria that most often cause UTIs are enteric in origin, with *Escherichia coli* being the most common [1].

Pathogenesis and basic science

Infection of the urinary tract occurs as a complex interaction of both bacterial virulence factors and impaired host defense. Routes of entry into the genitourinary (GU) tract are (in order of frequency) ascending infection via the urethra, direct hematogenous spread, and lymphatic spread.

Bacterial virulence factors increase the infectivity of a bacterial inoculum. The ability of bacteria to adhere to vaginal and urothelial epithelial cells is necessary for an infection to develop. Type 1 pili are expressed by *E. coli* and adhere to uroplakins on umbrella cells of the bladder epithelium. Studies have shown that inoculation of the urinary tract with type 1 piliated organisms results in increased colonization with those organisms. P pili are bacterial adhesins that bind glycolipid receptors in the kidney. The P stands for pyelonephritis, designated because of the high percentage of pyelonephrogenic *E. coli* that express these pili. Bacteria may downregulate the expression of pili once infection is established since pili increase phagocytosis of the organisms. The ability of bacteria to regulate the expression of their pili is known as *phase variation*.

Host defense factors decrease the likelihood of infection. Colonization of the vaginal introitus, urethra, and periurethral skin by non-uropathogenic bacteria provide a mechanical barrier to colonization. Normal voiding also washes away colonizing uropathogenic bacteria. There is genetic variation in the receptivity of epithelial cells to bacterial adhesion. There may be an association between adherence and a protective effect of the HLA-A3 allele. Complicating factors that increase infection risk are due to obstruction, anatomic abnormality, and epithelial cell receptivity. Obstruction or urinary stasis can increase host susceptibility to UTIs. Calculus disease, vesicoureteral reflux, benign prostatic hypertrophy, and neurogenic bladder all increase the susceptibility of the host to UTIs [1].

Interpreting the urinalysis

While urine culture is the gold standard for diagnosing UTIs, it is a test that takes 1–2 days to provide results and potentially longer for antibacterial sensitivity analysis. UA is more expeditious and can support the diagnosis made by history and physical. A UA often consists of two parts: a dipped UA and a microscopic UA. The dipped component tests for pH and the presence of leukocyte esterase (LE), nitrates, and blood. The microscopic component identifies red and white blood cells, red and white blood cells casts, granular casts, bacteria, and yeast.

- Pyuria: >5 WBC/hpf
- Leukocyte esterase (LE): an enzyme released by white blood cells. Positive LE correlates with pyuria
- Nitrite: Urine contains nitrates from protein catabolism. Gram-negative bacteria are able to reduce nitrate to nitrite creating a positive result. One notable exception is pseudomonas which although gram-negative, is associated with negative nitrite on UA.

A UA suggestive of infection typically has positive LE, pyuria, microscopic hematuria, and bacteria. Nitrite is present with gram-negative infection. The presence of epithelial cells can indicate contamination with vaginal flora and should prompt repeat midstream collected urine after adequate cleaning [1].

Bladder infections

Cystitis

Cystitis, or infection of the bladder, may be classified as uncomplicated or complicated. Factors that make cystitis complicated are infections in a male, the elderly, children, diabetics, the immunosuppressed, in the presence of anatomic abnormality, during pregnancy, after recent instrumentation, in the presence of a urinary catheter, and after recent antimicrobials or hospitalization. The typical presentation of cystitis includes symptoms of dysuria, frequency, urgency, ±suprapubic pain, and ±hematuria. Notably, constitutional symptoms including fever and chills are usually absent. This history is crucial in making diagnosis since as many as 50–90% of patients presenting with these symptoms will have cystitis. The diagnosis is supported by urinalysis findings of pyuria, bacteriuria, and the presence of nitrite and LE [1].

Treatment of uncomplicated UTI is dependent on availability, allergy, and local resistance patterns. The

Infectious Diseases Society of America (IDSA) guidelines recommend the following agents as first line: Nitrofurantoin macrocrystals 100 mg bid × 5 days, trimethoprim–sulfamethoxazole 160/800 mg bid × 3 days, or fosfomycin 3 g single dose. Second-line agents include fluoroquinolones or beta-lactams. Knowledge of institutional and community antibiograms should influence prescriber patterns [2].

Cystitis is considered complicated when it occurs in a compromised urinary tract. Treatment regimens are generally the same as for complicated UTI, but the duration is 7–14 days. Nitrofurantoin should not be used in complicated UTI as it has poor tissue penetration. Additionally, modifiable factors such as removal of foreign bodies including stones and indwelling urinary catheters should be considered if clinically indicated. Indwelling catheters in place for over 2 weeks associated with UTI should be changed [3, 4].

Asymptomatic bacteriuria

Asymptomatic bacteriuria is defined as bacteria in the urine in the absence of clinical signs of infection. It is more common in women than men, but increases in prevalence in both sexes with age. Patients with indwelling catheters, bladder reconstruction using bowel, and patients with neurogenic bladders almost always have bacteriuria. Asymptomatic bacteriuria should not be screened for nor treated with a few important exceptions. Pregnant women and patients undergoing urologic procedures should be screened and treated [5].

Recurrent UTI

Unresolved UTI refers to an infection that has not responded to antimicrobial therapy. This commonly occurs because of resistant bacteria or can occur in the case of other unrealized complicating factors (see section Cystitis).

Recurrent UTI is an infection that occurs after resolution of a previous infection. These infections may represent either reinfection or bacterial persistence. Reinfection designates a new event in which the same or different organism enters the urinary tract, or bacterial persistence. Persistence, on the other hand, is when the same bacteria reappear from a nidus such as infected stone or hardware. Reinfection is responsible for 80% of recurrent UTIs [1].

Pyocystis

Pyocystis is a condition in which purulent material is retained in the bladder. Typically, the bladder is defunctionalized as a result of urinary diversion or hemodialysis. Presenting symptoms include purulent discharge, fever, or suprapubic pain. Treatment begins with placing a catheter to drain the purulent material and antibiotics. Oral antibiotics may be used in nonseptic patients, while intravenous (IV) antibiotics should be chosen in ill patients. Additionally, intravesical instillation of an antibiotic or antiseptic may be considered as well as periodic self-catheterization and saline irrigation. Refractory cases warrant more aggressive management—including cystectomy, bladder sclerosis, or surgically created fistula (vaginal or perineal vesicostomy) [1].

Emphysematous cystitis

Emphysematous cystitis is a rare type of cystitis in which gas is found within the wall of the urinary bladder. It is caused by infection with gas-forming bacteria and most often presents in diabetics and elderly patients. Symptoms are essentially the same as in typical cystitis, and treatment consists of culture-specific antibiotics. This condition must be distinguished from air within the lumen of bladder, which is much more common, and often caused by urinary tract instrumentation, indwelling Foley catheter, or by colovesical or enterovesical fistula [1].

Kidney

Acute pyelonephritis

Diagnosis and workup

Acute pyelonephritis is a renal parenchymal infection that is usually caused by ascending infection from the bladder. *Escherichia coli* is the most common organism. The classic presentation is acute onset of fever, chills, and flank pain; however, presentation is variable and there is no *sine qua non* to make the diagnosis. Abdominal pain, nausea or vomiting often accompanies the condition. Physical examination often reveals costovertebral angle tenderness. Laboratory tests often reveal an elevated serum WBC count, while UA findings are similar to those found in acute cystitis. Figure 1.1 shows classic radiographic

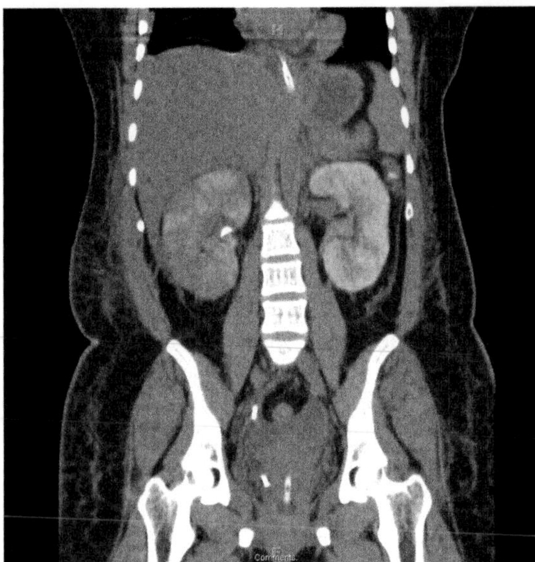

Figure 1.1 CT of pyelonephritis. Contrast CT of the abdomen and pelvis demonstrating enlarged right kidney with wedge-shaped areas of low attenuation, giving a "moth-bitten appearance" consistent with pyelonephritis. Right ureteral stent in place.

signs of acute pyelonephritis, including enlarged kidney, wedge-shaped areas of low attenuation giving a "moth-bitten appearance," and asymmetrical nephrogram [1].

Treatment

Treatment is dependent upon the severity of illness and comorbidities. Patients who are nonseptic and can tolerate oral antibiotics may be treated empirically with a fluoroquinolone as an outpatient after urine culture is obtained. Most patients will improve within 72 hours of antimicrobial initiation. Failure to improve warrants more aggressive therapy with hospitalization and broad spectrum antibiotics initiated if culture data are not available. Additionally, radiologic investigation is indicated to rule out obstruction or development of an abscess. Abscesses may require drainage, and obstruction should be relieved with a ureteral stent or percutaneous nephrostomy tube.

In septic patients, blood and urine cultures should be obtained and intravenous antibiotics should be initiated. Common regimens include third-generation cephalosporins (e.g., ceftriaxone), fluoroquinolones (e.g., levofloxacin or ciprofloxacin), or ampicillin plus gentamicin. Early radiologic investigation is warranted in these patients as well [1, 2].

Chronic pyelonephritis

Chronic pyelonephritis is an often asymptomatic condition caused by multiple bouts of acute pyelonephritis. It can result in renal insufficiency. The diagnosis is made with imaging, which demonstrates atrophic, scarred, and pitted kidneys. Management is to treat active infection and prevent future infections. The condition is rare in patients without underlying urinary tract disease but may occur in vesicoureteral reflux and other abnormalities [1].

Emphysematous pyelonephritis

Emphysematous pyelonephritis is an acute, necrotizing infection of the renal parenchyma resulting from infection with gas-producing organisms. It is more common in diabetic patients and in the presence of obstruction. Diagnosis is made by cross-sectional imaging, demonstrating air in the renal parenchyma. Treatment consists of IV antibiotics, relief of any obstruction, supportive care, and often nephrectomy. Despite aggressive treatment, the mortality rate is over 50% [1].

Renal abscess

Renal abscess (or renal carbuncle) is a collection of purulent material within and confined to the parenchyma. Gram-negative organisms from ascending infection are the most common causative organisms. Hematogenous spread can also occur and gram-positive organisms are often isolated in this mechanism. Risk factors include diabetes mellitus and recurrent UTIs. Presentation begins identical to pyelonephritis, but it does not respond to typical antimicrobial therapy. Failure to respond after 72 hours of therapy warrants imaging to rule out an abscess [1].

Treatment is directed by abscess size. Lesions of any size require parenteral antibiotics. Abscesses less than 3 cm may be observed in the patients that are not immunocompromised or severely ill. Abscesses, 3–5 cm, along with small abscesses that fail conservative therapy necessitate percutaneous drainage. Abscess greater than 5 cm and others failing percutaneous drainage may require surgical drainage [6].

Perinephric abscess

Perinephric abscess is a collection of purulence outside the kidney parenchyma but inside Gerota's fascia. Gram-negative organisms are usually causative, with *E. coli* being the most common. Clinical presentation, diagnosis, and treatment are similar to parenchymal infection. Up to 50% of blood cultures will be positive.

Treatment of perinephric abscess almost always requires drainage. Percutaneous drainage should be considered first line for smaller lesions. Larger abscess or those associated with a nonfunctioning kidney may require nephrectomy [1].

Infected hydronephrosis

Infected hydronephrosis is an infection in an obstructed, hydronephrotic kidney. It is a urologic emergency. Patients are typically very ill, often in urosepsis, with flank pain. It can lead to pyonephrosis or suppurative damage to renal parenchyma. Treatment consists of broad spectrum antibiotics and emergent drainage with either retrograde ureteral stent or percutaneous nephrostomy tube. In decompensating patients, percutaneous nephrostomy is preferred given that it may be performed under less sedation, and to avoid high pressure from irrigation on the collecting system. Drainage should be followed by 10–14 day course of culture-specific antibiotics [1, 7].

Xanthogranulomatous pyelonephritis

Xanthogranulomatous pyelonephritis (XGP) is a chronic, destructive renal infection. It is often associated with unilateral obstructing calculi. The end result is an enlarged, nonfunctioning kidney. The differential diagnosis includes renal cell carcinoma; consequently, this entity must be ruled out. The pathognomonic feature at the cellular level is the presence of lipid-laden macrophages. Treatment often requires nephrectomy [1].

Prostate

Prostatitis

The most common urologic diagnosis in men younger than 50 years is prostatitis and is most prevalent in men between aged 20 and 49 years. Enterobacteriaceae and *Enterococci* are the two most common pathogens. The NIH classifies prostatitis into four categories.

Category I: Acute bacterial prostatitis
Patients with acute bacterial prostatitis present with lower urinary tract symptoms, including dysuria, frequency and urgency, and often obstruction. It typically is associated with a profound systemic inflammatory response, including fever, chills, and malaise. Systemic symptoms include fever, chills, or perineal pain. Digital rectal examination demonstrates a swollen, exquisitely tender prostate.

Treatment should be tailored to cultures. Fluoroquinolones may be empirically started with duration of 4–6 weeks. Bladder obstruction has classically been treated with a suprapubic cystostomy tube, since indwelling Foley catheters are through to cause further obstruction of urethral ducts. However, straight catheterization to relive the initial obstruction is an appropriate first step [8].

Category II: Chronic bacterial prostatitis
The hallmark of chronic bacterial prostatitis is a history of recurrent UTIs. The traditional classification of chronic prostatitis relied on the Meares–Stamey four-glass test. This technique consists of collecting four samples of urine to distinguish urethral, bladder, and prostate infection. The voided bladder 1 (VB1) specimen is the first 10 mL of urine, representing the ureteral specimen. Voided bladder 2 (VB2) is a midstream specimen, representing the bladder specimen. Next, the prostate is massage, and the expressed prostatic secretions (EPSs) are collected. Finally, voided bladder 3 (VB3) is the first 10 mL of urine after massage. Each specimen is analyzed for leukocytes and microbes, as well as sent for culture. Alternatively, a two-cup test has been proposed that consists of collecting urine before and after massage. Chronic bacterial prostatitis will have both WBCs and positive cultures in both the EPS and VB3 specimens [8].

Category III: Chronic pelvic pain syndrome
Patients with chronic pelvic pain syndrome (CPPS) present with pain lasting greater than 3 months. The pain is most often in the perineum. Men often complain of pain associated with ejaculation. This category is subdivided into inflammatory (IIIa) and noninflammatory (IIIB) CPPS. This is distinguished by

the four-glass test that demonstrates WBCs in the EPS and VB3 in category IIIA, and no WBC in IIIB. Cultures are negative for both. More information about chronic pelvic pain can be found in Chapter 15 [8].

Category IV: Asymptomatic inflammatory prostatitis
This classification is reserved for asymptomatic patients who are found to have inflammation incidentally during prostate biopsy or fertility workup. Treatment is not warranted unless treating an elevated prostate-specific antigen (PSA) with a trial of antimicrobials [8].

Prostate abscess

Prostate abscesses typically evolve from cases of acute bacterial prostatitis. An abscess should be suspected when a patient with acute prostatitis fails to respond to antimicrobial therapy. The diagnosis is confirmed with transrectal ultrasound or computed tomography (CT). Treatment involves drainage of the abscess by one of several methods. Classically, transurethral incision has been used for most prostatic abscess, though transperineal incision and drainage may be required for abscesses that extend beyond the prostatic capsule. Percutaneous drainage may also be employed to drain a prostatic abscess and may offer a less morbid approach [8].

Testis and epididymis

Orchitis often presents with associated epididymitis, or *epididymo-orchitis*. The presence of orchitis alone suggests viral infection, such as mumps orchitis. More commonly, the combined epididymo-orchitis usually occurs via retrograde spread of bacteria through the ejaculatory ducts and vas deferens into the epididymis. The original source is often the bladder, urethra, or prostate. In prepubescent patients, a chemical etiology is more common than an infectious etiology and is related to the reflux of urine up the genital tract in dysfunctional voiders. In adults younger than 35 years, the most common cause of epididymitis is sexually transmitted infection, most common *Neisseria gonorrhoeae* and *Chlamydia trachomatis*. In men older than 35 years, the source is often coliform bacteria that have colonized the bladder or prostate, with *E. coli* being the most common.

Clinical presentation reveals tender epididymis and testis. The spermatic cord is often tender as well. Radiographic presentation with ultrasound demonstrates increased vascularity in the epididymis, testis, or both. Ultrasound should be obtained when the diagnosis is unclear to rule out torsion, which has decreased or no flow, as well as malignancy. Untreated epididymitis sometimes progresses to a paratesticular abscess or pyocele. Figure 1.2 demonstrates the appearance of pyocele on ultrasound. This requires open incision and drainage [8].

Treatment
Treatment of isolated orchitis is mainly supportive—scrotal support, bed rest, antipyretics. Antimicrobials may be used when a bacterial origin is presumed with fluoroquinolones being the agent of choice. There is no antiviral regimen for mumps orchitis. Treatment of epididymitis is dependent on age. The Center for Disease Control and Preventions guidelines recommend ceftriax-

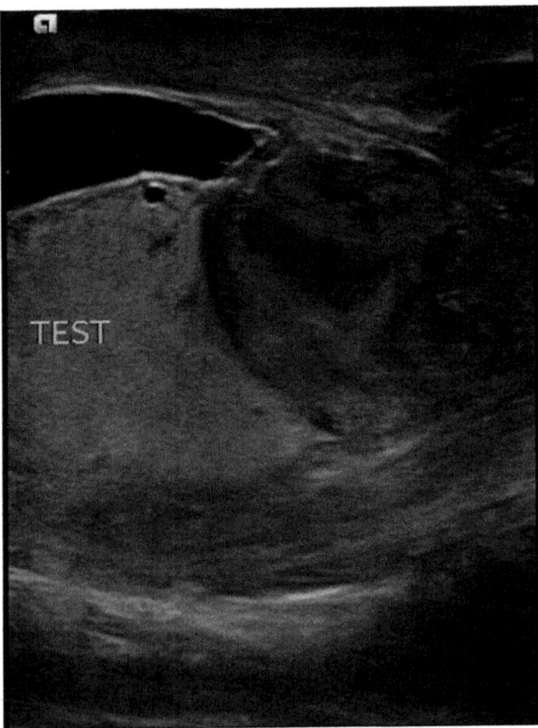

Figure 1.2 Ultrasound of pyocele. Scrotal ultrasound demonstrating heterogenous collection adjacent to testis found to be pus upon scrotal exploration.

one and doxycycline for men younger than 35 years and levofloxacin or ofloxacin for men older than 35 years. The antibiotic course is typically 10 days but may be longer if concomitant prostatitis is suspected [8].

Special infections

Genitourinary tuberculosis

While tuberculosis (TB) is most commonly a pulmonary process, 10% of cases occur in extrapulmonary sites. Of these, 30–40% of extrapulmonary TB occurs in the GU tract. Seeding of the GU tract occurs via hematogenous spread from the alveoli to hilar lymph nodes to the blood stream. The primary landing site is the kidney due to its high vascularity. Downstream infection of the bladder and urethra can occur. The epididymis may also be seeded due to hematogenous spread [9].

Fournier gangrene

Fournier Gangrene is necrotizing fasciitis of the perineum. It is a rapidly progressive, potentially life-threatening infection that is usually polymicrobial, consisting of gram-positive, gram-negative, and anaerobic bacteria. Because of the high morbidity and mortality (16–40%) associated with the infection, it must be ruled out in every case of soft tissue infection of the genitalia. Diabetes mellitus, peripheral vascular disease, alcoholism, and malnutrition are risk factors. Examination may demonstrate cellulitis, blisters, or frankly necrotic areas. Pain out of proportions to visible infection may indicate more extensive underlying infection. Treatment includes broad-spectrum parenteral antibiotics and extensive surgical debridement [1, 9].

Antimicrobial therapy

The goal of antimicrobial therapy is to eliminate microbial growth in the urinary tract. Table 1.1 lists the most common antibiotics used to treat infections of the urinary tract, along with the mechanism of action, spectrum, and common adverse reactions of each drug. Institutional antibiograms and regional resistance patterns should guide antimicrobial therapy [1].

Table 1.1 Common antimicrobials

Antimicrobials	Mechanism of Action	Spectrum	Adverse reactions/Cautions
Beta-lactams	Inhibition of bacterial cell wall synthesis	*Streptococcus*, *Staphylococcus saprophyticus*, *Enterococcus*, *Escherichia coli*, *Proteus*	• PCN allergy cross-reactivity • High prevalence of *E. coli* resistance in some regions • Disruption of normal vaginal flora • Frequent gasterointestinal intolerance and diarrhea • Acute interstitial nephritis
Cephalosporins	Inhibition of bacterial cell wall synthesis	Spectrum by generation: 1st: *Streptococcus*, methicillin-sensitive *Staphylococcus aureus*, some gram-negative rods 2nd: Strep, some gram-negative rods, some anaerobes. 3rd: Strep, most gram-negative rods, moderate Pseudomonas 4th: Most gram-negative rods, and good pseudomonal coverage	• 10% cross-reactivity with PCN allergy • Synergistic toxicity with aminoglycosides

(continued)

Table 1.1 *(Continued)*

Antimicrobials	Mechanism of Action	Spectrum	Adverse reactions/Cautions
Trimethoprim/ sulfamethoxazole (TMP/SMX)	Inhibition of bacterial folic acid metabolism required for DNA synthesis.	*Streptococcus*, *Staphylococcus*, gram-negative rods (not *Pseudomonas*), and atypical *Mycobacteria*	• Interacts with Coumadin to prolong INR • May be associated with hematological abnormalities (especially in G6PD and AIDS), nephrotoxicity, hepatotoxicity, and Stevens–Johnson syndrome • Avoid in pregnancy
Nitrofurantoin	Inhibits multiple bacterial enzymes. Sterilizes urine without affecting GI or vaginal flora	• *E. Coli* and *S. saprophyticus* • Achieves high urinary levels but poor tissue penetration—contraindicated in pyelonephritis.	• Neurotoxicity • Pulmonary fibrosis, interstitial pneumonitis • Hematologic abnormalities and frequent GI intolerance • Requires longer treatment course (7 days instead of 3) • Avoid in G6PD, renal failure
Aminoglycosides	Inhibition of protein synthesis	Gram-negative rods including *Pseudomonas*	• Ototoxicity (usually irreversible) • Nephrotoxicity (usually reversible, nonoliguric ARF after 5–10 days) • Avoid in pregnancy • Neuromuscular blockade (rare) • Once-daily dosing has less nephrotoxicity but similar ototoxicity
Fluoroquinolones	Inhibition of DNA gyrase	Gram-positives, most gram-negative rods including *Pseudomonas*, *N. gonorrhoeae*	• Avoid during pregnancy and in children • May cause false-positive urine opiate test • Peripheral neuropathy (rare) • Tendonitis/tendon rupture
Vancomycin	Inhibition of bacterial cell wall	Gram-positives, including MRSA	• Nephrotoxicity & ototoxicity • "Red-man syndrome": caused by histamine release caused by rapid infusion. Causes erythematous rash of the face, neck, or torso with pruritus. Severe cases cause hypotension
Clindamycin	Inhibition of protein synthesis	Gram-positives (including MRSA) and anaerobes	• Association with *Clostridium difficile* colitis

WHAT TO AVOID

- Avoid initiating antimicrobial therapy before obtaining cultures, except in cases where treatment delay could lead to patient harm.
- Avoid prescribing antimicrobials without considering renal or hepatic dose adjustments, drug interactions, and/or potential drug toxicities.
- Avoid the overuse and misuse of antimicrobials which can lead to bacterial resistance.

KEY WEB LINKS

Johns Hopkins Antibiotic Guide
http://www.hopkinsguides.com/hopkins/ub/index/Johns_Hopkins_ABX_Guide/All_Topics/A

Infectious Disease Society of America Practice Guidelines
http://www.idsociety.org/IDSA_Practice_Guidelines/

American Urological Association Clinical Guidelines
http://www.auanet.org/content/clinical-practice-guidelines

Multiple choice questions

1 Which of the following antimicrobials is not appropriate in the treatment of pyelonephritis?
  a Ciprofloxacin
  b Nitrofurantoin
  c Ceftriaxone
  d Trimethoprim/Sulfamethoxazole

2 Which of the following is the mechanism of action of levofloxacin?
  a Inhibition of cell wall synthesis
  b Inhibition of DNA gyrase
  c Inhibition of protein synthesis
  d Inhibition of folic acid synthesis

References

1 Schaeffer AJ, Schaeffer EM. Infections of the urinary tract. In: Wein AJ, Kavoussi LR, Novick AC, Partin AW, Peters CA, editors. *Campbell-Walsh Urology*. 10th ed. Philadelphia, PA: Saunders; 2011.
2 Gupta K, Hooton TM, Naber KG, et al. International clinical practice guidelines for the treatment of acute uncomplicated cystitis and pyelonephritis in women: A 2010 update by the Infectious Diseases Society of America and the European Society for Microbiology and Infectious Diseases. *Clin Infect Dis* 2011;52(5):e103–e120.
3 Hooton TM, Bradley SF, Cardenas DD, et al. Diagnosis, prevention, and treatment of catheter-associated urinary tract infection in adults: 2009 International Clinical Practice Guidelines from the Infectious Diseases Society of America. *Clin Infect Dis* 2010;50(5):625–663.
4 Johns Hopkins Antibiotic Handbook, 2012–2013. Johns Hopkins Hospital Antimicrobial Stewardship Program.
5 Nicolle LE, Bradley S, Colgan R, et al. Infectious Diseases Society of America guidelines for the diagnosis and treatment of asymptomatic bacteriuria in adults. *Clin Infect Dis* 2005;40(5):643–654.
6 Lee SH, Jung HJ, Mah SY, Chung BH. Renal abscesses measuring 5 cm or less: outcome of medical treatment without therapeutic drainage. *Yonsei Med J* 2010;51(4):569–573.
7 Mokhmalji H, Braun PM, Martinez Portillo FJ, Siegsmund M, Alken P, Köhrmann KU. Percutaneous nephrostomy versus ureteral stents for diversion of hydronephrosis caused by stones: a prospective, randomized clinical trial. *J Urol* 2001;165(4):1088–1092.
8 Nickel J. Prostatitis and related conditions, orchitis, and epididymitis. In: Wein AJ, editor. *Campbell-Walsh Urology.* 10th ed. Philadelphia, PA: Saunders; 2011.
9 Ghoneim I, Rabets J, Mawhorter S. Tuberculosis and other opportunistic infections of the genitourinary system. In: Wein A, Kavoussi L, Novick A, Partin A, Peters C, editors. *Campbell-Walsh Urology*. 10th ed. Philadelphia, PA: Saunders; 2011.

Answers to multiple choice questions

1 Nitrofurantoin is not appropriate for the treatment of pyelonephritis. The drug does not reach adequate tissue levels to irradiate parenchymal infection.
2 Fluoroquinolones inhibit the enzyme DNA gyrase, blocking the unzipping of double stranded DNA required for DNA replication.

Antimicrobial prophylaxis for urologic procedures

Jeffrey K. Mullins

The James Buchanan Brady Urological Institute and Department of Urology, The Johns Hopkins School of Medicine, Baltimore, MD, USA

KEY POINTS

- Antimicrobial prophylaxis is the administration of an antimicrobial agent before and for a limited duration after the procedure to prevent local or systemic infection.
- The risk of developing a surgical site infection is moderated by patients' past medical/surgical history, characteristics of the disease for which the procedure is being performed, and the technical details of the procedure itself.
- Ideal antimicrobial agents for procedural prophylaxis include agents that are efficacious against potential infecting bacteria, achieve acceptable blood and tissue concentrations, and are cost-effective.
- Antimicrobial agents should be administered within 30–60 minutes of incision or initiation of endoscopy. Vancomycin and fluoroquinolones should be administered within 120 minutes of incision. Prophylaxis is generally not extended past skin closure.
- Patients with total joint replacements may be at increased risk for hematogenous joint infections, and should be considered for additional prophylaxis after considering characteristics of the patient and the procedure.

CASE STUDY 1

A 45-year-old male presents to the operating theater to undergo left radical nephrectomy for an 8 cm hilar mass of the left kidney. His past medical history includes hypertension, hyperlipidemia, obesity (BMI = 32), and a smoking history. He has had no previous surgeries and has no known drug allergies.

His surgery is considered a clean procedure and he has a risk factor increasing his risk for a surgical site infection (smoking). Therefore, in accordance with the AUA Best Practice Guideline, he should receive antimicrobial prophylaxis. The ideal agent in this case would be a single dose of a first-generation cephalosporin.

CASE STUDY 2

A 68-year-old male was recently diagnosed with Gleason 3 + 4 = 7 adenocarcinoma of the prostate. After considering his various treatment options, he elected open radical retropubic prostatectomy. His past medical history is significant only for gastroesophageal reflux disease. He has had no previous surgeries and does not smoke. He has an allergy to penicillin which causes anaphylaxis.

Radical retropubic prostatectomy involves entry into the urinary tract and is considered a clean–contaminated case. All patients undergoing these procedures should receive antimicrobial prophylaxis. Given his severe penicillin allergy he should receive a single dose of ampicillin/sulbactam or a fluoroquinolone.

Handbook of Urology, First edition. J. Kellogg Parsons, John B. Eifler and Misop Han.
Published 2014 by John Wiley & Sons, Ltd.

CASE STUDY 3

An 81-year-old woman was diagnosed with a 1 cm left proximal ureteral stone after presenting to the emergency room with hematuria and left flank pain. She has no evidence of urinary tract or systemic infection. She was admitted to the hospital for pain control, and is scheduled for left ureteroscopy and laser lithotripsy of her stone. Past medical history is notable for hypertension, insulin-dependent diabetes mellitus, osteoarthritis, and coronary artery disease. She has a history of a total knee replacement 18 months ago. She has no other past medical history and is a nonsmoker. She has no allergies.

This woman has a total joint prosthesis and is undergoing a urologic procedure. The patient is at risk for hematogenous total joint infection given her diabetes and recent joint replacement (<2 years). Furthermore, she is undergoing a procedure with stone manipulation, which is considered to be a high-risk procedure for bacteremia. Therefore, she should receive antimicrobial prophylaxis to prevent hematogenous infection of her joint prosthesis. Acceptable agents would be a parenteral fluoroquinolone or ampicillin plus gentamicin.

Introduction

Infections occurring after surgery in the location of the body where the surgery was performed have been described as surgical site infections (SSI). These infections represent a major health concern in the United States, accounting for up to 20% of all healthcare-acquired infections and costing up to $10 billion annually [1, 2]. Rates of SSI are modulated by both risk factors germane to the patient as well as procedure-specific characteristics. Both meticulous adherence to sterile technique and appropriate procedural antimicrobial prophylaxis have been shown to reduce the risk of SSI. Despite the availability of procedure-specific antimicrobial prophylaxis guidelines in multiple specialties, there is wide variability in provider compliance to these recommendations [3]. In response to this, multiple medical societies and individual institutions have issued statements and guidelines on antimicrobial prophylaxis in an effort to improve patient safety.

In 2011, the American Urological Association (AUA) issued a Best Practice Statement on antimicrobial prophylaxis for urologic procedures providing procedure-specific recommendations for antimicrobial prophylaxis [4]. The following chapter discusses the risk factors for SSIs, the basic principles of antimicrobial prophylaxis, and AUA guidelines for antimicrobial prophylaxis for common urologic procedures.

Risk factors for infection

Host factors

Host factors are patient characteristics that (1) increase the risk of developing a SSI, (2) increase the negative sequelae of a SSI, and/or (3) increase the concentration or alter the flora of potential infectious organisms (Table 2.1) [4, 5]. These factors often exist along a spectrum and several may exist within the same patient. Therefore, careful consideration of the patient, their various comorbidities, and the proposed surgical procedure is imperative when determining a patient's risk for developing a SSI.

Surgical factors

Procedures are typically classified as clean, clean–contaminated, contaminated, or dirty. Definitions for the various procedures are listed in Table 2.2 [6]. The rates of infection increase with the amount of contamination present. A contemporary series estimated the risk of SSI after a clean, clean–contaminated, and

Table 2.1 Host factors increasing the risk of surgical site infection

Advanced age
Anatomic anomalies
Poor nutritional status
Smoking
Chronic corticosteroid use
Immunodeficiency
Chronic indwelling hardware
Infected endogenous/exogenous material
Distant coexistent infection
Prolonged hospitalization

Source: Schaeffer AJ and Schaeffer EM. Infections of the urinary tract. In:. AJ Wein, LR Kavoussi, AC Novick, AW Partin, CA Peters, editors. *Campbell-Walsh Urology*, 9th ed., Vol. 1. Philadelphia, PA: Saunders-Elsevier; 2007; pp. 223–303.

Table 2.2 Surgical wound classification [6]

Classification	Description
Clean	Uninfected operative site, with primary skin closure.
Clean–contaminated	Entry into respiratory, alimentary, genital, or urinary tracts.
Contaminated	Fresh accidental wounds, major break in sterile technique, gross spillage from gastrointestinal tract, or presence of acute but nonpurulent inflammation at the operative site.
Dirty–infected	Old accidental wound with devitalized tissue or presence of clinical infection or perforated viscera at the operative site. This definition implies that organisms that might cause postoperative infection were present at the operative site before surgery.

contaminated surgery as 1.2%, 7.8%, and 23.4%, respectively [7]. All GU procedures that enter the urinary tract are considered clean–contaminated.

Basic principles of antimicrobial prophylaxis

Definitions

There is an important distinction between antimicrobial prophylaxis and antimicrobial treatment. **Antimicrobial prophylaxis** is the administration of an antimicrobial agent before and for a limited duration after the procedure to prevent local or systemic infection. In contrast, **antimicrobial treatment** is therapy for an established local or systemic infection directed, ideally, at culture-documented organisms [4, 5].

General guidelines

According to the AUA Best Practice Statement, antimicrobial prophylaxis is indicated "only when the potential benefit exceeds the risks and anticipated costs" [4]. The benefit of antimicrobial prophylaxis is the prevention of SSIs, which have been associated with adverse patient outcomes and increased healthcare costs [8, 9]. The cost of antimicrobial prophylaxis includes financial, personal health, and public health costs. The financial cost is influenced by the agent chosen and the duration of administration. Personal health risks include allergic reactions and alterations of normal intestinal flora, predisposing patients to opportunistic infections (i.e., *Clostridium difficile*). Finally, public health risks of inappropriate antimicrobial prophylaxis include changes in bacterial resistance patterns within the community and the emergence of multidrug-resistant organisms. In general, the AUA recommends using the least expensive agent that is efficacious for the potential putative organisms for the shortest duration possible [4].

Administration

In patients where antimicrobial prophylaxis is indicated, correct administration depends on choosing the correct agent and administering it at the appropriate time. Choosing an appropriate agent for antimicrobial prophylaxis is dependent upon the procedure and the properties of the drug. The antimicrobial agent must be efficacious against potential infectious organisms, including gram-positive bacteria on the skin, gram-negative bacteria when the urinary tract is entered, and anaerobic bacteria when the gastrointestinal tract is entered. Furthermore, the agent must achieve tissue levels that exceed the minimal inhibitory concentration for these organisms, and must maintain these levels for a period during which the case can be completed [4].

Antimicrobial prophylaxis should be given within 60 minutes of surgical incision (or initiation of endoscopy). Intravenous fluoroquinolones and vancomycin are an exception to this rule and should be given within 120 minutes of incision. The antimicrobial agent should be redosed during the procedure if the procedure exceeds two half-lives of the given agent [4].

Duration of prophylaxis

It is generally not recommended that antimicrobial prophylaxis be extended past skin closure or cessation of endoscopy. Continuation of antimicrobial prophylaxis may be considered in the presence of an existing infection, placement of indwelling prosthetic material, and manipulation of an indwelling urinary catheter [4]. There is little literature providing guidance for the appropriate duration of antimicrobial prophylaxis when placing a prosthetic device (i.e., penile prosthesis or artificial urinary sphincter), and practices vary between operating urologists. In the presence of an existing infection or a colonized indwelling urinary catheter, every effort should be made to treat the infection prior to surgery. However, oftentimes this is not practical, and the goal of preoperative therapy is to suppress bacterial counts to minimize systemic spread of the infection perioperatively. Postoperatively, patients should be treated with an appropriate therapeutic course of a culture-specific antimicrobial. In the absence of a preexisting infection there is no evidence to suggest that antimicrobial prophylaxis should be extended solely due to the placement of a urinary catheter.

Procedure-specific recommendations

The section below details the use of antimicrobial prophylaxis for common genitourinary procedures. Within each section, the AUA Best Practice Guidelines are denoted in **bold text.** Several procedures refer to patients with risk factors. These risk factors are listed in Table 2.1.

Placement and removal of urinary catheters

In general, antimicrobial prophylaxis is not recommended for patients undergoing urethral catheterization. The rate of urinary tract infections (UTIs) after a one-time catheterization in healthy women has been reported as <2% [10, 11]. However, this risk may be greatly increased in hospitalized patients and those with risk factors for developing a UTI. Therefore, in hospitalized patients and those with risk factors (Table 2.1) one may consider oral trimethoprim-sulfamethoxazole (TMP-SMX) or a fluoroquinolone for prophylaxis [5]. No guidelines for routine urethral catheterization are provided by the AUA Best Practice Statement.

The rate of colonization of external urinary catheters has been reported as 5–10% per day of catheterization [12–14]. Despite this high rate of colonization, prophylactic antibiotics are not recommended for the duration of the catheterization given concerns about the effectiveness of this strategy and the promotion of resistant strands of bacteria [15]. However, in patients undergoing catheter removal after a prolonged catheterization, consideration should be given to antimicrobial *treatment* at the time of catheter removal. In fact, two randomized control trials found that cefotaxime administered before catheter removal after a transurethral procedure significantly reduced postoperative complications compared to controls who did not receive antibiotics before catheter removal [16, 17]. Given this data, **it is recommended that antimicrobial prophylaxis be given at the time of catheter removal in patients with risk factors** [4]. Alternatives to this approach include antimicrobial treatment directed at culture-specific bacteria or no antibiotics in the case of a negative urine culture.

Cystography and urodynamics

The evidence on the need for antimicrobial prophylaxis in these, typically outpatient procedures, is conflicting. On the one hand, a randomized control trial demonstrated a reduction in rates of posturodynamic UTIs from 14% to 1% with the use of a single dose of an oral fluoroquinolone [18]. However, other randomized control trials have demonstrated no benefit to antimicrobial prophylaxis when performing urodynamics [19, 20] or cystography [21]. **Therefore it is currently recommended that patients with risk factors undergo antimicrobial prophylaxis prior to these procedures** [4].

Transrectal prostate biopsy

Four separate randomized control trials have demonstrated a reduction in infection-related complications after transrectal prostate biopsy with the use of antimicrobial prophylaxis versus control [22–25]. Furthermore, these studies have shown that single-day or single-dose regimens of prophylaxis are as efficacious as antimicrobial prophylaxis spanning several days. **Therefore, antimicrobial prophylaxis is indicated in all patients undergoing transrectal prostate biopsy**[4].

Extracorporeal shock-wave lithotripsy

The reported rates of UTIs after shock-wave lithotripsy (SWL) range from 0% to28% [5]. A meta-analysis assessing relevant randomized control trials demonstrated a significant reduction of bacteriuria after SWL with the use of antimicrobial prophylaxis (5.7% vs. 2.1%) [26]. **Therefore, antimicrobial prophylaxis is indicated in all patients undergoing SWL** [4].

Cystourethroscopy with and without manipulation

Endoscopic procedures of the lower urinary tract can be considered as those with and without tissue manipulation. Simple cystourethroscopy, in which there is no tissue manipulation, has a 2–8% rate of culture-proven postprocedural UTIs without prophylaxis [27, 28]. In fact, two separate randomized control trials demonstrated significant reductions in the incidence of post-procedure positive urine cultures compared to placebo in patients receiving antimicrobial prophylaxis with either parenteral gentamicin (21% vs. 5%) [29] or oral TMP or Ciprofloxacin (9% vs. 5% vs. 3%) [30]. However, these findings have not been demonstrated in all studies. **Therefore, it is recommended that patients with risk factors receive antimicrobial prophylaxis before simple cystourethroscopy** [4].

Endoscopic procedures of the lower urinary tract with manipulation include, but are not limited to transurethral resection of the prostate (TURP), laser vaporization of the prostate, transurethral resection of bladder tumors (TURBT), cystolitholapaxy, direct vision internal urethrotomy, and foreign body retrieval. Extrapolating from data on TURP and TURBT which unequivocally show a reduction in bacteriuria and sepsis with antimicrobial prophylaxis versus control [31, 32], **it is recommended that all patients undergoing these procedures receive antimicrobial prophylaxis** [4].

Ureteroscopy

The incidence of bacteremia after routine ureteroscopy without antimicrobial prophylaxis has been estimated to be as high as 30%. This may cause a febrile UTI in up to 25% of patients undergoing ureteroscopy [33]. Given these data, it is not surprising that a randomized control trial of an oral fluoroquinolone versus no prophylaxis demonstrated a significant decrease in the incidence of postoperative bacteremia (2% vs. 13%) [34]. **Therefore, it is recommended that all patients undergoing ureteroscopy receive antimicrobial prophylaxis** [4].

Percutaneous renal surgery

There is a reported 35% incidence of postoperative UTIs after percutaneous renal surgery even in the setting of a sterile preoperative urine culture [35]. Therefore, despite the lack of randomized data, **it is recommended that all patients undergoing percutaneous renal surgery undergo antimicrobial prophylaxis** [4].

Vaginal surgery

There is a paucity of data on vaginal urologic surgery and antimicrobial prophylaxis. However, a recent meta-analysis on the use of antibiotic prophylaxis prior to vaginal hysterectomy unequivocally demonstrated a reduction in pelvic infections with the use of antimicrobial prophylaxis [36]. **It is recommended that all patients undergoing a vaginal urologic surgery receive antimicrobial prophylaxis** [4].

Open or laparoscopic procedures without entry into genitourinary tract

Urologic procedures on noninfected structures that do not enter the genitourinary or gastrointestinal tract are considered clean procedures. Studies on radical nephrectomy have shown a significant benefit to prophylaxis with a first-generation cephalosporin versus no prophylaxis [37, 38]. However, there is a robust body of literature on nonurologic clean procedures which have mixed results regarding the efficacy of antimicrobial prophylaxis. **Therefore, it is recommended that patients with risk factors receive prophylaxis** [4].

Entry into genitourinary tract

Urologic procedures with controlled entry into the urinary tract are considered clean–contaminated cases. Rates of febrile UTIs after such procedures have been reported to range from 5% to 10% [34]. Furthermore, a randomized control trial demonstrated a significant reduction in postradical prostatectomy infections in men receiving prophylaxis versus no prophylaxis [39]. **Therefore, prophylaxis is recommended in all patients undergoing urologic surgery with entry into the urinary tract** [4].

Entry into gastrointestinal tract

Urologic procedures with controlled entry into the gastrointestinal tract (i.e., urinary diversion) are considered clean–contaminated. Several meta-analyses of nonurologic procedures involving the bowel have demonstrated the benefits of antimicrobial prophylaxis [40, 41]. **Therefore, all patients undergoing urologic procedures involving the gastrointestinal tract should receive prophylaxis** [4].

Placement of indwelling prosthesis

There is a paucity of data regarding the use of antimicrobial prophylaxis in patients undergoing urologic procedures in which foreign material is implanted in the body. However, data from the general surgery and orthopedic literature suggest that prophylaxis is beneficial in the setting of implanting foreign material [42, 43]. **Therefore, all patients undergoing a procedure during which foreign material is implanted in the body should receive prophylaxis. Of note, the duration of such prophylaxis has not been established** [4].

Special considerations

Endocarditis prophylaxis

The American Heart Association currently does not recommend prophylactic antimicrobials before genitourinary procedures solely to prevent infective endocarditis. However, in patients at high risk for infective endocarditis who are receiving prophylactic antibiotics to prevent sepsis or wound infections or who have an established UTI, an agent with activity against *Enterococcus* should be considered (Amoxicillin, Ampicillin, Vancomycin) [44].

Orthopedic prosthetic joints

The AUA recommends antimicrobial prophylaxis to specifically reduce the risk of total joint infections in patients who are both at increased risk of a hematogenous joint infection and undergoing a procedure with an increased risk of bacteremia (Table 2.3). For patients not meeting these criteria, prophylaxis may be indicated as per the guidelines discussed in previous sections. Recommendations for prophylaxis in these patients include (1) systemic fluoroquinolone

Table 2.3 Patient- and procedure-related risk factors for hematogenous infection of total joint replacements. Patients meeting both criteria should receive antimicrobial prophylaxis to prevent hematogenous total joint infection [45]

Increased risk of hematogenous total joint infection	Increased risk of bacteremia associated with urologic procedures
Patients during the first 2 yr after prosthetic joint replacement	Any stone manipulation (includes shock-wave lithotripsy)
Immunocompromised patients with prosthetic joint replacements	Any procedure with transmural incision into urinary tract (does not include simple ligation with excision or percutaneous drainage procedure)
Inflammatory arthropathies (e.g., rheumatoid arthritis, systemic lupus erythematosus)	Any endoscopic procedures of upper tract (ureter and kidney)
Drug-induced immunosuppression	Any procedure that includes bowel segments
Radiation-induced immunosuppression	Transrectal prostate biopsy
Patients with prosthetic joint replacements and comorbidities	Any procedure with entry into the urinary tract (except for urethral catheterization) in individuals with higher risk of bacterial colonization
Previous prosthetic joint infections	Indwelling catheter or intermittent catheterization
Malnourishment	Indwelling ureteral stent
Hemophilia	Urinary retention
HIV infection	History of recent/recurrent urinary tract infection or prostatitis
Diabetes	Urinary diversion
Malignancy	

1–2 hours preoperatively or (2) ampicillin 2 g (or Vancomycin 1 g 1–2 hours preoperatively) + Gentamicin 1.5 mg/kg 30–60 minutes preoperatively [4].

WHAT TO AVOID

- Avoid administering antibiotics >1 hour prior to surgery except for vancomycin and fluoroquinolones.
- Avoid giving prophylaxis to patients with an infected wound. These patients should be treated.
- Avoid giving antimicrobial prophylaxis specifically for prevention of endocarditis.
- Avoid failing to give additional antimicrobial prophylaxis to patients at risk of hematogenous seeding of prosthetic joints.

KEY WEB LINK

http://www.auanet.org/content/clinical-practice-guidelines/clinical-guidelines.cfm#2

Multiple choice questions

1 Antimicrobial prophylaxis should generally be stopped at what time period?

a Antimicrobial prophylaxis should never be administered
b 24–48 hours after skin closure
c At the time of skin closure in noninfected cases
d When the patient shows no sign of continued infection

2 Ciprofloxacin should be administered within what time of incision?

a 30 minutes
b 60 minutes
c 120 minutes
d 240 minutes

3 The recommended antimicrobial to be given to a patient undergoing a radical retropubic prostatectomy who has a penicillin allergy is:

a Cephalexin
b Vancomycin
c Clindamycin
d Ampicillin/Sulbactam

4 Which patient undergoing simple office cystourethroscopy would require antimicrobial prophylaxis?

a 54-year-old male with prosthetic joint 3 years ago
b 23-year-old female with mitral valve prolapsed
c 65-year-old former smoker with insulin-dependent diabetes mellitus
d All of the above

5 True or False: The American Heart Association does not currently recommend antimicrobial prophylaxis prior to urologic procedures specifically to reduce the risk of infective endocarditis.

References

1 Scott R. The direct medical costs of healthcare-associated infections in U.S. hospitals and the benefit of prevention; 2009. Available at http://www.cdc.gov/HAI/pdfs/hai/Scott_CostPaper.pdf (Last accessed 13 June 2012).
2 Klevens RM, Edwards JR, Richards CL, Jr., et al. Estimating health care-associated infections and deaths in U.S. hospitals, 2002. *Public Health Rep* 2007;122:160–166.
3 Bratzler DW, Houck PM, Richards C, et al. Use of antimicrobial prophylaxis for major surgery: baseline results from the National Surgical Infection Prevention Project. *Arch Surg* 2005;140:174–182.
4 Wolf JS, Jr., Bennett CJ, Dmochowski RR, Hollenbeck BK, Pearle MS, Schaeffer AJ. *Best Practice Policy Statement on Urologic Surgery Antimicrobial Prophylaxis*. Bethesda, MD: American Urological Association Education and Research, Inc; 2012.
5 Schaeffer AJ, Schaeffer EM. Chapter 10: Infections of the urinary tract. In: Wein AJ, Kavoussi LR, Novick AC, Partin AW, Peters CA, editors. *Campbell-Walsh Urology*. 10th ed., Vol. 1. Philadelphia, PA: Saunders; 2011; pp. 274–285.
6 Mangram AJ, Horan TC, Pearson ML, Silver LC, Jarvis WR. Guideline for prevention of surgical site infection, 1999. Hospital Infection Control Practices Advisory Committee. *Infect Control Hosp Epidemiol* 1999;20:250–278; quiz 279–280.
7 Yamamoto S, Kanamaru S, Kunishima Y, Ichiyama S, Ogawa O. Perioperative antimicrobial prophylaxis in urology: a multi-center prospective study. *J Chemother* 2005;17:189–197.
8 Herwaldt LA, Cullen JJ, Scholz D, et al. A prospective study of outcomes, healthcare resource utilization, and costs associated with postoperative nosocomial infections. *Infect Control Hosp Epidemiol* 2006;27:1291–1298.

9 Leaper DJ, van Goor H, Reilly J, et al. Surgical site infection – a European perspective of incidence and economic burden. *Int Wound J* 2004;1:247–273.
10 Turck M, Goffe B, Petersdorf RG. The urethral catheter and urinary tract infection. *J Urol* 1962;88:834–837.
11 Thiel G, Spuhler O. [Catheter infection and so-called infectious (episomal) resistance]. *Schweiz Med Wochenschr* 1965;95:1155–1157.
12 van der Wall E, Verkooyen RP, Mintjes-de Groot J, et al. Prophylactic ciprofloxacin for catheter-associated urinary-tract infection. *Lancet* 1992;339:946–951.
13 Saint S, Lipsky BA. Preventing catheter-related bacteriuria: should we? Can we? How?. *Arch Intern Med* 1999;159:800–808.
14 Sedor J, Mulholland SG. Hospital-acquired urinary tract infections associated with the indwelling catheter. *Urol Clin North Am*.1999;26:821–828.
15 Niel-Weise BS, van den Broek PJ. Antibiotic policies for short-term catheter bladder drainage in adults. *Cochrane Database Syst Rev* 2005:CD005428.
16 Grabe M, Forsgren A, Hellsten S. A short antibiotic course given in conjunction with and after catheter removal consecutive to transurethral prostatic resection. *Scand J Urol Nephrol* 1984;18:193–199.
17 Duclos JM, Larrouturou P, Sarkis P. Timing of antibiotic prophylaxis with cefotaxime for prostatic resection: better in the operative period or at urethral catheter removal? *Am J Surg*. 1992;164:21S–23S.
18 Kartal ED, Yenilmez A, Kiremitci A, Meric H, Kale M, Usluer G. Effectiveness of ciprofloxacin prophylaxis in preventing bacteriuria caused by urodynamic study: a blind, randomized study of 192 patients. *Urology* 2006;67:1149–1153.
19 Cundiff GW, McLennan MT, Bent AE. Randomized trial of antibiotic prophylaxis for combined urodynamics and cystourethroscopy. *Obstet Gynecol* 1999; 93:749–752.
20 Peschers UM, Kempf V, Jundt K, Autenrieth I, Dimpfl T. Antibiotic treatment to prevent urinary tract infections after urodynamic evaluation. *Int Urogynecol J Pelvic Floor Dysfunct* 2001;12:254–257.
21 Tsugawa M, Monden K, Nasu Y, Kumon H, Ohmori H. Prospective randomized comparative study of antibiotic prophylaxis in urethrocystoscopy and urethrocystography. *Int J Urol* 1998;5:441–443.
22 Kapoor DA, Klimberg IW, Malek GH, et al. Single-dose oral ciprofloxacin versus placebo for prophylaxis during transrectal prostate biopsy. *Urology*. 1998;52:552–558.
23 Shigemura K, Tanaka K, Yasuda M, et al. Efficacy of 1-day prophylaxis medication with fluoroquinolone for prostate biopsy. *World J Urol* 2005;23:356–360.
24 Sabbagh R, McCormack M, Peloquin F, et al. A prospective randomized trial of 1-day versus 3-day antibiotic prophylaxis for transrectal ultrasound guided prostate biopsy. *Can J Urol* 2004;11:2216–2219.
25 Aron M, Rajeev TP, Gupta NP. Antibiotic prophylaxis for transrectal needle biopsy of the prostate: a randomized controlled study. *BJU Int* 2000;85:682–685.
26 Pearle MS, Roehrborn CG. Antimicrobial prophylaxis prior to shock wave lithotripsy in patients with sterile urine before treatment: a meta-analysis and cost-effectiveness analysis. *Urology* 1997;49:679–686.
27 Clark KR, Higgs MJ. Urinary infection following outpatient flexible cystoscopy. *Br J Urol* 1990;66:503–505.
28 Manson AL. Is antibiotic administration indicated after outpatient cystoscopy. *J Urol* 1988;140:316–317.
29 Rane A, Cahill D, Saleemi A, Montgomery B, Palfrey E. The issue of prophylactic antibiotics prior to flexible cystoscopy. *Eur Urol* 2001;39:212–214.
30 Johnson MI, Merrilees D, Robson WA, et al. Oral ciprofloxacin or trimethoprim reduces bacteriuria after flexible cystoscopy. *BJU Int* 2007;100:826–829.
31 Berry A, Barratt A. Prophylactic antibiotic use in transurethral prostatic resection: a meta-analysis. *J Urol* 2002;167:571–577.
32 Qiang W, Jianchen W, MacDonald R, Monga M, Wilt TJ. Antibiotic prophylaxis for transurethral prostatic resection in men with preoperative urine containing less than 100,000 bacteria per ml: a systematic review. *J Urol* 2005;173:1175–1181.
33 Knopf HJ, Graff HJ, Schulze H. Perioperative antibiotic prophylaxis in ureteroscopic stone removal. *Eur Urol* 2003;44:115–118.
34 Grabe M. Controversies in antibiotic prophylaxis in urology. *Int J Antimicrob Agents* 2004;23(Suppl 1):S17–S23.
35 Charton M, Vallancien G, Veillon B, Brisset JM. Urinary tract infection in percutaneous surgery for renal calculi. *J Urol* 1986;135:15–17.
36 Duff P, Park RC. Antibiotic prophylaxis in vaginal hysterectomy: a review. *Obstet Gynecol* 1980;55: 193S–202S.
37 Steiner T, Traue C, Schubert J. [Perioperative antibiotic prophylaxis in transperitoneal tumor nephrectomy: does it lower the rate of clinically significant postoperative infections?]. *Urologe A* 2003;42:34–37.
38 Montgomery JS, Johnston WK, 3rd, Wolf JS, Jr. Wound complications after hand assisted laparoscopic surgery. *J Urol* 2005;174:2226–2230.
39 Prokocimer P, Quazza M, Gibert C, et al. Short-term prophylactic antibiotics in patients undergoing prostatectomy: report of a double-blind randomized trial with 2 intravenous doses of cefotaxime. *J Urol* 1986;135:60–64.
40 Andersen BR, Kallehave FL, Andersen HK. Antibiotics versus placebo for prevention of postoperative infection after appendicectomy. *Cochrane Database Syst Rev* 2005:CD001439.

41 Song F, Glenny AM. Antimicrobial prophylaxis in colorectal surgery: a systematic review of randomized controlled trials. *Br J Surg* 1998;85:1232–1241.
42 Sanabria A, Dominguez LC, Valdivieso E, Gomez G. Prophylactic antibiotics for mesh inguinal hernioplasty: a meta-analysis. *Ann Surg* 2007;245:392–396.
43 Southwell-Keely JP, Russo RR, March L, Cumming R, Cameron I, Brnabic AJ. Antibiotic prophylaxis in hip fracture surgery: a metaanalysis. *Clin Orthop Relat Res* 2004;419:179–184.
44 Wilson W, Taubert KA, Gewitz M, et al. Prevention of infective endocarditis: guidelines from the American Heart Association: a guideline from the American Heart Association Rheumatic Fever, Endocarditis, and Kawasaki Disease Committee, Council on Cardiovascular Disease in the Young, and the Council on Clinical Cardiology, Council on Cardiovascular Surgery and Anesthesia, and the Quality of Care and Outcomes Research Interdisciplinary Working Group. *Circulation* 2007;116: 1736–1754.
45 American Urological Association; American Academy of Orthopaedic Surgeons. Antibiotic prophylaxis for urological patients with total joint replacements. *J Urol* 2003 ;169:1796–1797.

Answers to multiple choice questions

1 c
2 c
3 d
4 c
5 T

Section 2 Urinary lithiasis

3 Nephrolithiasis: etiology, stone composition, medical management, and prevention

Robert M. Turner II and Michelle Jo Semins
Department of Urology, University of Pittsburgh, Pittsburgh, PA, USA

KEY POINTS

- The lifetime risk of developing a kidney stone is 10% and the prevalence continues to rise.
- Calcium oxalate stones are the most common.
- Urine pH is the primary determinant of uric acid crystallization (pH < 5.5).
- Struvite stones, composed of magnesium ammonium phosphate, are referred to as infection stones because of their association with urease-producing urinary tract infections.
- Cystinuria is an autosomal recessive disorder characterized by a defect in transport of dibasic amino acids and typically presents in childhood.
- All stone formers should maintain a urine volume of 2 L/day, restrict salt intake, consume moderate animal protein, and consume the normal daily recommended allowance of calcium.
- A more extensive metabolic evaluation is indicated for recurrent stone formers, all children, and those with a solitary kidney, renal insufficiency, residual stone burden, and high risk for recurrence.

CASE STUDY

A 58-year-old female has recurrent calcium oxalate nephrolithiasis. She was started on a thiazide diuretic 2 years ago for hypercalciuria. Her laboratory results are normal with a serum potassium 3.5 mg/dL. Her 24-hour urine collections are reviewed:

	Baseline	3 months	2 years
Urine volume (L/day)	1.87	2.09	2.48
Urine calcium (mg/day)	286	216	113
Urine oxalate (mg/day)	38	35	38
Urine citrate (mg/day)	1157	809	300
Urine pH	6.933	6.129	5.987
Urine uric acid (mg/day)	551	581	630
Urine sodium (mg/day)	164	124	57

Her urine calcium decreases in response to the thiazide and she improves her urine volume. Both of these improvements decrease the urinary saturation of calcium-based salts. Her urinary citrate has decreased significantly. Thiazide-induced hypokalemia leads to intracellular acidosis, which promotes proximal tubular reabsorption of citrate and reduced citrate synthesis, leading to hypocitraturia. This patient should be continued on her thiazide with the addition of potassium citrate to treat the hypocitraturia.

Handbook of Urology, First edition. J. Kellogg Parsons, John B. Eifler and Misop Han.
Published 2014 by John Wiley & Sons, Ltd.

Epidemiology

Nephrolithiasis is a common urological condition, with the probability of having a stone varying according to age, sex, race, and geographic location. In the United States, the lifetime risk has been estimated at 10% and the prevalence is rising globally [1–3]. Recurrence rate is high with 30–50% of patients having a repeat stone event within 5 years of the initial episode [4, 5]. Geographically, the prevalence of stone disease has a north-south and west-east gradient and is highest in the Southeastern United States [6, 7]. Family history increases the risk 2.5-fold [8]. Some additional risk factors include obesity, diabetes, gout, primary hyperparathyroidism, renal tubular acidosis (RTA), intestinal disease or surgery, certain medications, and specific dietary habits [9].

Stone formation

Stones are essentially salts that precipitate out of urine. The underlying impetus for urine crystal formation is urinary supersaturation, or the ability of urine to keep ionic components, such as calcium and oxalate, in solution at higher-than-expected concentrations. Typically, when a salt concentration exceeds its thermodynamic solubility product (K_{sp}), it will precipitate unless conditions, such as temperature and pH, are changed. Urine allows salts to remain in solution at concentration products higher than K_{sp} because of the presence of inhibitors [10]. When urine contains a salt with a concentration product greater than its K_{sp}, it is considered to be metastable. At this concentration, new stone formation is limited by inhibitors, but growth of existing crystals may occur. If the salt concentration increases and exceeds its "upper limit of metastability" (ULM), crystallization is no longer prevented by inhibitors and *de novo* stone formation occurs [11]. Stone formation occurs in several phases, specifically nucleation, growth, aggregation, and retention [12]. Nucleation is the formation of the smallest crystal that does not dissolve. In homogenous nucleation, crystals form from salt components in pure solution. Heterogeneous nucleation, or epitaxy, refers to the formation of nuclei on a substrate such as epithelial cells, cell debris, or other crystals. Inhibitors include citrate, magnesium, pyrophosphate, glycosaminoglycans, nephrocalcin, Tamm-Horsfall protein, and uropontin [10, 13]. Following nucleation and initiation of crystal growth, stone formation relies on aggregation of crystals and development of particles that are too large to be excreted.

Stone composition

Calcium-based stones

Calcium stones (calcium oxalate and calcium phosphate) represent 75–80% of stones [14]. The most common stone type is calcium oxalate (60%). Underlying metabolic conditions that increase the risk of calcium stone formation include hypercalciuria, hypocitraturia, hyperoxaluria, hyperuricosuria, and gouty diathesis. RTA, topiramate, pregnancy, and pH > 7 are associated with calcium phosphate stones.

Hypercalciuria

Hypercalciuria (greater than 200 mg daily) occurs in 35–65% of stone formers [15]. It is classified by three subtypes: absorptive, renal, and resorptive. *Absorptive hypercalciuria* is characterized by intestinal hyperabsorption of calcium. The increase in calcium load decreases parathyroid hormone (PTH) secretion and increases the renal filtered load of calcium, thus increasing the excretion of urinary calcium. *Renal hypercalciuria* is caused by impaired renal tubular reabsorption of calcium. The resulting decrease in calcium load increases PTH secretion which results in an increase in intestinal calcium absorption and bone resorption (driven by enhanced 1,25-[OH]D synthesis). Due to the balance of renal calcium loss with calcium absorption and bone resorption, the serum calcium remains unchanged. Lastly, *resorptive hypercalciuria* is a consequence of primary hyperparathyroidism. Excess PTH secretion from a parathyroid adenoma or carcinoma leads to increased 1,25-[OH]D synthesis, increased calcium absorption, and increased bone resorption. This results in elevated serum calcium levels (>10.1 mg/dL) and treatment is parathyroidectomy. Less common causes of hypercalciuria include hypercalcemia of malignancy, sarcoidosis, and vitamin D toxicity.

Hypocitraturia

Hypocitraturia (less than 320 mg daily) is present in 20–60% of stone formers [16]. Urinary citrate is an important inhibitor of stone formation that forms a soluble complex with calcium. It directly inhibits crystallization and aggregation of calcium oxalate and calcium phosphate. Metabolic acidosis promotes proximal tubular reabsorption of citrate and reduces citrate synthesis, both of which lead to hypocitraturia. Pathologic states associated with acidosis and resulting hypocitraturia include distal RTA, chronic diarrhea, excess animal protein intake (Atkins diet), thiazide use, and vigorous exercise [15]. Idiopathic hypocitraturia can occur in the absence of an acidotic state.

Hyperoxaluria

Hyperoxaluria is defined as oxalate excretion greater than 40 mg daily. Oxalate absorption is inhibited by the presence of intestinal calcium. In the intestine, calcium binds oxalate to form a complex and reduces the amount of free oxalate available for absorption [17]. *Primary hyperoxaluria* is a rare autosomal recessive disorder caused by an inborn error of metabolism. Normal hepatic conversion of glyoxalate to glycine by alanine–glyoxalate aminotransferase (AGT) is affected, and glyoxalate is instead oxidized to oxalate. Systemic oxalosis and severe hyperoxaluria result in recurrent stones, nephrocalcinosis, and renal failure. Patients with end-stage renal disease often require combined liver–kidney transplantation [18]. *Enteric hyperoxaluria* occurs in patients with intestinal disease (i.e., inflammatory bowel disease or celiac sprue) or intestinal surgery (i.e., resection or bypass) that results in a malabsorptive state. Fat malabsorption leads to saponification of fatty acids with calcium. This reduces the calcium available for binding to oxalate and increases the amount of free oxalate available for intestinal absorption [19]. Malabsorptive states also lead to dehydration (low urine volume), bicarbonate loss (low urine pH), metabolic acidosis (hypocitraturia), and poor magnesium absorption (hypomagnesuria). *Dietary hyperoxaluria* occurs from the excessive dietary intake of oxalate-rich foods such as black tea, spinach, beets, rhubarb, chocolate, and nuts. Vitamin C is converted to oxalate and increases its excretion.

Hyperuricosuria

Hyperuricosuria (greater than 600 mg daily) is a common risk factor for both calcium and uric acid stones. At a urine pH > 5.5, soluble monosodium urate crystals act as a nidus for heterologous nucleation in calcium stone formation [20]. Monosodium urate also binds to and reduces the activity of urinary inhibitors [21]. Hyperuricosuria is most commonly caused by dietary intake of purine-rich foods. While some patients present with a history of gout and hyperuricemia, many present with a normal serum uric acid.

Uric acid stones

Uric acid stones are the most common radiolucent stones, representing 10% of the total stone occurrence in the United States, and have a higher prevalence in patients with diabetes and obesity [22, 23]. Uric acid is the product of purine degradation. Purines can be derived exogenously from dietary intake or endogenously through purine synthesis from nucleic acids or nonpurine precursors. Purine synthesis occurs in the liver, where excess guanine and hypoxanthine are converted to xanthine and then to uric acid by xanthine oxidase. In addition to a high-purine diet, hyperuricosuria can result from states of increased catabolism including myeloproliferative disorders, hemolytic anemia, and chemotherapy-induced tumor lysis. Rare enzymatic disorders that increase urinary excretion include Lesch–Nyhan syndrome, phosphoribosylpyrophosphate synthetase overactivity, and several glycogen storage diseases. These conditions are associated with hyperuricemia and often present during childhood. Uricosuric drugs such as probenecid, high-dose salicylates, radiocontrast agents, and losartan also promote hyperuricosuria [24]. Urine pH is the primary determinant of uric acid crystallization. Uric acid is a weak organic acid with a p*Ka* of 5.5. At a urine pH less than 5.5, the relatively insoluble uric acid predominates over the soluble base urate [25]. It should be noted that the solubility of urate depends on its associated cation. Monosodium urate is less soluble than monopotassium urate and plays a role in heterogeneous nucleation of calcium oxalate stones [26].

Struvite stones

Struvite stones, composed of magnesium ammonium phosphate, are referred to as infection stones because of their strong association with urinary tract infections (UTIs). The offending organisms are urease-producing bacteria including *Proteus* (most common), *Klebsiella*, *Pseudomonas*, and *Staphylococcus* species [27]. Although *Escherichia coli* is a common cause of

UTIs, only rare species of *E. coli* produce urease and thus are an infrequent cause of infection stones [28]. Struvite stones are notable for their large size and rapid growth, often presenting as "staghorn" calculi. Bacterial urease converts urinary urea to ammonium and carbon dioxide, which then hydrolyzes to ammonium ions and bicarbonate. Ammonium ions bind available magnesium and phosphate to form struvite. Magnesium ammonium phosphate is relatively insoluble in alkaline urine at a pH ≥ 7.2 [29]. Risk factors include recurrent urinary tract obstruction, chronic indwelling urinary catheter, urinary diversion, and neurogenic voiding dysfunction. If left untreated, staghorn calculi frequently lead to chronic renal insufficiency, septic complications, and death [30, 31].

Cystine stones

Cystine stones are rare, representing approximately 0.6–1% of all urinary stones, however, they comprise about 10% of stones reported in pediatric series [32]. They are caused by cystinuria, an inherited autosomal recessive disorder characterized by a defect in intestinal and renal tubular transport of dibasic amino acids, including cystine, ornithine, lysine, and arginine (COLA) [12, 22]. The result is diminished reabsorption of these amino acids in both the intestine and renal proximal tubule. Increased urinary excretion of cystine promotes supersaturation and crystal formation. Cystine is poorly soluble at physiologic pH values between 5 and 7, but pH values >8 lead to a 3-fold increase in cystine solubility [33]. Ornithine, lysine, and arginine are soluble at normal urinary pH and do not crystallize [32]. Two genes involved in the disease are *SLC3A1* (type A cystinuria) and *SLC7A9* (type B cystinuria). In Europe and the United States, reported mean incidence of cystinuria is 1 in 1000–17,000 and prevalence varies dramatically with ethnicity [34–36]. The age of onset ranges between 2 and 40 years, but the median is 12–15 years [37]. Men are affected earlier and have more stone events per year [32]. Fifty percent of asymptomatic individuals with cystinuria eventually develop symptomatic stones, and stones are bilateral in 75% of cases [32, 38]. Cystine stones are poorly radio-opaque and, on urinalysis, have a classic hexagonal shape, though this finding is only present in 20–25% of cases [36]. Patients excreting a cystine level of more than 1000 µmol/g of creatinine per day are considered homozygous [39].

Other rare stones

Xanthine and 2,8-dihydroxyadenine (2,8-DHA) stones are radiolucent stones that are often confused with uric acid stones. Lesch–Nyhan syndrome and allopurinol use increase the risk of xanthine stones, whereas 2,8-DHA stones are seen in patients with a deficiency in adenine phosphoribosyltransferase (APRT). Matrix stones, predominantly composed of mucoprotein and mucopolysaccharide, are also radiolucent. Ammonium acid urate stones are associated with laxative abuse, recurrent UTI, and inflammatory bowel disease. They are an endemic cause of bladder calculi in developing countries [12]. Medications that directly promote stone formation include indinivir and triamterene. Indinivir, a protease inhibitor used in the management of HIV, forms stones that are radiolucent on plain radiograph and computed tomography.

Medical evaluation

Comprehensive metabolic evaluation identifies abnormalities in 75–90% of stone formers, and the institution of preventative dietary and medical measures has resulted in substantial reduction in stone recurrence rates [15].

Screening evaluation

All patients with kidney stone disease should undergo a screening evaluation to assess for underlying systemic syndromes. This begins with a thorough history and physical examination. Medical history should identify patients with intestinal disease, pathologic fractures, osteoporosis, recurrent UTIs, gout, and family history of nephrolithiasis. Dietary habits (including fluid intake) and medications should be reviewed carefully. Basic laboratory screening should be done (Table 3.1). These can identify systemic problems including primary hyperparathyroidism (high serum calcium, low serum phosphorus), distal RTA (low potassium, low carbon dioxide), and gouty diathesis (high uric acid). A simple clean catch urinalysis can be informative and should be performed in all stone formers. A persistently elevated urinary pH (>7.0) is associated with RTA or infection lithiasis while a persistently low urinary pH (<5.5) increases

Table 3.1 Initial evaluation of all stone formers

Serum tests
Electrolytes (potassium, bicarbonate, and phosphorus)
Creatinine
Calcium, vitamin D levels
Intact parathyroid hormone
Uric acid
Urine tests
Urinalysis (specific gravity, pH, nitrites, leukocyte esterase)
Urine sediment (crystals)
Urine culture

uric acid stone risk. UTI is supported by the presence of nitrites, leukocyte esterase, and bacteria and can be confirmed by culture. The presence of urea-splitting organisms such as *Proteus*, *Klebsiella*, and *Pseudomonas* is associated with the formation of struvite stones. Urine sediment can reveal crystals that predict the stone composition [40]. Calcium oxalate dihydrate and calcium oxalate monohydrate crystals have tetrahedral envelope and hourglass appearances, respectively. Rectangular "coffin lid" crystals indicate struvite calculi, and hexagonal crystals are pathognomonic for cystinuria. An abdominal radiograph can document stone burden. Radio-opaque stones include calcium oxalate, calcium phosphate, struvite, and cystine (poorly), whereas uric acid, triamterene, and xanthine stones are radiolucent. Stone should be analyzed to determine composition.

Metabolic evaluation

Select patients should undergo a more extensive metabolic evaluation (Table 3.2). The 24-hour urine collection is the mainstay of this evaluation (Table 3.3). Due to disparities of serial collections that may alter management in up to 70% of cases, two 24-hour urine collections on initial evaluation are advised to maximize the diagnostic yield [41, 42]. These collections should be deferred until the patient has recovered from an acute stone episode, surgical intervention, and/or UTI [43]. The amount of creatinine in the sample can determine adequacy of collection. Men should have 20–25 mg/kg/day and women should have 15–20 mg/kg/day. Urine collections include both stone-specific and dietary risk factors including volume, calcium, oxalate, uric acid, sodium, phosphate, magnesium, and supersaturations of the various stone compositions.

Table 3.2 Indications for complete metabolic evaluation

Recurrent stone formers
Select first-time stone formers
Strong family history of nephrolithiasis
Solitary kidney, anatomic abnormalities
Renal insufficiency
Poor health (would not tolerate recurrent stone episodes)
High risk for recurrence
Intestinal disease (chronic diarrhea)
Osteoporosis, pathologic skeletal fractures
History of gout
Cystine, uric acid, or struvite stones
All children

Table 3.3 Key components of a 24-hour urine collection

Stone risk factors
Urine volume
Urine calcium
Urine oxalate
Urine citrate
Urine pH
Urine uric acid
Dietary factors
Urine sodium
Urine magnesium
Adequacy of collection
Urine creatinine

Medical management

General recommendations

There are general recommendations that all stone formers should follow to decrease stone recurrence rates. All patients should maintain a urine volume of 2 L/day [44]. Low urine volume is the most common metabolic abnormality found in patients and increases the supersaturation of crystal components [45]. A strict low-salt diet is also advised, as elevated urinary sodium excretion can induce or exacerbate hypercalciuria. Moderate animal protein intake is recommended as a high-protein intake increases urinary calcium, oxalate, and uric acid excretion [46–48]. Lastly, a normal recommended daily allowance of calcium (1200 mg/day) is advised as a low-calcium diet can induce a hyperoxaluria and increase stone risk [5].

Specific recommendations

Hypercalciuria (>200 mg/day)

Hypercalciuria in a patient with normal serum calcium may be considered idiopathic. If urine sodium is also elevated, dietary management with salt restriction can be first attempted to decrease urinary calcium. Patients with severe hypercalciuria (urinary calcium >275 mg/day) or mild hypercalciuria and reduced bone mineral density may be treated with a thiazide as it will increase renal tubular reabsorption of calcium [15]. Chronic thiazide use can lead to hypokalemia, metabolic acidosis, and hypocitraturia. These secondary metabolic derangements can be treated with concomitant potassium citrate supplementation. Resorptive hypercalciuria secondary to primary hyperparathyroidism requires parathyroidectomy.

Hypocitraturia (<320 mg/day)

Potassium citrate restores normal urinary citrate, inhibits the crystallization of calcium salts, and significantly reduces stone recurrence rates [49]. This therapy also corrects the metabolic acidosis, hypokalemia, and profound hypocitraturia found in patients with distal RTA [50]. In patients with chronic diarrheal states, a liquid preparation of potassium citrate has better absorption in the setting of rapid intestinal transit time [40]. Potassium citrate supplementation treats thiazide-induced hypocitraturia [51]. Dietary modifications with lemonade and other citrus juices can also increase citrate in the urine [52].

Hyperoxaluria (>40 mg/day)

Enteric hyperoxaluria rarely occurs as an isolated metabolic derangement on account of associated intestinal fluid losses and malabsorption. These patients often present with concomitant low urine volume, metabolic acidosis, hypocitraturia, and hypomagnesuria. In addition to hydration and potassium citrate, the dietary restriction of oxalate is required. Calcium supplementation may be given to bind oxalate in the intestine, but this benefit may be offset by a rise in urinary calcium. Repeat urine collection is recommended 4–6 weeks after initiation of therapy [53]. Magnesium supplementation also binds intestinal oxalate and corrects the associated hypomagnesuria but often provokes further diarrhea [40].

Hyperuricosuria (>600 mg/day)

First-line treatment of patients with hyperuricosuric calcium oxalate or uric acid nephrolithiasis is hydration and reduction in intake of animal protein (red meat, fish, and poultry). Patients with moderate to severe hyperuricosuria and pH < 6 who have failed dietary modification can be treated with alkalinization of the urinary milieu such that uric acid remains in a dissolved state [54]. Potassium citrate can be administered to raise the urine pH to ≥6.1. Citrate supplementation also raises urinary citrate levels and inhibits crystallization of calcium salts. While potassium citrate is preferred due to the relative solubility of monopotassium urate, sodium citrate or sodium bicarbonate are alternatives in patients with intolerance to potassium, hyperkalemia, and/or renal insufficiency [23]. Alkalinization of the urine to a pH > 7.0 should be avoided as this increases the risk of calcium phosphate stone formation. If serum uric acid is high or if hyperuricosuria and uric acid lithiasis persist despite alkalinization, allopurinol can be used [55]. Allopurinol is generally well tolerated but can cause irreversible liver enzyme elevation. Because of the risk of Stevens–Johnson syndrome, report of a skin rash should prompt immediate cessation of the drug [15].

Cystinuria (>30 g/day)

The primary goal in the treatment of cystinuria is to improve the solubility of cystine. Initial treatment is aggressive hydration to produce a urine volume of 3 L/day in children and 4–5 L/day in adults [36]. Urinary alkalinization to raise the urine pH to 6.5–7.0 brings the pH value closer to 8.3, the p*K*a of cystine [40]. Excessive alkalinization should be avoided to avoid the risk of calcium phosphate stone formation. A low-salt diet is effective in reducing the excretion of cystine [56, 57]. Dietary restriction of methionine, a precursor to cystine, requires strict protein restriction which is often difficult for adults and should be avoided in children [36]. The next line of therapy involves the use of chelating agents like D-penicillamine or α-mercaptopurine (Thiola). They cleave the disulfide bond of cystine to produce cysteine, which is 50 times more soluble [58]. D-penicillamine is associated with frequent side effects including nephrotic syndrome, dermatitis, and pancytopenia. It induces pyridoxine depletion that requires supplementation [36]. α-Mercaptopurine (Thiola) is slightly less efficacious but better tolerated [40, 58]. Common side effects include rash, arthralgia, thrombocytopenia, polymyositis, proteinuria, and nephritic syndrome [36].

Lastly, the angiotensin-converting enzyme captopril, which contains a free sulfahydryl group, is well tolerated and has been used in the treatment of cystinuria. However, the data regarding its efficacy are mixed [40].

Struvite stones
Surgery and antibiotics are the main treatment for this stone type. Patients that are not surgical candidates can be considered for treatment with acetohydroxamic acid, a urease inhibitor, and/or irrigation with an acidic solution, but severe side effects are common.

WHAT TO AVOID/KEY PITFALLS

- Creatinine in the sample can determine adequacy of collection. Men should have 20–25 mg/kg/day and women should have 15–20 mg/kg/day.
- High sodium intake will offset the effect of thiazide therapy patients with hypercalciuria.
- Urine alkalinization to pH > 7.0 will increase the risk of calcium phosphate stone formation.
- Thiazide use promotes hypocitraturia that can be treated with potassium citrate.
- Penicillamine use leads to vitamin B6 deficiency that can be prevented with pyridoxine.

KEY WEB LINKS

A Simple Step-by-Step Approach to the Diagnosis and Prevention of Nephrolithiasis
http://abcsofstonedisease.com/index.aspx

An Example of a Commercial Provider of 24-Hour Urinary Stone Risk Profiles
http://www.litholink.com/en/PhysicianLitholinkStone

Multiple choice questions

1 A 58-year-old male with Crohn's disease presents with recurrent calcium oxalate stones. His laboratory results are normal. A 24-hour urine was obtained:

Urine volume (L/day)	2.29
Urine calcium (mg/day)	103
Urine oxalate (mg/day)	78
Urine citrate (mg/day)	283
Urine pH	5.58
Urine uric acid (mg/day)	294
Urine sodium (mg/day)	103

The mechanism of this patient's metabolic derangement is
a Increased intestinal absorption of calcium.
b Increased secretion of oxalate in the distal convoluted tubule.
c Increased colonic absorption of free oxalate.
d Decreased intestinal absorption of citrate.
e Increased reabsorption of citrate in the proximal convoluted tubule.

2 Select all of the following that are TRUE regarding cystinuria.
a The pattern of inheritance is autosomal dominant.
b It is characterized by a defect in intestinal and renal tubular transport of dibasic amino acids.
c Initial treatment involves aggressive hydration, urine alkalinization, and a low-salt diet.
d Chelating agents cleave the disulfide bond of cystine to produce soluble lysine.
E D-penicillamine is better tolerated than α-mercaptopurine (Thiola) and is preferred in patients requiring drug therapy for cystinuria.

References

1 Johnson CM, Wilson DM, O'Fallon WM, Malek RS, Kurland LT. Renal stone epidemiology: a 25-year study in Rochester, Minnesota. *Kidney Int* 1979;16(5):624–631.
2 Stamatelou KK, Francis ME, Jones CA, Nyberg LM, Curhan GC. Time trends in reported prevalence of kidney stones in the United States: 1976–1994. *Kidney Int* 2003;63(5):1817–1823.
3 Romero V, Akpinar H , Assimos DG. Kidney stones: a global picture of prevalence, incidence, and associated risk factors. *Rev Urol* 2010;12(2–3):e86–e96.
4 Ettinger B, Pak CY, Citron JT, Thomas C, Adams-Huet B, Vangessel A. Potassium-magnesium citrate is an effective prophylaxis against recurrent calcium oxalate nephrolithiasis. *J Urol* 1997;158(6):2069–2073.
5 Borghi L, Schianchi T, Meschi T, et al. Comparison of two diets for the prevention of recurrent stones in idiopathic hypercalciuria. *N Engl J Med* 2002;346(2):77–84.
6 Soucie JM, Thun MJ, Coates RJ, McClellan W, Austin H. Demographic and geographic variability of kidney stones in the United States. *Kidney Int* 1994; 46(3):893–899.
7 Curhan GC, Rimm EB, Willett WC, Stampfer MJ. Regional variation in nephrolithiasis incidence and prevalence among United States men. *J Urol* 1994;151(4): 838–841.

8 Curhan GC, Willett WC, Rimm EB, Stampfer MJ. Family history and risk of kidney stones. *J Am Soc Nephrol* 1997;8(10):1568–1573.
9 Curhan GC. Epidemiology of stone disease. *Urol Clin North Am* 2007;34(3):287–293.
10 Fleisch H. Inhibitors and promoters of stone formation. *Kidney Int* 1978;13(5):361–371.
11 Asplin JR, Parks JH , Coe FL. Dependence of upper limit of metastability on supersaturation in nephrolithiasis. *Kidney Int* 1997;52(6):1602–1608.
12 Pearle MS, Yair L. Chapter 45: Urinary lithiasis: etiology, epidemiology, and pathogenesis. In: Wein AJ, Kavoussi LR, Novick AC, Partin AW, Peters CA, editors. *Campbell-Walsh Urology*. Philadelphia, PA: Elsevier Saunders; 2011.
13 Marangella M, Bagnis C, Bruno M, Vitale C, Petrarulo M, Ramello A. Crystallization inhibitors in the pathophysiology and treatment of nephrolithiasis. *Urol Int* 2004. 72(Suppl 1):6–10.
14 Pak CY. Etiology and treatment of urolithiasis. *Am J Kidney Dis* 1991;18(6):624–637.
15 Park S, Pearle MS. Pathophysiology and management of calcium stones. *Urol Clin North Am* 2007;34(3): 323–334.
16 Hamm LL, Hering-Smith KS. Pathophysiology of hypocitraturic nephrolithiasis. *Endocrinol Metab Clin North Am* 2002;31(4):885–893, viii.
17 Liebman M, Chai W. Effect of dietary calcium on urinary oxalate excretion after oxalate loads. *Am J Clin Nutr* 1997;65(5):1453–1459.
18 Cochat P, Fargue S, Harambat J. Primary hyperoxaluria type 1: strategy for organ transplantation. *Curr Opin Organ Transplant* 2010;15(5):590–593.
19 Dobbins JW Binder HJ. Effect of bile salts and fatty acids on the colonic absorption of oxalate. *Gastroenterology* 1976;70(6):1096–1100.
20 Grover PK, Marshall VR, Ryall RL. Dissolved urate salts out calcium oxalate in undiluted human urine in vitro: implications for calcium oxalate stone genesis. *Chem Biol* 2003;10(3):271–278.
21 Pak CY, Holt K, Zerwekh JE. Attenuation by monosodium urate of the inhibitory effect of glycosaminoglycans on calcium oxalate nucleation. *Invest Urol* 1979;17(2):138–140.
22 Mandel NS, Mandel GS. Urinary tract stone disease in the United States veteran population. II. Geographical analysis of variations in composition. *J Urol* 1989;142(6):1516–1521.
23 Cameron MA, Sakhaee K. Uric acid nephrolithiasis. *Urol Clin North Am* 2007;34(3):335–346.
24 Maalouf NM, Cameron MA, Moe OW, Sakhaee K. Novel insights into the pathogenesis of uric acid nephrolithiasis. *Curr Opin Nephrol Hypertens* 2004;13(2):181–189.
25 Coe FL, Strauss AL, Tembe V, Le Dun S. Uric acid saturation in calcium nephrolithiasis. *Kidney Int* 1980;17(5):662–668.
26 Wilcox WR, Khalaf A, Weinberger A, Kippen I, Klinenberg JR. Solubility of uric acid and monosodium urate. *Med Biol Eng* 1972;10(4):522–531.
27 Silverman DE, Stamey TA. Management of infection stones: the Stanford experience. *Medicine (Baltimore)* 1983;62(1):44–51.
28 Bichler KH, Eipper E, Naber K, Braun V, Zimmermann R, Lahme S. Urinary infection stones. *Int J Antimicrob Agents* 2002;19(6):488–498.
29 Healy KA, Ogan K. Pathophysiology and management of infectious staghorn calculi. *Urol Clin North Am* 2007;34(3):363–374.
30 Koga S, Arakaki Y, Matsuoka M, Ohyama C. Staghorn calculi—long-term results of management. *Br J Urol* 1991;68(2):122–124.
31 Teichman JM, Long RD, Hulbert JC. Long-term renal fate and prognosis after staghorn calculus management. *J Urol* 1995;153(5):1403–1407.
32 Rogers A, Kalakish S, Desai RA, Assimos DG. Management of cystinuria. *Urol Clin North Am* 2007;34(3): 347–362.
33 Dent CE, Senior B. Studies on the treatment of cystinuria. *Br J Urol* 1955;27(4):317–332.
34 Cabello-Tomas ML, Garcia-Gomez AM, Guillen-Dominguez ML. Pilot screening programme for cystinuria in the Valencian community. *Eur J Epidemiol* 1999;15(7):681–684.
35 Schon R, Thalhammer O. [Routine screening for inborn errors using urine filter paper specimens at age 4–5 weeks (author's transl)]. *Padiatr Padol* 1976;11(1):319–325.
36 Knoll T, Zöllner A, Wendt-Nordahl G, Michel MS, Alken P. Cystinuria in childhood and adolescence: recommendations for diagnosis, treatment, and follow-up. *Pediatr Nephrol* 2005;20(1):19–24.
37 Font-Llitjos M, Jiménez-Vidal M, Bisceglia L, et al. New insights into cystinuria: 40 new mutations, genotype-phenotype correlation, and digenic inheritance causing partial phenotype. *J Med Genet* 2005;42(1):58–68.
38 Purohit RS, Stoller ML. Laterality of symptomatic cystine calculi. *Urology* 2003;62(3):421–424.
39 Guillen M, Corella D, Cabello ML, García AM, Hernández-Yago J. Reference values of urinary excretion of cystine and dibasic amino acids: classification of patients with cystinuria in the Valencian Community, Spain. *Clin Biochem* 1999;32(1):25–30.
40 Farrandino MN, Pietrow PK, Preminger GM. Chapter 46: Evaluation and medical management of urinary lithiasis. In: Wein AJ, Kavoussi LR, Novick AC, Partin AW, Peters CA, editors. *Campbell-Walsh Urology*. Philadelphia, PA: Elsevier Saunders; 2011.

41 Parks JH, Goldfisher E, Asplin JR, Coe FL. A single 24-hour urine collection is inadequate for the medical evaluation of nephrolithiasis. *J Urol* 2002; 167(4):1607–1612.
42 Semins MJ, Matlaga BR. Medical evaluation and management of urolithiasis. *Ther Adv Urol* 2010;2(1):3–9.
43 Begun FP, Foley WD, Peterson A, White B. Patient evaluation. Laboratory and imaging studies. *Urol Clin North Am* 1997;24(1):97–116.
44 Porena M Guiggi P, Micheli C. Prevention of stone disease. *Urol Int* 2007;79(Suppl 1):37–46.
45 Yagisawa T, Chandhoke PS, Fan J. Comparison of comprehensive and limited metabolic evaluations in the treatment of patients with recurrent calcium urolithiasis. *J Urol* 1999;161(5):1449–1452.
46 Pak CY, Barilla DE, Holt K, Brinkley L, Tolentino R, Zerwekh JE. Effect of oral purine load and allopurinol on the crystallization of calcium salts in urine of patients with hyperuricosuric calcium urolithiasis. *Am J Med* 1978;65(4):593–599.
47 Fellstrom B, Danielson BG, Karlström B, Lithell H, Ljunghall S, Vessby B. The influence of a high dietary intake of purine-rich animal protein on urinary urate excretion and supersaturation in renal stone disease. *Clin Sci (Lond)* 1983;64(4):399–405.
48 Breslau NA, Brinkley L, Hill KD, Pak CY. Relationship of animal protein-rich diet to kidney stone formation and calcium metabolism. *J Clin Endocrinol Metab* 1988;66(1):140–146.
49 Barcelo P, Wuhl O, Servitge E, Rousaud A, Pak CY. Randomized double-blind study of potassium citrate in idiopathic hypocitraturic calcium nephrolithiasis. *J Urol* 1993;150(6):1761–1764.
50 Preminger GM, Sakhaee K, Skurla C, Pak CY. Prevention of recurrent calcium stone formation with potassium citrate therapy in patients with distal renal tubular acidosis. *J Urol* 1985;134(1):20–23.
51 Pak CY, Peterson R, Sakhaee K, Fuller C, Preminger G, Reisch J. Correction of hypocitraturia and prevention of stone formation by combined thiazide and potassium citrate therapy in thiazide-unresponsive hypercalciuric nephrolithiasis. *Am J Med* 1985;79(3):284–288.
52 Zuckerman JM, Assimos DG. Hypocitraturia: pathophysiology and medical management. *Rev Urol* 2009;11(3):134–144.
53 Barilla DE, Notz C, Kennedy D, Pak CY. Renal oxalate excretion following oral oxalate loads in patients with ileal disease and with renal and absorptive hypercalciurias. Effect of calcium and magnesium. *Am J Med* 1978;64(4):579–85.
54 Pak CY Peterson R. Successful treatment of hyperuricosuric calcium oxalate nephrolithiasis with potassium citrate. *Arch Intern Med* 1986;146(5):863–867.
55 Ettinger B, Tang A, Citron JT, Livermore B, Williams T. Randomized trial of allopurinol in the prevention of calcium oxalate calculi. *N Engl J Med* 1986;315(22): 1386–1389.
56 Jaeger P, Portmann L, Saunders A, Rosenberg LE, Thier SO. Anticystinuric effects of glutamine and of dietary sodium restriction. *N Engl J Med* 1986;315(18): 1120–1123.
57 Rodriguez LM, Santos F, Málaga S, Martínez V. Effect of a low sodium diet on urinary elimination of cystine in cystinuric children. *Nephron* 1995;71(4):416–418.
58 Pak CY, Fuller C, Sakhaee K, Zerwekh JE, Adams BV. Management of cystine nephrolithiasis with alpha-mercaptopropionylglycine. *J Urol* 1986;136(5):1003–1008.

Answers to multiple choice questions

1 c
2 b, c

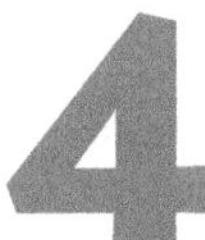

Nephrolithiasis: evaluation and surgical treatment

Bishoy A. Gayed and Michelle Jo Semins
University of Pittsburgh Medical Center, Pittsburgh, PA, USA

KEY POINTS

- Meticulous history and physical examination are required during evaluation.
- Classic presentation of an acute stone event includes flank pain radiating to the ipsilateral lower abdomen and groin, nausea/vomiting, hematuria, lower urinary tract symptoms, and/or fever.
- Imaging and labs help guide treatment.
- Noncontrast computed tomography (CT) scan is the gold standard for diagnosis.
- Acute management includes intravenous (IV) fluids, pain control, antiemetics, and antibiotics if infection is suspected.
- If fever or hemodynamic instability is present, urgent decompression with ureteral stent or nephrostomy tube is required.
- Expectant management with medical expulsive therapy (MET) can be first-line therapy for the appropriate patient.
- Stone size, location, composition, and patient factors guide treatment type.
- Ureteroscopy (URS), percutaneous nephrolithotomy (PNL), and shock wave lithotripsy (SWL) are the surgical options for treatment.
- Ultrasound is the first-line imaging choice for pregnant patients.

CASE STUDY

A 32-year-old pregnant female in her third trimester presents to the emergency department with complaints of nausea, vomiting, and right flank pain for 1 day. Temperature is 38.3°C. Other vital signs are normal. Laboratory values reveal a white blood cell count (WBC) 18 and creatinine 2.0. Renal ultrasound reveals marked hydronephrosis with a 1.3 cm obstructing proximal ureteral stone. She is given IV antibiotics and taken to the operating room for decompression with a ureteral stent. This is placed with ultrasound guidance. Definitive stone management occurs 2 weeks postpartum with URS and laser lithotripsy.

This patient has signs of infection (elevated WBC and fever) associated with obstruction. Urgent decompression is required. Definitive management is contraindicated at this time due to the presence of infection. Pregnancy itself is not a contraindication for definitive management, but complex stones in pregnancy (i.e., large stone burden, abnormal anatomy) are best treated in the postpartum phase. Ultrasound is utilized as the diagnostic modality of choice in the pregnant patient.

Handbook of Urology, First edition. J. Kellogg Parsons, John B. Eifler and Misop Han.
Published 2014 by John Wiley & Sons, Ltd.

Introduction

Nephrolithiasis is a common malady that affects 10% of the population during their lifetime. Recurrence rate is high at 30–50% within 5 years. As such, it is important to be aware of the evaluation and the surgical management of these patients.

Evaluation

History

The discovery of kidney stones may be related to acute onset of symptoms or an incidental finding on imaging studies. Acute presentation generally involves symptoms of renal colic. Classically, the patient experiences significant acute onset flank pain that radiates to the ipsilateral abdomen and groin. The pain typically waxes and wanes, but may be continuous. Often, these patients are unable to find a comfortable position. Other common symptoms include nausea, vomiting, lower urinary tract symptoms, hematuria, and sometimes fever. Distal stones can present with ipsilateral groin, testicular, and vulvar pain. The physician must be aware that this presentation can mimic the symptoms of testicular torsion or epididymitis.

Evaluation begins with a meticulous history and careful physical examination. A thorough past medical history determines risk factors for stone formation including a history of nephrolithiasis. Medical comorbidities that predispose to an increased rate of stone formation include inflammatory bowel disease, small bowel resection, gastric bypass, colectomy, recurrent urinary tract infections (UTIs), sarcoidosis, hyperparathyroidism, and gouty diathesis. Distal renal tubular acidosis (type I) is an important risk factor for stone formation. It is characterized by metabolic acidosis, hypokalemia, and a urinary pH > 6. This metabolic derangement is associated with the formation of calcium phosphate stones. Urological problems that can alter the transport of urine and increase the risk of stone formation include ureteropelvic junction (UPJ) obstruction, history of bladder reconstruction, prostatic obstruction, history of UTIs, and medullary sponge kidney.

A good dietary history is helpful including inquiries regarding fluid, calcium, oxalate, salt, and animal protein intake and hydration status. Medications are also important and many contribute to stone formation (Table 4.1).

Table 4.1 Medications associated with kidney stone formation

Drug	Type of stone/ metabolic derangement
Steroids	Hypercalciuria
Loop diuretics	Hypercalciuria
Colchicine	Hyperuricosuria
Vitamin D	Hypercalcemia
Indinivir	Radiolucent stones
Triamterene	Radiolucent stones

A social and family history is also important to elicit. Patients with a family history of stones have an increased risk of stone formation [1]. A sedentary lifestyle and immobility also carry an increased risk.

Physical examination

A thorough physical examination may aid in the diagnosis and localization of stone disease. Vitals signs are reviewed for temperature, heart rate, blood pressure, and respirations to screen for infection and impending sepsis. Examination of the abdomen and flank region can help localize the stone. A complete genitourinary examination is required particularly when groin, testicular, or vulvar pain is present. A thorough examination helps narrow the differential diagnosis to urologic and exclude gastrointestinal and gynecologic etiologies.

Laboratory studies

Urinalysis and urine culture are required. Microscopic hematuria is usually present, although in 15% of patients it is absent [1]. Leukocytes may also be present and can suggest inflammation. The presence of nitrites in the urine suggests infection. Urine pH is a critical aspect of urinalysis that can aid in determination of stone composition and therefore possible treatment. A pH of <5.5 suggests uric acid stone composition. A pH of >6.0 with associated metabolic acidosis, and hypokalemia could signify renal tubular acidosis and calcium phosphate stones. A pH of >6.0 with a positive urine culture with ureolytic bacteria suggests that a struvite stone may be present. Lastly, urine sediment should be analyzed for crystals (Table 4.2).

Table 4.2 Stone composition and crystal shape

Stone composition	Crystal shape
Calcium oxalate	Dumbbell/hourglass/bipyramidal
Calcium phosphate	Needle shaped/amorphous
Uric acid	Amorphous/rosettes
Struvite	Coffin lid
Cystine	Hexagonal (benzene ring)

Serum studies such as complete blood count (CBC) and complete metabolic panel (CMP) should be drawn to evaluate white blood cell count, electrolytes, creatinine, and calcium levels. Phosphate and uric acid may also be useful. If calcium is elevated, intact parathyroid hormone (PTH) and vitamin D levels should be evaluated as well.

Imaging

The gold standard for stone diagnosis is computed tomography (CT) scan of the abdomen and pelvis without contrast. Over 99% of stones, including those that are radiolucent on plain film radiography, will be seen on CT scan [2]. In addition to visualization of the stone, CT reveals other important signs including hydronephrosis, hydroureter, perinephric stranding, and nephromegaly. Sites of obstruction are typically the UPJ, pelvic brim, and ureterovesical junction [2]. Other imaging modalities that are used to evaluate stones are plain radiography (KUB) and ultrasound. Less commonly used are magnetic resonance imaging and nuclear scans. Intravenous (IV) pyelograms were historically used but are rarely used today for evaluation of stones. KUB can be challenging in the primary diagnosis of stones, particularly in the pelvis, as they can be difficult to distinguish from phleboliths. Stones are usually irregular in shape while pelvic phleboliths are round. KUB can assist in following a stone if it is radio-opaque; if it is radiolucent on KUB, uric acid composition is likely.

Ultrasound is first line for evaluating stones in pregnant patients and the pediatric population. Its diagnostic utility however is limited with ureteral stones. Transvaginal ultrasound can sometimes be helpful for distal ureteral stones. Magnetic resonance urography is also a noncontrast alternative that shows good sensitivity and specificity compared to CT [3].

Management of acute stone event

The acute management of renal colic begins with supportive measures. IV fluids are crucial to hydrate a patient who presents with nausea and vomiting. Antiemetics can be used if nausea persists. Pain control can be achieved with oral and IV analgesics. A combination of narcotics and nonsteroidal anti-inflammatories (NSAIDs) helps alleviate pain in the majority of patients but are contraindicated in patients with renal dysfunction, bleeding diathesis, peptic ulcer disease, and gastroesophageal reflux disease. If infection is suspected, antibiotics should also be administered.

Indications for admission include uncontrolled pain, inability to tolerate food or liquid, renal insufficiency, solitary kidney, bilateral obstruction, suspicion of obstructed pyelonephritis (leukocytosis and/or fever), or multiple comorbidities. If infection is present, urgent decompression with a nephrostomy tube or ureteral stent is required, and definitive management should be deferred until the antibiotic course is completed to reduce the risk of sepsis perioperatively. Choice of decompression depends on several factors including stone location and size, anatomical abnormalities, presence of hydronephrosis, available resources, and surgeon preference. Clinical deterioration may be rapid with obstructed pyelonephritis, and the choice of ureteral stent or nephrostomy tube may involve which may be placed more expeditiously.

Healthy patients with no evidence of infection, no renal insufficiency, well-controlled pain, ability to tolerate food and liquid, and stones <1 cm in size may be placed on expectant management with a trial of passage and treated with medical expulsive therapy. Urine should be strained and stone sent for analysis, if passed.

Expectant management

Expectant management consists of medical expulsive therapy and pain medications for a maximum of 4 weeks. Alpha-blockers, steroids, and calcium channel blockers have all been used for medical expulsive therapy. In general, stones <4 mm have a 90% chance of passage, 4–6 mm have a 60% chance of passage, and >6 mm have a 20% chance of passage with expectant management.

Alpha-blockers inhibit alpha receptors located on the terminal ureter, decreasing ureteral tone. In a prospective trial, Wang et al. demonstrated a 78–81%

expulsion rate when comparing alpha-blockers to placebo for lower ureteral stones <10 mm [4]. Parsons et al. conducted a meta-analysis evaluating the efficacy of alpha-blocker therapy for aid in the expulsion of ureteral stones. Eleven randomized trials were reviewed with 911 participants. Their results show that the use of alpha-blockers was associated with a 44% higher chance of spontaneously expelling the stone versus conservative therapy alone [5].

Steroids may aid in decreasing inflammation and ureteral spasms. Porpiglia et al. prospectively examined the effects of alpha-blockers given with corticosteroids in the treatment of symptomatic distal ureteral stones. Their published results show a significantly higher expulsion rate with the use of combined corticosteroids with alpha-blockers compared to either one alone and placebo. Furthermore, their combined use was associated with a significant decrease in analgesic consumption [6].

The role of calcium channel blockers during expectant management of stones has also been studied. Studies show that calcium channel blockers decrease ureteral muscle spasms and help with stone passage when combined with steroids [7, 8]. The EAU/AUA guidelines for management of ureteral calculi recommend expectant management as an option for patients with stones <10 mm, with alpha-blockers preferred over calcium channel blockers for medical expulsive therapy [9].

Surgical planning

If expectant management fails, if the stone is >1 cm, or if there is another indication for treatment as discussed above, then the next course of action is surgical treatment. Shock wave lithotripsy (SWL), ureteroscopy (URS), and percutaneous nephrolithotomy (PNL) are the current surgical techniques utilized. Herein, we discuss each modality, their indications, and their potential complications. Regardless of which modality is chosen, culture-specific antibiotics are imperative to a safe and effective operation [10].

Extracorporeal SWL

SWL utilizes external energy in the form of sound waves to fragment stones in a minimally invasive fashion. At the time of SWL, the stone is visualized using fluoroscopy or ultrasound while the patient is under general anesthesia or sedation. Potential long-term renal effects of SWL include renal injury/scar and hypertension. There is a transient decrease in renal blood flow. Immediate complications include hematoma (<1%), UTI/sepsis, or obstruction (steinstrasse). Although extremely rare, injury to adjacent nearby organs can occur. Contraindications to the use of SWL include pregnancy, calcified aneurysm, morbid obesity, and bleeding diathesis.

Success of SWL depends on patient selection with several factors associated with a poor outcome. Contraindications include stone burden >2 cm and staghorn calculi. Stone composition also affects success rate. Patients with stones composed of brushite, matrix, cystine, calcium oxalate monohydrate, or that are high density on imaging (>750 HU) have been associated with worse outcomes. Obese patients, abnormal renal anatomy, and stones in lower pole calyces and diverticuli also portend lower success rates [11].

There are several factors that help optimize the success rate of SWL. Technical factors that can increase stone-free rate include slow shock wave delivery (60 shocks per minute) and "ramping up" shock wave energy. Ramping up the energy can also help decrease renal injury [12]. Several clinical trials comparing IV sedation versus general anesthesia revealed significantly superior outcomes with general anesthesia (78–87% vs. 51–55%) [12–14]. Lastly, optimizing coupling between the SWL device and the patient is important. Using large amounts of coupling medium (gel or oil) and proper application can help optimize coupling and decrease the amount of air pockets created [11].

Postoperative follow-up should include a KUB in 2–4 weeks to assess stone fragmentation and passage. Patients should also be monitored for hypertension.

Ureteroscopy

URS allows for direct visualization and manipulation of the stone. Significant advances in endourologic technology have resulted in miniaturization of both scopes and instruments. Additionally, deflection capabilities have improved significantly. This allows for increased maneuverability, better visualization, and an increased safety profile. Available devices to be used in adjunct with URS have grown as well. As a result of these developments, URS has become safer, more efficient, and more efficacious. Potential complications include infection, stent discomfort, ureteral injury, and ureteral stricture.

Percutaneous nephrolithotomy

Indications for the use of PNL include a stone burden >2 cm, stones in a calyceal diverticulum, proximal ureteral stone burden >1 cm, and failure of other methods. Major complications from PNL occur in 1–7% of patients and include bleeding, organ injury, perforation, hydrothorax, or pneumothorax [9]. Minor complications also occur at 11–25% [9]. A multi-institutional review of findings on routine postoperative CT after PNL in 197 patients revealed a variety of thoracic complications including atelectasis (44.7%), pleural effusion (8.6%), pneumothorax (1.5%), hemothorax (1%), and hydrothorax (0.5%). Renal complications were observed as well with perinephric hematoma (7.6%) and collecting system perforation (2%) being the most common [15]. Urologists often obtain a CT scan postoperatively to evaluate residual stone burden.

Renal stone treatment

Stones <2 cm

As discussed before, expectant management with medical expulsive therapy (MET) is a viable option for stones <1 cm in size. Additionally, nonobstructing asymptomatic stones <2 cm that are diagnosed incidentally can be observed. However, many stones in the kidney will increase in size, and up to 50% will become symptomatic within 5 years. If the stone composition is uric acid, a trial of alkalinizing agents can be attempted for dissolution.

For symptomatic stones <2 cm, both SWL and URS are the viable options. Success rates of SWL have been reported by size: <1 cm, 80%; 1.1–2 cm, 65%; and >2 cm, 50%; but these vary based on location as well [16]. The use of ureteral stent prior to SWL has not been shown to be effective and will increase lower urinary tract symptoms. Hard stones composed of cystine, calcium oxalate monohydrate, and HU >750 have poor fragmentation rates with SWL and should be treated with URS. Obesity will also hinder stone fragmentation with SWL.

URS with laser lithotripsy is a very effective modality for the treatment of stones <2 cm in size. Stone-free rates have been reported to be >90% in expert hands [17].

Opinions regarding treatment of lower pole stones <2 cm are mixed. Pearle et al. conducted a prospective randomized multicenter trial that evaluated the use of SWL versus URS in 78 patients with lower pole stones <1 cm. At 3 months follow-up, patients who underwent SWL and URS had radiograph stone-free rates of 35% and 50%, respectively. However, their results were not statistically significant [18]. Comparing SWL to PNL, stone-free rates for <1 cm lower pole stones are 70% and 100% for SWL and PNL, respectively [19, 20].

For lower pole stones 1–2 cm, many factors must be taken into account to determine the optimal treatment modality. Factors should be stone composition, renal anatomy, and patient preference.

For stones <2 cm, PNL is reserved for stones that have failed SWL and/or URS, are in a narrow infundibulum (<4 mm), are within a calyx with an acute infundibulopelvic angle (<90°), are in a calyceal diverticulum, and for patients with any anatomic abnormality that may compromise the effectiveness of SWL or URS.

Stones >2 cm

PNL should be employed for stones >2 cm in size as first-line therapy. Stone-free rates have been shown to be 90% for PNL and 30% for SWL [19, 20]. Staged URS can be considered if the patient is morbidly obese, coagulopathic, or other conditions are present that would complicate PNL. Open or laparoscopic anatrophic nephrolithotomy is rarely done, but is reserved as a last option if all other therapies have failed.

Staghorn calculi are complex stones that can be partial or complete in nature. A partial staghorn extends into two or more calyces. A complete staghorn extends into all calyces. Management of staghorn calculi can be handled using several approaches. PNL is the first-line therapy and the main treatment modality. AUA guidelines state that PNL monotherapy should be the treatment of choice. Furthermore, PNL results in superior stone-free rates when compared to SWL [21].

"Sandwich therapy" is a term reserved for the treatment of staghorn calculi and consists of three stages: PNL, SWL, and then flexible nephroscopy (or second PNL). Stages are separated by a minimum of 1–2 days. CT imaging should be done to evaluate for residual stone burden after each stage. Residual stone fragments can also be treated with flexible URS [21]. SWL monotherapy for staghorn calculi is not recommended and can result in postoperative complications that include steinstrasse (several small stones along the ureter and causing obstruction—literally, stone street), renal colic, sepsis, and perinephric hematoma. If SWL monotherapy must be performed, a percutaneous nephrostomy tube or ureteral stent is mandatory, but again only in cases in which PNL is contraindicated [21]. PNL stone-free rates for the treatment of staghorn calculi are around 78%. Sandwich therapy has been reported at 66%, SWL 54%, and open surgery 71% [21]. Complication rates for PNL, sandwich therapy, SWL, and open surgery have been reported at 15%, 14%, 19%, and 13%, respectively [21].

Anatomic variants

Treatment of stones in patients with anatomic variants can be challenging. Patients with stones in calyceal diverticulum should be managed with PNL (stone-free rate 90%). The use of PNL allows for ablation of the diverticulum as well as incision of the calyceal neck. URS can be attempted for the management of small stones in these diverticuli, however, this can be challenging and stone-free rate is low.

Management of stones in patients with horseshoe kidneys can usually be done with either SWL or PNL. SWL is usually reserved for smaller stones while PNL is mainly for larger stones, patients who have failed SWL, or those who have contraindications for SWL. Percutaneous access is achieved in the upper pole into a posterior calyx.

Finally, patients with a concomitant UPJ obstruction can be managed with combined PNL and endopyelotomy.

Ureteral stone treatment

Stones <1 cm: proximal

Stones <5 mm have over a 50% chance of passing on their own [14]. If expectant management is not preferred, both SWL and URS are reasonable options. Stone-free rates using SWL and URS are reported as 90% and 80%, respectively [9].

Stones >1 cm: proximal

Any of the described modalities (SWL, URS, and PNL) are acceptable options. Stone- free rates are 68%, 79%, and 74%, respectively [9].

Stones <1 cm: distal

Small stones in the distal ureter have a spontaneous passage rate over 50% [14]. If MET fails or treatment is required for another indication, typically they can be managed with either SWL or URS. Stone-free rates are high using either modality at 86% and 90%, respectively [9]. The limiting factor for SWL is good visualization on radiography.

Stones >1 cm: distal

SWL and URS are both options with stone-free rates reported to be 74% and 93%, respectively [9].

Stone fragmentation techniques

There are several stone fragmentation methods that are currently utilized. Electrohydraulic, electromagnetic, and piezoelectric are the different SWL devices that have been utilized. Holmium:YAG laser, pneumatic, and ultrasonic devices are used for URS and PNL.

Metabolic stone evaluation

Once the acute stone event is resolved, a metabolic stone evaluation may be warranted. Please see Chapter 3: *Nephrolithiasis: etiology, stone composition, medical management, and prevention* for a more thorough explanation of a metabolic stone evaluation [22, 23].

Stones during pregnancy

There are several changes that occur during pregnancy that alter the risk profile of nephrolithiasis. Hydronephrosis occurs secondary to increased progesterone and mechanical compression by the enlarged uterus inducing urinary stasis. Pregnancy is also associated with hypercitraturia, hypermagnesuria, hyperuricosuria, and hypercalciuria [24].

Renal colic during pregnancy poses a diagnostic challenge, as radiation exposure must be minimized. Ultrasound is the first-line modality of choice for but can have limited utility for ureteral stones. Transvaginal ultrasound may assist with visualization of distal ureteral stones [25]. Magnetic resonance imaging is emerging as a new noncontrast radiation-free technique that is safe in pregnancy and shows similar diagnostic yield to CT [3].

With conservative management, spontaneous passage rate is high (75%). Obstructing stones can be managed as in nonpregnant patients, but with the use of ultrasound, to place a stent or nephrostomy tube. Ureteral stents must be changed every 4–8 weeks in pregnant patients due to increased tendency to encrust.

With recent advances in endourologic technology, treatment of the stone with URS and laser is now an acceptable option in experienced hands [26, 27]. A recent meta-analysis evaluating the safety of URS in pregnant patients showed no significant difference in pregnant versus nonpregnant patients [28]. Both SWL and PNL are contraindicated.

WHAT TO AVOID/KEY PITFALLS

- Nephrolithiasis can have an atypical presentation. A low threshold for obtaining CT scan is necessary, particularly if infection is suspected.
- Differential diagnosis for nephrolithiasis is broad, and a thorough examination and evaluation is required.
- Gastrointestinal and gynecologic etiologies should be excluded.
- Other possible urologic causes include, but are not limited to, pyelonephritis, testicular torsion, and epididymitis
- Observation of an obstructing stone with associated infection can lead to life-threatening sepsis
- Special considerations must be made for anatomical variations, such as UPJ obstruction, horseshoe kidneys, and changes related to pregnancy

KEY WEB LINKS/RECOMMENDED READING

AUA website

www.auanet.org

Clinical Guidance:

- Staghorn Calculi—Report on the Management of Staghorn Calculi (2005) (Reviewed and validity confirmed 2009.)
- Ureteral Calculi—Management of Ureteral Calculi: EAU/AUA Nephrolithiasis Panel (2007). (Reviewed and validity confirmed 2010.)

Other AUA Clinical Guidance Documents:

- Shock Wave Lithotripsy—White Paper: Current Perspective on Adverse Effects in Shock Wave Lithotripsy (2009).

Multiple choice questions

1 Which of the following is most consistent with renal tubular acidosis type 1?

a Calcium phosphate stones; urine pH > 6; metabolic acidosis; hypokalemia
b No formation of stones; pH > 6; metabolic alkalosis; hypokalemia
c pH < 6; metabolic acidosis; hypokalemia
d Calcium phosphate stones; pH > 6; metabolic acidosis; hyperkalemia
e pH < 6; metabolic alkalosis; hyperkalemia

2 Which imaging modality is considered first line for the diagnosis of stones in pregnancy?

a Intravenous pyelogram
b Magnetic resonance imaging
c Renal ultrasound
d CT scan
e Plain radiography

3 The following are all metabolic derangements found in pregnant patients *except:*

a Hypercitraturia
b Hypermagnesuria
c Hypercalciuria
d Hyperoxaluria

4 For stones in a calyceal diverticulum the best modality for clearing the stone is

a URS
b SWL
c PNL
d URS followed by SWL
e Do nothing

References

1 Menon M. Urinary lithiasis: etiology, diagnosis, and medical management. In: Campbell MF, Walsh PC, Retik AB, editors. *Campbell's Urology.* 8th ed. Philadelphia, PA: Elsevier Saunders; 2002.

2 Smith RC, Coll DM. Helical computed tomography in the diagnosis of ureteric colic. *BJU Int* 2000;86(Suppl 1): 33–41.

3 Regan F, Kuszyk B, Bohlman ME, Jackman S. Acute ureteric calculus obstruction: unenhanced spiral CT versus HASTE MR urography and abdominal radiograph. *Br J Radiol* 2005;78(930):506–511.

4 Wang CJ, Huang SW, Chang CH. Efficacy of an alpha1 blocker in expulsive therapy of lower ureteral stones. *J Endourol* 2008; 22(1):41–46.

5 Parsons JK, Hergan LA, Sakamoto K, Lakin C. Efficacy of alpha-blockers for the treatment of ureteral stones. *J Urol* 2007;177(3):983–987; discussion 987.

6 Porpiglia F, Vaccino D, Billia M, et al. Corticosteroids and tamsulosin in the medical expulsive therapy for symptomatic distal ureter stones: single drug or association? *Eur Urol* 2006;50(2):339–344.

7 Borghi L, Meschi T, Amato F, et al. Nifedipine and methylprednisolone in facilitating ureteral stone passage: a randomized, double-blind, placebo-controlled study. *J Urol* 1994;152(4):1095–1098.

8 Porpiglia F, Destefanis P, Fiori C, Fontana D. Effectiveness of nifedipine and deflazacort in the management of distal ureter stones. *Urology* 2000;56(4):579–582.

9 Preminger GM, Tiselius HG, Assimos DG, et al. 2007 guideline for the management of ureteral calculi. *J Urol* 2007;178(6):2418–2434.

10 Pearle MS. Prevention of nephrolithiasis. *Curr Opin Nephrol Hypertens* 2001;10(2):203–209.

11 Matlaga BR, Semins MJ. How to improve results with extracorporeal shock wave lithotripsy. *Ther Adv Urol* 2009;1(2):99–105.

12 Semins MJ, Trock BJ, Matlaga BR. The effect of shock wave rate on the outcome of shock wave lithotripsy: a meta-analysis. *J Urol* 2008;179(1):194–197; discussion 197.

13 Sorensen C, Chandhoke P, Moore M, Wolf C, Sarram A. Comparison of intravenous sedation versus general anesthesia on the efficacy of the Doli 50 lithotriptor. *J Urol* 2002;168(1):35–37.

14 Eichel L, Batzold P, Erturk E. Operator experience and adequate anesthesia improve treatment outcome with third-generation lithotripters. *J Endourol* 2001;15(7):671–673.

15 Semins MJ, Bartik L, Chew BH, et al. Multicenter analysis of postoperative CT findings after percutaneous nephrolithotomy: defining complication rates. *Urology* 2011;78(2):291–294

16 Lingeman JE, Lifshitz DA, Evan AP. Surgical management of urinary lithiasis. In: Campbell MF, Walsh PC, Retik AB, editors. *Campbell's Urology*. Philadelphia, PA: Elsevier Saunders; 2002.

17 Fabrizio MD, Behari A, Bagley DH. Ureteroscopic management of intrarenal calculi. *J Urol* 1998;159(4): 1139–1143.

18 Pearle MS, Lingeman JE, Leveillee R, et al. Prospective randomized trial comparing shock wave lithotripsy and ureteroscopy for lower pole caliceal calculi 1 cm or less. *J Urol* 2008;179(5 Suppl):S69–S73.

19 Lingeman JE, Siegel YI, Steele B, Nyhuis AW, Woods JR. Management of lower pole nephrolithiasis: a critical analysis. *J Urol* 1994;151(3):663–667.

20 Albala DM, Assimos DG, Clayman RV, et al. Lower pole I: a prospective randomized trial of extracorporeal shock wave lithotripsy and percutaneous nephrostolithotomy for lower pole nephrolithiasis—initial results. *J Urol* 2001;166(6):2072–2080.

21 Preminger GM, Assimos DG, Lingeman JE, et al. Chapter 1: AUA guideline on management of staghorn calculi: diagnosis and treatment recommendations. *J Urol* 2005;173(6):1991–2000.

22 Consensus Conference. Prevention and treatment of kidney stones. *JAMA* 1988;260(7):977–981.

23 Lifshitz DA, Shalhav AL, Lingeman JE, Evan AP. Metabolic evaluation of stone disease patients: a practical approach. *J Endourol* 1999;13(9):669–678.

24 McAleer SJ, Loughlin KR. Nephrolithiasis and pregnancy. *Curr Opin Urol* 2004;14(2):123–127.

25 Shokeir AA, Mahran MR, Abdulmaaboud M. Renal colic in pregnant women: role of renal resistive index. *Urology* 2000;55(3):344–347.

26 Watterson JD, Girvan AR, Beiko DT, et al. Ureteroscopy and holmium:YAG laser lithotripsy: an emerging definitive management strategy for symptomatic ureteral calculi in pregnancy. *Urology* 2002;60(3): 383–387.

27 Kavoussi LR, Jackman SV, Bishoff J.T. Re: Renal colic during pregnancy: a case for conservative treatment. *J Urol* 1998;160(3 Pt 1):837–838.

28 Semins MJ, Trock BJ, Matlaga BR. The safety of ureteroscopy during pregnancy: a systematic review and meta-analysis. *J Urol* 2009;181(1):139–143.

Answers to multiple choice questions

1 a Renal tubular acidosis (RTA) type 1 (distal) is associated with formation of calcium phosphate stones. It is the *only RTA* that is associated with kidney stones. Hypocitraturia is the main culprit leading to stone formation in RTA type 1. The main cause of development of RTA type 1 is impaired secretion of hydrogen ions in the distal nephron. Manifestations include urine pH > 6 and hypokalemia. Definitive diagnosis is marked by reduced urinary ammonium excretion (measured by urine anion gap).

Renal tubular acidosis type II (proximal) is a result of a defect in bicarbonate reabsorption. Initially, urine pH is elevated, but later normalizes. In contrast to type 1, citrate excretion is normal. Hence, nephrolithiasis is uncommon. Type II is associated with hypokalemia due to metabolic acidosis.

Renal tubular acidosis type IV (hypoaldosteronism) is seen in patients with renal disease and diabetic nephropathy. Nephrolithiasis is also uncommon in this type of RTA. Patients usually have hyperkalemic, hyperchloremic metabolic acidosis.

2 **c** Detecting and diagnosing nephrolithiasis in pregnancy can be challenging. The main point is to limit the radiation exposure to the fetus. AUA guidelines state that the *initial* modality of choice for diagnosing kidney stones during pregnancy is renal ultrasound. If this fails to diagnose, limited intravenous urogram or magnetic resonance imaging has historically been used. Magnetic resonance HASTE urogram without contrast is a newer modality that appears to be comparable to CT scans in the diagnosis of nephrolithiasis and is safe during pregnancy.

3 **d** There are several metabolic derangements found in pregnant patients. However, overall there is *no change in risk* of stone formation. This is due to the net effect of promoters and inhibitors being excreted. Increased calcium excretion results from increased vitamin D levels and increased GFR. Pregnancy also causes increased urinary excretion of inhibitors of crystal formation (magnesium and citrate). Hyperoxaluria does not occur in pregnancy.

4 **c** PNL is the most optimal and efficacious treatment for stones in a calyceal diverticulum with a stone-free rate of 90%. The use of PNL allows for ablation of the diverticulum as well as incision of the calyceal neck. URS can be attempted for the management of small stones, however, this can be challenging and stone-free rate is low.

Section 3 Reproductive and sexual function

5 Male infertility

Ahmed Magheli

Universitätsmedizin Charité Berlin, Berlin, Germany

KEY POINTS

- Among couples with normal fertility parameters, 20–25% will typically conceive within 1 month, 75% within 6 months, and 90% within 1 year.
- Fifteen percent of US couples are infertile: male factor infertility accounts up to 50% of infertility.
- Initial evaluation of male factor infertility includes history, physical examination, and semen analysis.
- Further evaluation and treatment depends upon semen analysis results. Patients may have low volume or absent ejaculate, azoospermia, oligospermia, asthenospermia (abnormalities of sperm movement), sperm morphological defects, and/or combinations of these abnormalities.
- Of infertile couples, 25–35% will conceive by intercourse alone without treatment.
- Intracytoplasmic sperm injection (ICSI) is an efficacious treatment modality.

CASE STUDY

A 36-year-old male patient and his 32-year-old female partner were seen in the outpatient clinic for evaluation of infertility. The couple had 2 years of unprotected sexual intercourse. However, no pregnancy was induced. The female partner has been recently thoroughly evaluated and female factor infertility seems unlikely. The patient stated that he had induced a pregnancy in another partner about 10 years ago. Furthermore, he commented that semen volume decreased over the past years following an epididymal infection. Otherwise, he is in good health and there is no prior urological or surgical history. On physical examination, the external genitalia were with no pathological findings with regular-sized testes of normal consistency. His laboratory tests including FSH, LH, prolactin, and TSH were within normal limits. On scrotal ultrasound the testes were normal, however, transrectally the left seminal vesicle was dilated and there was no right seminal vesicle. Semen analyses showed azoospermia. A diagnosis of left ductal aplasia and postinfectious secondary right ductal obstruction was made. The couple was recommended to undergo either testicular biopsy, and in the case of regular spermatogenesis, vasovasostomy or MESA and ICSI. The couple elected to undergo MESA and ICSI which resulted in sufficient sperm retrieval and induction of a pregnancy.

Introduction

Infertility is defined as the inability of a couple to successfully conceive after 1 year of unprotected sexual intercourse. It is estimated that about 15% of couples suffer from this condition. However, there are significant differences in infertility rates around the world and in the majority of countries the prevalence of infertility is not documented [1]. Traditionally, predominantly female factors were considered as the

Handbook of Urology, First edition. J. Kellogg Parsons, John B. Eifler and Misop Han.
Published 2014 by John Wiley & Sons, Ltd.

main cause. However, more recent evidence indicates that ~35% of infertilities are due to female factors alone, while 30% and 20% are considered due to male and combined factors, respectively. In 15% of cases, infertility lacks a clinically detectable cause and is categorized as unexplained or idiopathic infertilities. Among couples with normal fertility parameters, 20–25% will typically conceive within 1 month, 75% within 6 months, and 90% within 1 year [2].

The conditions associated with male infertility are numerous and can be found on a variety of pathophysiological levels. Generally, the etiology is categorized as acquired or congenital, and as pretesticular, post-testicular, or testicular. Since male infertility can be diagnosed with simple noninvasive means and little costs in the majority of cases, its detection or exclusion should be undertaken prior to more invasive examinations of the female partner. It has been shown that 70–80% of male factor infertilities can be diagnosed with history, physical examination, and hormonal/sperm analyses alone. One has to take into account that male and female partner age, as well as frequency of intercourse and timing of the intercourse, plays a significant role [3, 4].

Treatment options for male infertility could be as simple as antibiotic therapy for pyospermia up to complex microsurgical vasovasostomy for deferent duct obstruction, immunosuppression in patients with immunoinfertility, or advanced assisted reproduction techniques (ART).

Depending on the underlying conditions, diagnosis and therapy should be as less invasive as possible with an understanding attitude toward the challenging psychosocial aspects of infertility for a young couple.

Physiology and pathophysiology of male reproduction

Hypothalamus–pituitary–testicular axis

Gonadal and sexual functions are controlled by the hypothalamus–pituitary–testicular axis via the secretion of gonadotropin-releasing hormone (GnRH) by the hypothalamus in a pulsatile fashion (q90–120 minutes, highest in the morning and seasonally in the spring), which leads to the secretion of luteinizing hormone (LH) and follicular-stimulating hormone (FSH) from the anterior pituitary gland. The half-life of GnRH is 2–5 minutes. It is a closed-loop system with feedback control from the testis with the hypothalamus as the primary integration center. The GnRH-secreting neurons receive signals from multiple sites in the brain, including the amygdala and the olfactory and the visual cortex. Its release is stimulated by melatonin from the pineal gland and inhibited by testosterone, inhibin, corticotropin-releasing hormone, opiates, illness, and stress. Failure of GnRH-secreting cells to migrate properly during embryogenesis results in Kallmann syndrome (congenital hypogonadotropic hypogonadism), which is associated with anosmia and midline defects.

In the testes LH stimulates the Leydig cells to produce testosterone, while inhibin is produced by the Sertoli cells, which are stimulated via FSH. Inhibin and testosterone feedback on the anterior pituitary and inhibit FSH and LH secretions, respectively. FSH has a lower plasma concentration and a longer half-life than LH. For clinical purposes it is important to notice that the hypothalamus also releases thyrotropin-releasing hormone (TRH) and vasoactive intestinal peptide (VIP), which stimulate the secretion of prolactin from the anterior pituitary. Dopamine, which is also released from the hypothalamus, inhibits prolactin release. Excessive prolactin secretion may lead to gynecomastia, erectile dysfunction, and inhibition of GnRH and LH/FSH production, resulting in low testosterone levels (hypogonadism) and impaired spermatogenesis.

Anatomy of the testes

Normal testes have a volume of 15–25 mL and are covered by the tunica albuginea. The length is 4.5–5 cm. The arterial supply is by the internal spermatic artery, the deferential artery, and the cremasteric artery, while venous drainage is through the pampiniform plexus, which drains into the gonadal vein. Countercurrent exchange of heat lowers testicular temperature by 2–4°C, which is important for sufficient spermatogenesis. Varicocele formation, the dilatation and tortuosity of the pampiniform plexus, could lead to impaired spermatogenesis through the elevation of the testicular temperature.

The specific cellular content of the testes is composed of germ cells, Leydig cells, and Sertoli cells. The seminiferous tubules, which are surrounded by peritubular and myoid cells, contain the germ and Sertoli cells, while the Leydig cells are located in the interstitium between the seminiferous tubules.

Spermatogenesis, sperm maturation, and emission

Spermatogenesis is the development of early germ cells, spermatogonia, to spermatozoa in the seminiferous tubules. In the normal human testis there are 600–1200 seminiferous tubes, which are divided by fibrous septa from the tunica albuginea into 250 pyramidal lobes.

Spermatogonia, which are precursors of spermatozoa, are derived from the gonadal ridge and migrate as gonadocytes to the testes prior to testicular descent. During spermatogenesis, a process that takes 74 days, spermatogonia develop to primary and secondary spermatocytes and finally spermatids as they progress closer to the lumen of the seminiferous tubule. While the primary spermatocyte (46N) undergoes meiosis, secondary spermatocytes (23N) undergo cell division.

The role of the Sertoli cells, which are in contrast to germ cells nondividing, is to support spermatogenesis in the seminiferous epithelium. Furthermore, they form the blood–testis barrier with tight junctions between adjacent cells [5, 6].

The mature spermatids or spermatozoa migrate through the tubuli recti, rete testis, and ductuli efferentes into the epididymis. During the passage through the epididymis maturation of the spermatozoa takes place and fertilization capacity is acquired. Several substances, such as glycerophosphorylcholine, sialic acid, and carnitine are secreted by the epididymis to aid in sperm protection and nutrition.

After the maturation process in the epididymis, sperm enters the deferent duct or vas deferens, which is an ~30 cm long muscular tube. It is divided into the following segments: convoluted, scrotal, inguinal, retroperitoneal, and ampullary section. At the ampullary portion, the vas joins with the seminal vesicles and empties into the prostatic urethra at the verumontanum. Ejaculation is initiated by rhythmic contractions of the vas deferens smooth muscle and an interaction of the bulbourethral and a number of additional pelvic muscles.

Seminal fluid, sperm characteristics

The seminal fluid consists of secretions from the testis, epididymis, Cowper's bulbourethral glands, periurethral gland of Littre, prostate (acidic), and seminal vesicles (alkaline). Initially, the seminal fluid is a coagulum due to the seminal vesicle fluid which is high in fructose. After ~10–15 minutes, liquefaction occurs secondary to prostate-derived proteases (PSA and plasminogen activator). The seminal fluid volume is typically between 2 and 5 mL. Abnormally low volumes could be caused by ejaculatory duct obstruction (acidic pH, low fructose), androgen deficiency (acidic, low fructose), retrograde ejaculation, sympathetic denervation, agenesis of the vas deferens and/or seminal vesicles (acidic pH, low fructose, lack of coagulation), or drug therapy.

Ejaculate reference limits have recently changed (Table 5.1).

Sperm motility is categorized as follows: progressive motility (PR)—spermatozoa moving actively, either linearly or in a large circle, regardless of speed; nonprogressive motility (NP)—all other patterns of motility with an absence of progression, that is, swimming in small circles, the

Table 5.1 Characteristics of normal semen (WHO 1999 and WHO 2010) [32, 33]

Parameter	Lower reference limit (WHO 2010)	Lower reference limit (WHO 1999)
Semen volume	1.5 mL	2 mL
Total sperm number (10^6 per ejaculate)	39	40
Sperm concentration (10^6 per mL)	15	20
Total motility (PR-NR, %)	40	50
Progressive motility (PR, %)	32	25
Vitality (live spermatozoa, %)	58	75
Sperm morphology (normal forms, %)	4	15
Other consensus threshold values		
pH	≥7.2	≥7.2
MAR test (motile spermatozoa with bound particles, %)	<50	50
Immunobead test (motile spermatozoa with bound beads, %)	<50	50

flagellar force hardly displacing the head or when only a flagellar beat can be observed; and immotility (IM)—no movement [7].

Normal sperm morphology is defined as follows: head—oval shaped (5–6 × 2.5–3.5 microns), acrosome (40–70% of head); midpiece—1.5× head length, <1 micron wide; tail—uncoiled, free from kinks, ~45 microns long; cytoplasmic droplets—in midpiece only and <1/2 of the head area. The normal ranges for various parameters of semen quality are shown in Table 5.1.

Etiology of male infertility

There are a number of ways to categorize male infertility. One popular way is to categorize into pre-, intra-, and post-testicular etiology of infertility. In a nice overview, Nagler presented data on etiology of male infertility in the United States (see Table 5.2).

The details on the respective conditions leading to male infertility are presented in the diagnosis/clinical investigation section.

Pretesticular etiology

Pretesticular causes for infertility or secondary testicular failure are typically endocrinological diseases which alter testicular function.

Table 5.2 Etiology of male infertility in the United States

Category	Percent
Varicocele	42.2
Idiopathic	22.7
Obstruction	14.3
Normal/female factor	7.9
Cryptorchidism	3.4
Immunologic	2.6
Ejaculatory dysfunction	1.3
Testicular failure	1.3
Drugs/radiation	1.1
Endocrinopathy	1.1
Others	2.1

Source: Nagler HM, Martinis FG. Varicocele. In: Lipshultz LI, Howards S, editors. *Infertility in the Male*. St. Louis, MO: Mosby Year Book; 1997; pp. 336–59.

Hypogonadotropic hypogonadism

Hypogonadotropic hypogonadism is caused by inadequate GnRH secretion, which could be acquired or idiopathic.

Acquired: CNS abnormalities, head trauma, pituitary tumors, autoimmunologic, radiation, Cushing disease (through negative feedback of cortisol on the hypothalamus → GnRH↓).

Idiopathic: insufficient GnRH secretion, idiopathic, with Kallmann syndrome (hypogonadotropic hypogonadism plus anosmia, cleft palate), or Prader–Willi syndrome (hypotonia, obesity, cryptorchidism, short stature, mental retardation).

Hyperprolactinemia

Hyperprolactinemia is associated with erectile dysfunction, low serum testosterone, and decreased libido. Often, this condition is idiopathic or caused by stress and/or medications. However, a pituitary tumor has to be ruled out. The most effective modality in this context is an MRI of the head.

Other causes

Other potential causes for pretesticular infertility are hemochromatosis (iron deposits in testes (primary failure)/pituitary (secondary)), estrogen-producing tumors (adrenocortical, Sertoli cell tumor), or Noonan syndrome (male counterpart to Turner syndrome + cryptorchidism).

Intratesticular etiology

Klinefelter syndrome (47, XXY)

Klinefelter syndrome is the most common chromosomal cause of male infertility. It is estimated to occur in 1:500–1:1000 live births [8]. The syndrome has a broad variation of clinical presentation and is typically associated with eunuchoid appearance and delayed puberty.

46, XX male syndrome

Less frequent than Klinefelter syndrome (1:20,000). Presentation with gynecomastia, azoospermia, shorter stature, and hypospadias.

Down syndrome (trisomy 21)

Patients with Down syndrome typically present with impaired cognitive ability and physical growth, testicular dysfunction, and elevated LH and FSH levels.

Varicocele
Varicoceles are very common findings and affect up to 15% of the male population. They represent the most common attributable cause of male infertility and are a dilatation of the pampiniform plexus which leads to an increased testicular temperature and consecutive impairment of spermatogenesis [9]. Additional explanations for impaired spermatogenesis with varicoceles are reflux of toxic renal and adrenal metabolites to the testis and hypoxia of the testis through impaired venous outflow and associated oxidative stress [10]. Most commonly, a varicocele is found on the left side due to the drainage of the left scrotal vein to the renal vein which is considered to cause more turbulences than the direct drainage of the right testicular vein to the caval vein. Treatment is recommended if the varicocele is palpable on clinical examination, the couple has infertility, the female partner has normal fertility, and the male partner has abnormal findings on semen analysis (Best Practice Committee of the American Society for Reproductive Medicine).

Cryptorchidism
Cryptorchidism or undescended testis is a common finding in up to 2.7% of newborns, but <1% in 1-year olds. These patients are at high risk for infertility, even if the undescended testis is surgically brought to the scrotum. Impaired spermatogenesis is typically associated with elevated FSH and reduced inhibin levels. However, fertility rates are reported to be up to 89% in unilateral, 93% in age-matched controls, and 65% in patients with a history of bilateral cryptorchidism [11].

Trauma
Testicular trauma is a common cause for acquired infertility, either directly through the damage of testicular tissue or/and through the formation of antisperm antibodies (ASA).

Chemotherapy/radiation therapy
Radiation and chemotherapy are highly toxic to the testicular germ cells. Leydig cells, however, are more resistant and testicular testosterone production might be preserved. Even after radiation therapy with shielded testis, infertility might be caused by reactive oxygen-free radicals.

Sickle cell disease
Sickle cell disease could cause infertility as a consequence of microembolisms to the testis and secondary testicular scarring.

Other toxins
Alcohol, cigarettes, and marijuana use have been associated with infertility.

Post-testicular etiology

Vas deferens obstruction
Obstruction of the vas deferens might be congenital or acquired. Congenital obstruction has been reported in men whose mothers were exposed to DES. Furthermore, the congenital bilateral absence of the vas deferens (CBAVD) is a very common finding in cystic fibrosis.

Acquired obstruction of the vas deferens could be caused by surgery (inguinal hernia surgery, vasectomy) or prior infections (chlamydia, gonorrhea, tuberculosis)

Ejaculatory duct obstruction
Patients with ejaculatory duct obstruction typically present with normal FSH/LH, azoospermia, low ejaculatory volume, and bilaterally normal palpable vasa deferentia. Transrectal ultrasound usually leads to the diagnosis by the presence of dilated seminal vesicles.

Retrograde ejaculation
Retrograde ejaculation could be caused by a number of conditions, such as previous bladder neck surgery, retroperitoneal lymph node dissection, transurethral surgery, medications (alpha-antagonists, antidepressants), diabetes, spinal cord injury, and others. The consequence is demission of the semen into the bladder.

Management

Diagnosis and clinical investigations

History
Obtaining a thorough medical history is key to identify potential reasons for infertility. It is important to specifically ask for the duration of infertility, previous induced pregnancies, previous pregnancies of the female partner, and the results of potential previous

fertility assessments. Furthermore, seemingly trivial questions about libido, sexual habits, timing of intercourse, and the use of contraceptive methods have to be elucidated. Furthermore, developmental defects have to be evaluated. Evaluation should be undertaken for history of abnormal testicular descent, testicular surgery, abnormal puberty, loss of body hair, or decrease in frequency of shaving. Furthermore, any learning disabilities suggestive of Klinefelter syndrome and other childhood conditions, such as testicular torsion, orchitis, and hypospadias repair should be specifically asked about. Urological surgeries in the past should also be evaluated.

The presence of chronic medical conditions, such as diabetes, neurological disorders, renal, or liver disease could be important reasons for infertility. With regard to the urological history, previous infections of the urinary tract, sexually transmitted diseases (STD), previous testicular trauma, or testicular cancer should also be elucidated.

The social history could be important if there is evidence for cigarette and marijuana smoking and the regular use of alcohol as they could lead to decreased sperm count and/or motility/morphology and hypogonadism, respectively.

There are a number of medications, such as spironolactone, ketoconazole, and others which exhibit an antiandrogenic action. Others, such as sulfasalazine, colchicine, and methotrexate lead to impairment of sperm quality on many levels.

Furthermore, there are a number of substances and conditions which could cause infertility simply by environmental exposure. These include heat exposure and exposure to certain pesticides and other toxic substances in agriculture and several industrial branches.

The level of knowledge in the majority of couples regarding timing of the intercourse and the use of potentially sperm-harming substances (lubrication) is highly overestimated by many physicians and should be specifically asked about.

Physical examination

General Physical examination should be comprehensive with a special focus on the genital examination. However, possible endocrinological imbalances and/or genetic syndromes could be suspected from the general examination. A special focus should be on the level of virilization, gynecomastia, and eunuchoid proportions, which could be caused by low serum testosterone, adrenal dysfunction, irregularities in the estrogen–testosterone ratio, or Klinefelter syndrome.

Genital
Generally, the genital examination is started with an examination of the penis. Abnormalities, such as phimosis, hypospadias, or Peyronie's disease should be excluded. The testes should be examined in the supine and standing position in a warm room to prevent contraction of the cremasteric muscles. The testes should be palpated between the thumb, the index, and the third finger. The examiner has to evaluate size and consistency. To estimate the testicular volume, a Prader orchidometer or alternatively ultrasound measurement should be used. Normal testicular measurements have been established to be 20 mL in volume [12]. Since the majority of testicular volume (~85%) is considered to be involved in spermatogenesis, impaired spermatogenesis is likely with significantly reduced testicular size. On the other hand, testicular swelling could be caused by orchitis, testicular neoplasms, or other conditions requiring medical or surgical therapy.

Laboratory testing

Semen analysis—abnormal findings
Semen analysis is the cornerstone of the diagnostic workup for male infertility. It should be performed at a certified and experienced andrological laboratory to prevent misdiagnosis. The analysis of the semen includes macro- and microscopic evaluation, biochemical and immunological testing. The sample is usually collected through masturbation. However, if this is not an option for the patient, a special nonspermicidal condom can be used in order to collect the sample during intercourse. If patients prefer to obtain the sample at home, transportation to the laboratory within 30 minutes at body temperature should be guaranteed. Sexual abstinence is recommended for a period of 3 days, but not longer than 5 days. There should be two sperm analyses performed with a minimum of 7 days in between. The details on normal sperm count findings are described above and in Table 5.1. The following diagnoses could be established from this investigation.

Aspermia Aspermia is defined as the absence of any ejaculate. Potential reasons for this condition are medications, retroperitoneal or bladder neck surgery, ejaculatory duct obstruction, diabetes, spinal cord injury, psychological disturbances, or idiopathic.

Azoospermia Azoospermia is the absence of sperm in the ejaculate. It could be caused by congenital or acquired obstruction or absence of the vas deferens or spermatogenic arrest. Previous vasectomy is one of the most common reasons for azoospermia. One has to consider the following differential diagnoses.

Hypogonadotropic hypogonadism, Kallmann syndrome, pituitary tumor with hormonal imbalances, spermatogenic–chromosomal abnormalities, Y-chromosome microdeletions, gonadotoxins, varicocele, viral orchitis, torsion, idiopathic.

Ductal obstruction—CBAVD, vasal obstruction, epididymal obstruction, ejaculatory duct obstruction

Oligospermia Oligospermia is defined as a sperm concentration below the lower reference limit of 15 million/mL. Reasons for this condition are numerous and include the following:

varicocele (most common), cryptorchidism, idiopathic, drugs/heat/toxins, systemic infection, endocrinopathy.

Asthenospermia Asthenospermia is present if the percentage of motile sperm is below the lower reference limit for this characteristic (<40% overall motility or <32% progressive motility). This condition could be caused by a number of factors such as spermatozoal structural defects, prolonged sexual abstinence, idiopathic, genital tract infection, and ASA.

Teratospermia Teratospermia describes defects in sperm morphology. According to the latest WHO handbook for the evaluation of the ejaculate, at least 4% of the sperm should exhibit regular morphology.

Combinations of the aforementioned conditions are frequent. If a patient shows a low sperm count with reduced motility, the condition is called oligoasthenospermia.

Advanced sperm analyses

Postcoital test In the postcoital or sperm–mucus interaction test, the capability of sperm to transverse the cervix and the cervical mucus is evaluated. This *in vitro* test is performed 2–8 hours after regular intercourse utilizing a mucus migration assay. Generally, 10–20 sperms per high power field (HPF) are considered normal. Abnormal testing could be caused by ASA or inappropriate timing of the test as well as abnormal semen parameters and/or poor cervical mucus quality [13].

Acrosome reaction This test is rarely performed in clinical practice. The acrosome is a membrane-bound organelle at the sperm head which is crucial for successful sperm penetration into the ovum through the zona pellucida. Normal sperm shows a spontaneous acrosome reaction rate of <5%. However, if stimulation is performed during testing, the induced acrosome reaction rates are between 15% and 40%. Lower rates could be caused by sperm head malformations.

Hamster egg penetration assay In this assay, the functional capacity of sperm to fertilize an oocyte is determined. It is performed with zona pellucida free hamster eggs and allows observing the capability of spermatozoa to undergo capacitation, acrosome reaction, membrane fusion with oocytes, and chromatin condensation. Poor test results could explain unfavorable IVF results [14].

Sperm chromatin and DNA assays With the increased use of IVF, a number of tests for sperm DNA damage have been established. Spermatozoal chromatin is packed in the nuclear head in order to prevent stress and breakage. Its damage has multiple reasons, such as oxidative stress, tobacco use, chemotherapy, testicular cancer, and others [15]. Defects in sperm chromatin could explain low success rates of IVF. However, test results depend on many factors and show great intra- and interindividual variations.

Computer-aided semen analysis

Computer-aided semen analysis (CASA) was first applied in the 1980s to make sperm analyses more objective. With CASA a camera is linked to a computer and sperm concentration and movements are semiautomatically evaluated. In addition to curvilinear velocity, straight-line velocity and path velocity are measured. CASA is used very rarely in daily practice due to the immense technical expenditure with no direct clinical consequences. However, for research purposes, CASA is an interesting tool [16].

Antisperm antibody test Normally, the immune system does not have any contact with postmeiotic germ cells due to the blood–testis barrier established by the Sertoli cells. However, if there has been an infection, vasectomy, testicular torsion, or testicular trauma, the barrier is violated and ASA formation may result. The effect of the antibodies on the spermatozoa could be agglutinating, immobilizing, or spermotoxic. The impact on the presence of ASA on male infertility has not been entirely understood. However, if ASA is present and the postcoital test is abnormal, intracytoplasmic sperm injection (ICSI) should be preferred over IVF. The most commonly specific method to date to evaluate ASA is the immunobead test.

Endocrine analysis It is estimated that only 3% of infertile man have endocrinopathies [17]. Routine hormonal testing includes FSH, LH, testosterone, and prolactin. Although testing is recommended by international committees only in cases of low sperm concentration, impaired sexual function, or other findings indicating endocrinological irregularities, many physicians perform hormonal analyses routinely in all men complaining of subfertility.

One has to consider that testing for testosterone should be performed in the morning due to its physiologic decline during the day. Elevations in FSH could be caused by spermatogenic defects, such as primary testicular failure presenting with hypergonadotropic hypogonadism. Obstructive conditions typically present with normal FSH and oligo- or azoospermia. Hypogonadism (low serum testosterone) could be caused primarily by testicular failure or hypothalamic of pituitary imbalances.

Low FSH and LH could be an indicator for Kallmann syndrome and require advanced endocrinological evaluation.

Elevation in estrogen levels could present with erectile dysfunction, gynecomastia, libido problems, and low testosterone. The most common causes are obesity and aromatization of testosterone to estradiol in adipocytes.

Hyperprolactinemia typically presents with low serum testosterone and elevated LH. While mildly elevated prolactin levels could be caused by stress, medications, or idiopathically, significantly elevated levels need further work-up to rule out prolactinoma.

Rarely, other endocrinopathies such as congenital adrenal hyperplasia (CAH) and thyroid dysfunction are causes for subfertility.

Imaging

Transrectal ultrasound

Transrectal ultrasound (TRUS) provides detailed information on the prostate and seminal vesicles. Abnormal findings of the vas deferens ampulla and ejaculatory ducts could also be detected. TRUS is especially helpful in patients with oligo- or azoospermia, in whom ejaculatory duct obstruction is suspected. This condition typically presents with enlarged seminal vesicles (width 12–15 mm) or dilated ejaculatory duct diameter (>2.3 mm) [18].

Seminovesiculography

Seminovesiculography is performed by TRUS-guided injection of radiopaque contrast into the seminal vesicles. Thereafter, radiographs are done to evaluate the anatomy of the seminal vesicles and ejaculatory ducts.

Scrotal ultrasonography

Scrotal ultrasound is an effective and simple way to evaluate testicular and epididymal anatomy. Testicular cancer, which may be associated with infertility, could be detected. Furthermore, infections like epididymitis and other conditions such as epididymal cysts which could cause obstruction are easily identified. The presence of a varicocele could be verified by utilizing Doppler ultrasound during the Valsalva maneuver.

Vasography

Vasography is the method of choice to test for assessing the patency of the ductal system. A typical patient would present with azoospermia and normal findings on testicular biopsy. Vasography is mainly performed at the time of anticipated surgical reconstruction due to the fact that scarring might occur at the vasogram site [19].

Testicular biopsy

Testicular biopsy is indicated in azoospermic patients with normal endocrine studies to evaluate spermatogenesis. Obstructive versus nonobstructive azoospermia could be differentiated that way. Additionally, sperm may be retrieved for future ICSI. Typically, testicular biopsy is an outpatient procedure under local anesthesia. It is of greatest importance to preserve the samples properly (Bouin's solution, Zenker's solution) to prevent distortion artifacts into the specimen with formalin perseveration. There are several scores established to quantify spermatogenic failure. One of the most commonly used is the Johnsen score [20].

Histological findings

Normal: adequate number of germ cells with regular maturation to elongated spermatids and spermatozoa.

Hypospermatogenesis: decreased number of all germ cells; if no obstruction is present it correlates with sperm count findings.

Maturation arrest: spermatogenesis is blocked at a specific stage, for example, spermatogonia or spermatocytes I.

Sertoli cell only syndrome: small seminiferous tubules without any germ cells.

Treatment

Surgical therapy

Vasovasostomy/vasoepididymostomy

If vas deferens obstruction or discontinuation is proven, microsurgical correction is indicated. With advances in clinical experience and surgical technique, excellent patency rates can be achieved for vasovasostomy [21]. However, even with patency rates >90%, pregnancy rates are still significantly lower and vary between 30% and 70%. One of the most important factors in this setting is the age of the female partner [22]. Vasoepididymostomy is technically very challenging and should be performed by experienced surgeons. The patency results are inferior compared to vasovasostomy.

Varicocelectomy

There have been several surgical techniques described for varicocelectomy. One of the latest approaches introduced in the 1990s is the scrotal one where the veins of the varicose plexus are ligated. However, there is a great risk of testicular artery injury and secondary testicular atrophy.

In the retroperitoneal approach, the dilated testicular veins are clipped or ligated with a small abdominal incision. The advantage is that the testicular veins are ligated at a level where only two or three branches are present and the testicular artery has not yet branched. Therefore, separation of the veins and preservation of the artery are easier. The laparoscopic approach is similar to the retroperitoneal one with the difference that access to the testicular vein is transperitoneally with the need of peritoneal incision over the testicular vessel.

To date, the preferred method is an inguinal or a subinguinal approach. The inguinal approach has the advantage of fewer vascular branches encountered compared to the subinguinal approach. With microsurgical equipment, individual veins are ligated. A recent meta-analysis suggests that varicocelectomy leads to statistically significant improvements of sperm count and sperm motility with the inguinal approach yielding the highest pregnancy rates [23].

Sperm retrieval

There are several ways to retrieve sperm for further therapy.

The easiest way is via percutaneous epididymal sperm aspiration (PESA), which offers the advantage of local anesthesia and better sperm motility, but has high variability of success in retrieving sperm and typically allows only small quantities of sperm retrieval. Furthermore, epididymal obstruction may occur.

Microsurgical epididymal sperm aspiration (MESA) yields large numbers of sperm with good motility and has a low complication rate. However, it requires anesthesia in some cases and microsurgical skills are needed. Similar to PESA it is not indicated for nonobstructive azoospermia.

Testicular sperm aspiration (TESA) provides sperm with poorer motility than PESA, but could be applied in cases of nonobstructive azoospermia. However, due to the little—if any—amount of sperm retrieved, it is rarely performed.

Testicular sperm extraction (TESE) with microsurgical dissection and intraoperative evaluation of suitable areas of sperm retrieval is the preferred technique in cases of nonobstructive azoospermia. It requires anesthesia in some cases.

Transurethral resection of the ejaculatory ducts
Transurethral resection of the ejaculatory ducts (TURED) is recommended in patients with proven obstruction of the ejaculatory ducts. It could be performed as an outpatient procedure and harbors the risk of retrograde ejaculation, epididymitis, and bleeding. It is typically performed as an excision of the verumontanum. Success rates vary widely in the literature. It has been reported that up to 100% of men with partial ejaculatory duct obstruction benefit from TURED with respect to improvement of postoperative sperm count measures, while the majority of patients with complete obstruction of the ejaculatory ducts (~77%) seem not to benefit [24, 25].

Electroejaculation
Electroejaculation is performed under general anesthesia and in patients with spinal cord injury. A rectal probe is inserted and stimulations are begun at 5 V against the posterior seminal vesicles. The voltage is increased as necessary. Sperm retrieval rates are generally >80% [26, 27].

Alternatively, a penile vibrator stimulator could be applied with less side effects and no need for general anesthesia but lower rates of sperm retrieval.

Medical therapy

Medical therapy for the treatment of male infertility is very limited.

Antisperm antibodies
In patients with high ASA titers (>1:32), medical therapy with glucocorticoids might be effective (prednisone 40–80 mg/day for up to 6 months). However, one has to consider the potential side effects including Cushing syndrome.

Retrograde ejaculation
The most effective medications to treat retrograde ejaculation are alpha-sympathomimetics. However, there is a low evidence level in the literature. The substance of choice is imipramine. Overall mean response rate in terms of antegrade ejaculation is 65% for imipramine, while other substances, such as brompheniramine and ephedrine yield response rates of 38% and 20%, respectively [28]. Alternatively, sperm could be retrieved from the urine after ejaculation and used for ICSI.

Endocrine disorders
Patients with hypogonadotropic hypogonadism typically benefit from GnRH therapy. If hypogonadism is secondary to hyperprolactinemia/pituitary adenoma, prolactin concentrations should be lowered by the discontinuation of offending medications and potentially dopamine agonists (cabergoline, pergolide, bromocriptine). For macroadenomas of the pituitary gland, surgery is the treatment of choice.

Genital infections/leukospermia
For genital infections and/or leukospermia, antimicrobial therapy is recommended (erythromycin/bactrim/quinolone for 10 days).

Prognosis

Of infertile couples, 25–35% will conceive by intercourse alone without treatment [29]. While intrauterine insemination is only effective with mild male infertility, *in vitro* fertilization—with sperm concentration <5 million/mL and poor motility—provides pregnancy rates of <10%. ICSI—fertilization rate has a rate of ~60%, with a pregnancy rate of ~20% (multiple pregnancy rate: 29–38%) [30, 31]. Testicular spermatozoa with maturation arrest, defective spermiogenesis, deletion of the DAZ gene from Klinefelter syndrome, and long-standing azoospermia after chemotherapy have the ability to fertilize human oocytes. Thus, ICSI has revolutionized the treatment and improved the prognosis for fertility of men with the above mentioned conditions. Approximately 70% of men will have improvement in semen parameters (motility, then count and morphology) after varicocelectomy.

Conclusion

Infertility is a common medical problem with an almost equal distribution of male and female factor infertility. A variety of potential causes have to be thoughtfully evaluated through history, physical examination, and a variety of simple, and if necessary, highly advanced tests. Despite these efforts, a huge proportion of male factor infertilities remain idiopathic. However, treatment options are numerous and need the full support of a multidisciplinary team.

WHAT TO AVOID/KEY PITFALLS

- Extensive female infertility evaluation is typically invasive and costly. Evaluation of the male partner should be performed first in infertile couples.
- Accuracy of sperm count measures highly depends on the experience of the respective laboratory. Standardized methods should be guaranteed.
- Sperm count measures could vary intraindividually. Confirm abnormal sperm count measures at least once.

KEY WEB LINKS

http://andrologysociety.org/resources/Handbook/
http://www.auanet.org/content/media/optimalevaluation2010.pdf
http://www.uroweb.org/gls/pdf/15_Male_Infertility_LR%20II.pdf
http://www.nice.org.uk/nicemedia/pdf/CG011niceguideline.pdf
http://guideline.gov/content.aspx?id=4807
http://www.cdc.gov/std/infertility/default.htm

Multiple choice questions

1 A diagnosis of obstructive azoospermia can be confirmed by
 a Abnormal FSH and LH levels
 b Abnormal scrotal ultrasound
 c Abnormal prolactin levels
 d Evidence of vas deferens obstruction on vasography
 e None of the above

2 Vasectomy reversal is typically
 a A simple, technically not challenging procedure
 b An alternative treatment to TESE and ICSI
 c A microsurgical procedure with high patency rates
 d A microsurgical procedure with similar patency and pregnancy rates
 e The treatment of choice for CBAVD

3 Which of the following are typical features shown by patients with Klinefelter syndrome
 a The most common karyotype is 47 XXYY
 b Patients typically present with a short stature
 c The syndrome is commonly associated with azoospermia
 d The syndrome is commonly associated with increased gonadotropin levels
 e Treatment for infertility is successful in the majority of cases

4 Varicocele typically presents
 a With impaired sperm analysis
 b Bilaterally
 c With a painful swelling
 d In advanced ages
 e On the left side

References

1 Templeton A. Infertility-epidemiology, aetiology and effective management. *Health Bull (Edinb)* 1995;53(5):294–298.

2 Spira A. Epidemiology of human reproduction. *Hum Reprod* 1986;1(2):111–115.

3 Wilcox AJ, Weinberg CR, Baird DD. Timing of sexual intercourse in relation to ovulation. Effects on the probability of conception, survival of the pregnancy, and sex of the baby. *N Engl J Med* 1995;333(23):1517–1521.

4 Stewart AF, Kim ED. Fertility concerns for the aging male. *Urology* 2011;78(3):496–499.

5 Dym M. The fine structure of monkey Sertoli cells in the transitional zone at the junction of the seminiferous tubules with the tubuli recti. *Am J Anat* 1974;140(1):1–25.

6 Dym M, Fawcett DW. The blood-testis barrier in the rat and the physiological compartmentation of the seminiferous epithelium. *Biol Reprod* 1970;3(3):308–326.

7 World Health Organization. WHO Laboratory Manual for the Examination and Processing of Human Semen. 5th ed. 2010.

8 Simpson JL, de la Cruz F, Swerdloff RS, et al. Klinefelter syndrome: expanding the phenotype and identifying new research directions. *Genet Med* 2003;5(6):460–468.

9 Khera M, Lipshultz LI. Evolving approach to the varicocele. *Urol Clin North Am* 2008;35(2):183–189, viii.

10 Ito H, Fuse H, Minagawa H, Kawamura K, Murakami M, Shimazaki J. Internal spermatic vein prostaglandins in varicocele patients. *Fertil Steril* 1982;37(2):218–222.

11 Lee PA. Fertility after cryptorchidism: epidemiology and other outcome studies. *Urology* 2005;66(2):427–431.

12 Charny CW. The spermatogenic potential of the undescended testis before and after treatment. *J Urol* 1960;83:697–705.

13 Guzick DS, Overstreet JW, Factor-Litvak P, et al. Sperm morphology, motility, and concentration in fertile and infertile men. *N Engl J Med* 2001;345(19):1388–1393.

14 Liu DY, Baker HW. High frequency of defective sperm-zona pellucida interaction in oligozoospermic infertile men. *Hum Reprod* 2004;19(2):228–233.

15 Zini A, Libman J. Sperm DNA damage: clinical significance in the era of assisted reproduction. *CMAJ* 2006;175(5):495–500.
16 Amann RP, Katz DF. Reflections on CASA after 25 years. *J Androl* 2004;25(3):317–325.
17 Sigman M, Jarow JP. Endocrine evaluation of infertile men. *Urology* 1997;50(5):659–664.
18 Smith JF, Walsh TJ, Turek PJ. Ejaculatory duct obstruction. *Urol Clin North Am* 2008;35(2):221–227, viii.
19 Payne SR, Pryor JP, Parks CM. Vasography, its indications and complications. *Br J Urol* 1985;57(2):215–217.
20 Johnsen SG. Testicular biopsy score count—a method for registration of spermatogenesis in human testes: normal values and results in 335 hypogonadal males. *Hormones* 1970;1(1):2–25.
21 Magheli A, Rais-Bahrami S, Kempkensteffen C, Weiske WH, Miller K, Hinz S. Impact of obstructive interval and sperm granuloma on patency and pregnancy after vasectomy reversal. *Int J Androl* 2010;33(5):730–735.
22 Hinz S, Rais-Bahrami S, Kempkensteffen C, Weiske WH, Schrader M, Magheli A. Fertility rates following vasectomy reversal: importance of age of the female partner. *Urol Int* 2008;81(4):416–420.
23 Schauer I, Madersbacher S, Jost R, Hubner WA, Imhof M. The impact of varicocelectomy on sperm parameters: a meta-analysis. *J Urol* 2012;187(5):1540–1547.
24 Yurdakul T, Gokce G, Kilic O, Piskin MM. Transurethral resection of ejaculatory ducts in the treatment of complete ejaculatory duct obstruction. *Int Urol Nephrol* 2008;40(2):369–372.
25 El-Assmy A, El-Tholoth H, Abouelkheir RT, Abou-El-Ghar ME. Transurethral resection of ejaculatory duct in infertile men: outcome and predictors of success. *Int Urol Nephrol* 2012;44(6):1623–1630.
26 Perkash I, Martin DE, Warner H, Speck V. Electroejaculation in spinal cord injury patients: simplified new equipment and technique. *J Urol* 1990;143(2):305–307.
27 Ohl DA, Bennett CJ, McCabe M, Menge AC, McGuire EJ. Predictors of success in electroejaculation of spinal cord injured men. *J Urol* 1989;142(6):1483–1486.
28 Kamischke A, Nieschlag E. Update on medical treatment of ejaculatory disorders. *Int J Androl* 2002;25(6): 333–344.
29 Collins JA, Wrixon W, Janes LB, Wilson EH. Treatment-independent pregnancy among infertile couples. *N Engl J Med* 1983;309(20):1201–1206.
30 Schlegel PN, Girardi SK. Clinical review 87: in vitro fertilization for male factor infertility. *J Clin Endocrinol Metab* 1997;82(3):709–716.
31 Tarlatzis BC, Bili H. Intracytoplasmic sperm injection. Survey of world results. *Ann N Y Acad Sci* 2000;900:336–344.
32 World Health Organization. WHO Laboratory Manual for the Examination and Processing of Human Semen. 5th ed. 2009.
33 World Health Organization. WHO Laboratory Manual for the Examination of Human Semen and Sperm–Cervical Mucus Interaction. 4th ed. Cambridge University Press; 1999.

Answers to multiple choice questions

1 d
2 c
3 c, d
4 a, e

Erectile dysfunction and Peyronie's disease

Jeffrey K. Mullins

The James Buchanan Brady Urological Institute and Department of Urology, The Johns Hopkins School of Medicine, Baltimore, MD, USA

KEY POINTS

- Obtaining an erection sufficient for sexual activity requires a complex interplay between the central and peripheral nervous system and functional anatomic structures of the penis.
- It is generally accepted that nitric oxide represents the primary neurotransmitter mediating erection.
- The etiology of erectile dysfunction (ED) includes psychogenic, neurogenic, vasculogenic, endocrinologic, and drug-induced.
- Evaluation of the patient with ED is based primarily on the history and physical examination.
- Duplex penile ultrasound is the initial radiographic study for evaluating vasculogenic ED.
- Oral phosphodiesterase type 5 (PDE5) inhibitors are the first-line therapy for most men with ED.
- Oral PDE5 inhibitors should not be used in men taking nitrates for chest pain.
- Intraurethral alprostadil suppositories and intracavernous injections with a combination of alprostadil, papaverine, and phentolamine are other effective medical therapies for ED.
- Penile prosthesis surgery is an effective therapy for men with ED refractory to medical therapy.
- Peyronie's disease is a localized connective tissue disorder of the tunica albuginea.
- Peyronie's disease is characterized by a dorsal plaque and associated penile deformity.
- There is a strong association between Peyronie's disease and ED.
- Various oral and intralesional injection therapies exist for Peyronie's disease which have varying degrees of success.
- Surgical management of Peyronie's disease should only be performed after plaque stability.
- Penile prosthesis surgery for Peyronie's disease should only be performed in the setting of severe ED.

CASE STUDY 1

A 63-year-old male presents to his urologist with a chief complaint of ED. He states he is unable to have an erection for the past 6 months, and noted a decreased quality of his erections over the past year. He denies penile pain or loss of libido. He does not have any recent psychosocial stresses, and the condition is troublesome to him and his wife of 30 years. His past medical history is significant for hypertension, type-2 diabetes, hyperlipidemia, and obesity. He denies any past surgical history and has not had any major trauma in his life. Medications include propranolol, simvastatin, lantus, and aspirin. He has no allergies.

This patient has ED which is causing significant distress. Risk factors for the development of ED in this patient include age, hypertension, diabetes, obesity, and the use of a nonselective β-blocker. Initial management includes general lifestyle recommendations including weight loss, exercise, and proper diet. Additionally, changing of his antihypertensive should be considered if possible. This should be done under the direction of his primary care physician. Finally, this patient may consider therapy with an oral PDE5 inhibitor. He has no absolute contraindications to this medication as he is not on nitrates.

Handbook of Urology, First edition. J. Kellogg Parsons, John B. Eifler and Misop Han. © 2014 by John Wiley & Sons, Ltd. Published 2014 by John Wiley & Sons, Ltd.

After changing his antihypertensive to an ACE inhibitor, implementing lifestyle changes, and initiating sildenafil 50 mg daily on demand, he has experienced a marked return of erectile function. The patient and his wife are satisfied with their current sexual relationship. This case highlights the importance of a thorough history when evaluating a patient with ED.

CASE STUDY 2

A 69-year-old male has a history of significant ED secondary to long-standing diabetes and hypertension. He had a three-piece inflatable penile prosthesis placed 3 years ago. The left corporal cylinder eroded 8 months ago requiring explanation of the left cylinder. This was replaced 5 months ago. Since then, the device has been working well, and he and his partner are satisfied with the result. The patient reports to your office with a history of scrotal pump tenderness and erythema of the scrotum. On physical examination, the patient has a fever of 101.9°F, a pulse of 110, and a blood pressure of 108/72. His scrotum is very tender to palpation with induration and erythema extending to his left groin. Routine laboratory tests are sent which reveal a white blood cell count of 20,000.

This patient clearly has an infected penile prosthesis. His risk factors include multiple surgeries and diabetes. Given his local and systemic symptoms, he should be admitted to the hospital, broad spectrum antibiotics administered, and plans made for urgent prosthesis removal. It is important to remember that the entire device should be considered infected and explanted. After removal of the device and several days of intravenous antibiotics, the patient improved. He was discharged to home with wound care and a 2-week course of antibiotics. This case highlights the importance of identifying a patient with an infected penile prosthesis and the general management of these patients.

CASE STUDY 3

A 53-year-old male presents to your office with an 8-week history of penile pain and deformity. The process started without any single inciting event and has been progressing over the past 8 weeks. He describes a 30° upward bend of the penis which impairs his ability to have sexual intercourse with his girlfriend. A picture diary of his erect penis confirms these findings. The couple had previously enjoyed a vigorous sexual relationship. He denies any ED associated with the condition, but feels he is unable to have intercourse due to the functional bend of his penis. On physical examination, the patient has a palpable area of induration on the dorsal aspect of his penis.

Over the next 4 months, the patient is treated with oral vitamin E and intralesional injections of verapamil. His symptoms did not progress, but did not improve either. After 7 months of symptom onset, the patient reports no pain and a stable penile deformity interfering with sexual activity. He is interested in surgical management. He chooses to undergo a Nesbit plication. Postoperatively, his deformity is corrected, and he is able to enjoy a normal sexual relationship. Although not interfering with his sex life, he is slightly troubled by a perceived loss of penile length after the operation. This case highlights the important diagnostic and management issues in patients presenting with Peyronie's disease.

Erectile dysfunction

Introduction

Erectile dysfunction (ED) is the persistent inability of man to obtain and maintain an erection sufficient for sexual activity. The prevalence of ED increases with age and may be due to an alteration of the normal anatomic, neurologic, vasculogenic, or psychogenic mechanisms necessary for successful erection. Diagnosis and treatment consist of identifying possible etiologies and initiating patient-directed care. The following chapter reviews the evaluation and treatment of a man presenting with ED.

Normal erectile physiology

Obtaining an erection sufficient for sexual activity relies on a complex interplay between the central and peripheral nervous system and anatomic structures of the penis. The three structures in the penis that become engorged with blood during erection are the paired corpora cavernosa and corpus spongiosum. The corpora cavernosa, the primary erectile bodies of the penis, are composed of a network of sinusoids which fill with blood during erection. The cavernosal bodies are covered by a collagen-rich layer called the tunica albuginea which provides rigidity to the blood-filled erect penis. The corpus spongiosum has an incomplete tunica albuginea which allows for a low pressure urethra during erection [1].

The internal pudendal artery provides the main blood supply to the penis. However, up to 35% of men will have an accessory pudendal artery which may represent the main blood supply to the penis [2]. The internal pudendal artery terminates in the cavernosal arteries which run through the center of the corpora cavernosa and represent the main inflow of blood during erection. Venous drainage of the erectile bodies is via a subtunical venous plexus which drains into the deep dorsal vein of the penis. The paired cavernous nerves carry parasympathetic (S2–S4), sympathetic (T11–L2), and nonadrenergic/noncholinergic (NANC) fibers, and represent the main autonomic innervation of the cavernosal bodies [1].

In the flaccid state, the smooth muscle in the cavernosal bodies and arterial walls are tonically contracted resulting in a low flow state. Sexual stimulation results in the release of neurotransmitters from cavernous nerve terminals as well as the endothelial lining of the corporal sinusoids. Although acetylcholine is released from cholinergic nerve terminals, it is generally accepted that nitric oxide (NO) represents the primary neurotransmitter mediating erection [3, 4]. The release of NO results in smooth muscle relaxation, arterial dilation, and an increase in penile blood flow. This smooth muscle relaxation is mediated by NO interacting with cGMP resulting in an increase in intracellular calcium via cGMP-dependent protein kinases. The incoming blood is trapped within the sinusoids of the cavernosal bodies. As the corporal bodies become engorged, the subtunical venous plexus becomes compressed under the tunica albuginea and venous drainage is prevented. The trapped blood within the cavernosal bodies in conjunction with support from the tunica albuginea results in penile tumescence and rigidity [1].

Table 6.1 Risk factors for the development of erectile dysfunction

Advanced age
Poor general health status/chronic disease
Diabetes mellitus
Obesity
Cardiovascular disease
Chronic renal failure
Prostate disease
Dyslipidemia
Low socioeconomic status
Smoking
Psychiatric disorders
Medications
Pelvic surgery/trauma

Epidemiology and etiology of ED

The incidence of ED worldwide has been estimated to range from 10% to 20% [5]. However, this incidence varies significantly with age. Data from the Massachusetts Male Aging Study (MMAS) reported the incidence of complete, moderate, and mild ED among 40-year-old men was 5.1%, 15%, and 17%, respectively. Among 70-year-old men, rates increased to 15%, 34%, and 17%, respectively [6]. Additional risk factors for the development of ED are listed in Table 6.1.

The etiology of ED can roughly be subdivided into two main groups: organic and psychogenic. Organic ED can be further subdivided into vasculogenic, neurogenic, and endocrinologic. Psychogenic ED can be subdivided into generalized and situational ED. A final category includes drug-induced ED which may account for up to 25% of cases (Table 6.2) [7].

Table 6.2 Common medications associated with erectile dysfunction

Thiazide diuretics
Nonselective β-blockers
α-Blockers
Methyldopa
Antipsychotic medications
Tricyclic antidepressants
Selective serotonin reuptake inhibitors
Antiandrogens
5α-reductase inhibitors
Highly active retroviral therapy
Large quantities of alcohol

Determining the etiology of a patient's ED is imperative for optimal management. However, in many patients, ED is a mixed condition with several contributing risk factors.

Vasculogenic ED may be secondary to impairment in the arterial inflow to the cavernosal bodies or failure of the veno-occlusive mechanism. Arteriogenic ED is due to decreased pressure and flow into the cavernosal bodies. The most common etiologies include diffuse atherosclerotic disease or occlusion of the hypogastric, pudendal, or cavernosal arteries after pelvic trauma. Risk factors for atherosclerotic disease include hypertension, diabetes, dyslipidemia, smoking, and pelvic radiation. Failure of the veno-occlusive mechanism results in a venous leak and failure to retain blood in the penis during erection. Common etiologies of veno-occlusive failure include degenerative changes/traumatic injury to the tunica albuginea, structural changes of cavernosal trabeculae and smooth muscle, and acquired venous shunts [1].

Neurogenic ED can result from a multitude of diseases involving the brain, spinal cord, or peripheral nerves. Up to 19% of all ED has been attributed to a neurogenic etiology [1]. Disorders of the central nervous system commonly associated with ED include Parkinson's disease, stroke, Alzheimer's disease, dementia, and trauma. Notably, up to 95% of patients with upper spinal cord lesions have reflexogenic erections compared to only 25% of men with lower spinal cord injuries [8]. Damage to the pudendal or cavernous nerves via pelvic or surgical trauma commonly results in ED. In addition, damage to peripheral nerves associated with diabetes mellitus is a frequent cause of ED. In fact, 35–75% of men with diabetes experience some degree of ED [9].

Endocrinopathies including hypogonadism, hyperprolactinemia, and hyper- and hypothyroidism can be associate with ED. Approximately, 5–10% of cases of organic ED are attributed to endocrinopathies [10]. Importantly, low serum testosterone levels have been associated with decreases in libido and sexual activity but not with the ability to obtain a stimulated erection.

ED not attributable to the above organic categories is typically assumed to be psychogenic in nature. Psychogenic ED may be generalized to all sexual encounters, situational, or partner specific. The two mechanisms that have been attributed to psychogenic ED include inhibition of the spinal erection center by the brain and excessive sympathetic outflow [11, 12].

Evaluation and diagnosis

History and physical

A thorough sexual, medical, and psychosocial history followed by a complete physical examination is the first step in the evaluation of ED. The sexual history should ascertain the onset, duration, severity, and circumstances surrounding the altered erectile function. Additionally, the presence of morning erections should be assessed. Sexual history details that may suggest a psychogenic etiology include a sudden onset, complete and immediate loss of erection, situational ED, and the presence of morning erections. A complete past medical and surgical history should be obtained to document risk factors for ED. Finally, a complete physical examination should include a general assessment of the patient (body habitus, BMI, etc.), genital, cardiovascular, and neurologic examinations.

Laboratory and specialized assessment

The general laboratory assessment for the patient with ED should include fasting glucose, lipid profile, serum total testosterone, a complete blood count, and serum chemistries. A low serum total testosterone should be further analyzed with a serum-free testosterone and luteinizing hormone. Finally, prolactin and TSH are optional tests that may be ordered at the physician's discretion.

Although specialized assessment is not routinely performed on all patients, these tests may be very useful in complex cases. Commonly used tests and the physiologic component of the erection pathway tested are listed in Table 6.3. Duplex ultrasound quantifies arterial inflow and identifies veno-occlusive dysfunction and is often the first specialized test used to evaluate penile hemodynamics. It is indicated in young patients with pelvic trauma or likely arteriogenic ED. The evaluation is performed after pharmacostimulation and includes the penis and the perineum. The quality of erection at the time of evaluation should be evaluated, and poor erection quality may prompt redosing of the intracavernosal injection. Peak systolic velocity (PSV) >35 cm/s is considered normal while PSV < 25 cm/s is suggestive of cavernosal arterial insufficiency. Veno-occlusive dysfunction is suspected

Table 6.3 Specialized tests of erectile dysfunction and the physiologic component of the erection pathway tested

Test	Assessment
Intracavernous injection pharmacotesting	Vascular status of penis
Duplex ultrasound	Quantification of penile blood flow and veno-occlusive dysfunction
Penile angiography	Surgically correctable vascular lesions
Cavernosography	Site-specific veno-occlusive dysfunction
Nocturnal penile tumescence and rigidity testing	Psychogenic etiology

by persistently high PSV (>25 cm/s), high end diastolic velocity (EDV; >5 cm/s), and a restrictive index (PSV/EDV) < 0.75. Full discussion of all specialized testing is beyond the scope of this chapter [13].

Treatment

General lifestyle changes including weight loss, exercise, cessation of cigarette smoking, and change in diet have been shown to improve erectile function in certain risk groups. Medications that may be associated with ED should be changed or the dose changed if medically feasible. Hormonal or endocrine imbalances detected on initial workup should be corrected. Finally, psychosexual therapy may be a therapeutic strategy especially in those with psychogenic ED. General pharmacologic and surgical therapies are discussed below. Patients treated for ED should be healthy enough to undergo intercourse. Men with severe cardiac disease (e.g., inability to climb a flight of stairs without becoming short of breath) should undergo a cardiology evaluation prior to treatment.

Medications

The mainstay of oral pharmacotherapy are phosphodiesterase type 5 (PDE5) inhibiters. PDE5 is responsible for the degradation of cGMP, which is an intracellular mediator of NO-induced smooth muscle relaxation necessary for erection. Therefore, PDE5 inhibitors augment erections initiated by NO release from the endothelium in response to sexual stimulation [13]. The three main PDE5 inhibitors available include sildenafil (Viagra), vardenafil (Levitra), and tadalafil (Cialis). These medications differ in their half-lives, timing of action, and side effects as detailed in Table 6.4. Generally, all three agents are effective and allow men to achieve erections sufficient for intercourse in approximately 70% [14]. Success rates differ based on the etiology with the highest rates achieved in patients with spinal cord injuries and lower rates in patients with ED secondary to diabetes or radical prostatectomy (40–50%) [15, 16]. Men taking sildenafil and vardenafil should be counseled to take the medication on an empty stomach as a high-fat meal may delay systemic absorption [17]. Nitrate

Table 6.4 Properties of the four commercially available PDE5 inhibitors

	$T_{1/2}$ (h)	T_{max} (h)	Cross-reactivity	Side effects	Medication interactions
Sildenafil	3–5	0.8	PDE6	Visual disturbances Headache Flushing/rhinitis Dyspepsia	Nitrates
Vardenafil	4–5	0.7–0.9	–	Headache Flushing/rhinitis Dyspepsia	Nitrates α-Blockers Antiarrhythmics (precaution)
Tadalafil	17.5	2	PDE11	Myalgias/back pain Headache Flushing/rhinitis Dyspepsia	Nitrates α-Blockers

use is an absolute contraindication to taking any PDE5 inhibitors due to the risk of severe hypotension. Patients should not receive nitrates within 24 hours of taking sildenafil or vardenafil and within 48 hours of taking tadalafil [18]. Additionally, caution should be exercised when taking α-blockers and vardenafil and tadalafil due to risk of hypotension. Patients should delay taking α-blockers beyond 4 hours for sildenafil (doses > 25 mg) [13].

Intracavernous injections

Intracavernous injection therapy involves self-injection of vasoactive agents directly into the corporal bodies immediately before intercourse. The three most common agents in commercially available preparations include alprostadil, papaverine, and phentolamine. These agents may be given as monotherapy or in combination as a "bi-mix" or "tri-mix." Alprostadil is a synthetic form of prostaglandin E which increases intracellular cAMP leading to smooth muscle relaxation. The typical dose is 10–20 µg. The most troublesome side effect specific to alprostadil is painful erections as well as pain at the injection site. Papaverine is a nonspecific PDE5 inhibitor which increases intracellular cGMP and cAMP. Typical dose is 5–20 mg. Common disadvantages include increased risk for priapism and penile fibrosis with long-term use. Phentolamine is a nonselective α-blocker administered at a dose of 1 mg. Its use in monotherapy is limited, and potential side effects include hypotension, congestion, and dyspepsia [13].

Proper use of these agents results in a successful erection in 70–90% of patients [13, 19, 20]. Patients are typically started at a low dose, and titrated up as tolerated to achieve a successful erection. Contraindications to intracavernous injection therapy include psychological instability, history of priapism, severe coagulopathy, severe cardiovascular disease, physical inability to perform injections, and the use of monoamine oxidase inhibitors.

Intraurethral injection therapy

The only available intraurethral suppository available is MUSE (alprostadil). This medication is supplied as a suppository which is introduced to the external urethral meatus by an applicator devise. With proper use, the reported success rate is around 70% [21]. Common side effects include penile pain and urethral irritation/bleeding (30%).

Vacuum constriction devices

Vacuum erection devices mechanically engorge the penis with blood via negative pressure. Proper use of the device requires placement of a constricting ring at the base of the penis in order to maintain the erection. Although success rates range from 67% to 90%, patient satisfaction with the device is noticeably lower (34–68%) [22]. The advantages of the device include its noninvasive nature. Possible side effects include penile ischemia (if constricting band left in place for >30 minutes), pain, and impaired ejaculation.

Penile prostheses

Penile prosthesis surgery is generally considered for men with ED refractory to medical therapy, men unwilling to participate in medical therapy, and those with penile structural deformities occurring in association with ED. Penile prostheses function by providing mechanical support to the two corpora cavernosa. The two general types of devices available are the semi-rigid and inflatable penile prostheses.

The semi-rigid device is composed of a malleable, firm material which is bent up for intercourse and bent down when not in use. Advantages include low mechanical failure rates and ease of use. Disadvantages include risk of erosion and constant penile rigidity. The inflatable penile prosthesis is supplied as either a two- or three-piece device. These devices function by transferring fluid from a reservoir to inflatable cylinders in the corpora cavernosa via a scrotal pump before intercourse. The three-piece penile prosthesis is the device that best allows the patient to maintain normal penile flaccidity and erection.

Inflatable penile prostheses are a successful treatment modality for ED with patient and partner satisfaction rates exceeding 75% [23]. The most worrisome complications of penile prosthesis surgery include infection, erosion, and mechanical failure. The incidence of infection is reported at 1–3% with rates increasing for patients with diabetes mellitus and those requiring reimplantation [24, 25]. The treatment for an infected device is the removal of the entire device. Erosion occurs in <5% of patients [26]. The treatment consists of removal of the eroded cylinder or the entire device (if erosion has been present for prolonged time). Mechanical failure occurs in 5–20% of patients by 5 years depending on the device implanted [27]. The treatment should be directed at the malfunctioning component.

Peyronie's disease

Introduction

Peyronie's disease is a connective tissue disorder localized to the tunica albuginea. The disease is characterized by the development of a fibrous plaque most commonly on the dorsal aspect of the penis that alters penile anatomy. Generally, the disease occurs in two phases: the active and quiescent phases. The active phase is characterized by painful erections and changing of the dorsal plaque and associated penile deformity. This phase typically lasts 6–18 months. The quiescent phase typically appears after the active phase and is characterized by painless erections with stabilization of the plaque and associated deformity. Up to a third of patients with Peyronie's disease will present with a painless deformity [28, 29]. The following chapter will discuss the diagnosis and management of patients with Peyronie's disease.

Epidemiology and etiology

Peyronie's disease most commonly affects men in their 50's and has an estimated symptomatic incidence of 1%. However, the incidence of Peyronie's disease is thought to be increasing with current estimates approaching 5% [30]. There are well-documented associations with Peyronie's disease including Dupuytren's disease, Ledderhose disease, and tympanosclerosis [29]. Specifically, 30–40% of men with Peyronie's disease will also have Dupuytren's disease [31]. ED is closely associated with Peyronie's disease. The nature of ED may be psychogenic, functional, or vasculogenic. Approximately 20–40% of patients with Peyronie's disease have ED [32].

It is generally accepted that trauma is the inciting event in the development of Peyronie's disease. Specifically, buckling trauma during sexual intercourse is thought to cause trauma where the tunica albuginea inserts into the penile septum. After the inciting trauma, it has been proposed that high concentrations of proinflammatory cytokines (TGF-β) and failure to inhibit antiscarring enzymes (matrix metalloproteinases) contribute to plaque formation [29].

Evaluation and diagnosis

Men with Peyronie's disease typically present with penile pain, deformity, penile shortening, and presence of a plaque. The evaluation begins with a thorough medical history, sexual history, and physical examination. The history should ascertain the onset of the disorder, duration of symptoms, presence of associated diseases (e.g., Depuytren's contracture), and the presence of ED. Some experts advocate obtaining pictures of the patient's erect penis to quantify the severity of the disorder. On physical examination, the vast majority of patients will have a palpable plaque on the dorsal aspect of their penis.

The use of radiographic studies in the workup of Peyronie's disease is variable among providers. Approximately a third of cases will develop dystrophic calcifications within the plaque which can be visualized with ultrasound or plain film radiography. This may be helpful for determining the size of the plaque when monitoring the patient or planning for surgery. Vascular testing of the penis is often considered in patients interested in surgical therapy. This is done to better inform patients and providers regarding the risk of postoperative ED.

Treatment

Medical therapy

Medical therapy may be implemented at any stage of a patient's disease, but is more efficacious early in the disease process [33]. Although many medical therapies have been described, there is a paucity of high-level data supporting one therapy over another. Common oral and intralesional therapies are listed in Table 6.5. In general, the use of oral vitamin E or acetyl-L-carnitine and intralesional injection of verapamil or collagenase are reasonable treatment options during the active phase of the disease. However, the rates of success are unknown, and patients should be counseled as such [29].

Surgical therapy

Surgical therapy is reserved for patients who are in the quiescent phase of their disease and who have a severe deformity interfering with sexual activity. Considering that some patients with Peyronie's disease will improve spontaneously, it has been suggested that surgical intervention be delayed until 12–18 months after the onset of symptoms. Surgical options can be grouped into three categories: (1) tunical shortening procedures, (2) tunical lengthening procedures, and (3) prosthetic procedures [29].

Table 6.5 Commonly utilized oral and intralesional injection therapies for Peyronie's disease

Oral therapy	Intralesional injection therapy
Vitamin E	Saline
Potassium Aminobenzoate	Steroids
Tamoxifen	Verapamil
Colchicine	Interferon α 2b
Acetyl-L-carnitine	Collagenase

Tunical shortening procedures include corporoplasties and plication procedures that function to shorten the tunica opposite the Peyronie's plaque [34]. These are especially useful in men with associated ED as erectile function may be better preserved with these procedures. Numerous tunical lengthening procedures have been described, but most involve incising or excising the plaque with the placement of a graph in the resultant deformity. Penile prostheses should be reserved for patients with Peyronie's disease and severe ED or penile vascular impairment [35]. Incising or excising the plaque or penile modeling may be performed to correct the deformity at the time of prosthesis. Patients undergoing surgical management of Peyronie's disease should be counseled on common side effects including penile shortening, ED, glans anesthesia, pain, urethral injury, and further deformity.

WHAT TO AVOID

- Do not administer PDE5 inhibitors to men taking nitrates for chest pain.
- Do not remove a single component of a penile prosthesis in the setting of infection.
- Do not offer surgical management to patients with Peyronie's disease in the active stage.
- Do not offer prosthesis surgeries to all patients with Peyronie's disease.

KEY WEB LINKS

http://www.smsna.org/default.aspx

Multiple choice questions

1 The neurotransmitter most responsible for mediating physiologic erections is:
  a Acetylcholine
  b VIP
  c NO
  d Norepinephrine

2 What structure should be spared during radical prostatectomy in order to preserve erectile function?
  a Cavernous nerves
  b Accessory pudendal arteries
  c Endopelvic fascia
  d Superficial dorsal vein
  e A and b
  f All of the above

3 Cross reactivity with what structure or enzyme is responsible for back pain in patients taking tadalafil?
  a PDE11
  b PDE6
  c Myosin light chain
  d Matrix metalloproteinases

4 The component of tri-mix intracavernous injection therapy for ED most associated with penile pain is:
  a Papaverine
  b Phentolamine
  c Alprostadil
  d Sildenafil

5 All of the following are therapeutic options in men with Peyronie's disease in the active phase except:
  a Intralesional collagenase
  b Intralesional verapamil
  c Oral vitamin E
  d Tamoxifen
  e Nesbit plication

References

1 Lue TF. Chapter 23: Physiology of penile erection and pathophysiology of erectile dysfunction. In: Wein AJ, Kavoussi LR, Novick AC, Partin AW, Peters CA, editors. *Cambell-Walsh Urology*. Vol. 1. Philadelphia, PA: Saunders; 2011. pp. 688–720

2 Nehra A, Kumar R, Ramakumar S, Myers RP, Blute ML, McKusick MA. Pharmacoangiographic evidence of the presence and anatomical dominance of accessory pudendal artery(s). *J Urol* 2008;179:2317–2320

3 Burnett AL, Lowenstein CJ, Bredt DS, Chang TS, Snyder SH. Nitric oxide: a physiologic mediator of penile erection. *Science* 1992;257:401–403

4 Burnett AL, Tillman SL, Chang TS, et al. Immunohistochemical localization of nitric oxide synthase in the autonomic innervation of the human penis. *J Urol* 1993;150:73–76

5 Derogatis LR, Burnett AL. The epidemiology of sexual dysfunctions. *J Sex Med* 2008;5:289–300

6 Johannes CB, Araujo AB, Feldman HA, Derby CA, Kleinman KP, McKinlay JB. Incidence of erectile dysfunction in men 40 to 69 years old: longitudinal results from the Massachusetts male aging study. *J Urol* 2000;163:460–463

7 Keene LC, Davies PH. Drug-related erectile dysfunction. *Adverse Drug React Toxicol Rev* 1999;18:5–24

8 Biering-Sorensen F, Sonksen J. Sexual function in spinal cord lesioned men. *Spinal Cord* 2001;39:455–470

9 Hakim LS, Goldstein I. Diabetic sexual dysfunction. *Endocrinol Metab Clin North Am* 1996;25:379–400

10 Miralles-Garcia JM, Garcia-Diez LC. Specific aspects of erectile dysfunction in endocrinology. *Int J Impot Res* 2004;16 (Suppl 2):S10–S12

11 Steers WD. Neural pathways and central sites involved in penile erection: neuroanatomy and clinical implications. *Neurosci Biobehav Rev* 2000;24:507–516

12 Kim SC, Oh MM. Norepinephrine involvement in response to intracorporeal injection of papaverine in psychogenic impotence. *J Urol* 1992;147:1530–1532

13 Burnett AL. Chapter 24: Evaluation and management of erectile dysfunction. In: Wein AJ, Kavoussi LR, Novick AC, Partin AW, Peters CA, editors. *Campbell-Walsh Urology*. 10th ed. Vol. 1. Philadelphia, PA: Saunders; 2011. pp. 721–748

14 Carson CC, Lue TF. Phosphodiesterase type 5 inhibitors for erectile dysfunction. *BJU Int* 2005;96:257–280

15 Fonseca V, Seftel A, Denne J, Fredlund P. Impact of diabetes mellitus on the severity of erectile dysfunction and response to treatment: analysis of data from tadalafil clinical trials. *Diabetologia* 2004;47:1914–1923

16 Hatzimouratidis K, Hatzichristou DG. A comparative review of the options for treatment of erectile dysfunction: which treatment for which patient? *Drugs* 2005;65:1621–1650

17 Barada JH. Optimizing outcomes of oral therapy for patients with erectile dysfunction. *Rev Urol* 2003; 5 (Suppl 7):S28–S34

18 Cheitlin MD, Hutter AM, Jr., Brindis RG, et al. ACC/AHA expert consensus document. Use of sildenafil (Viagra) in patients with cardiovascular disease. American College of Cardiology/American Heart Association. *J Am Coll Cardiol* 1999;33:273–282

19 Floth A, Schramek P. Intracavernous injection of prostaglandin E1 in combination with papaverine: enhanced effectiveness in comparison with papaverine plus phentolamine and prostaglandin E1 alone. *J Urol* 1991;145:56–59

20 Linet OI, Neff LL. Intracavernous prostaglandin E1 in erectile dysfunction. *Clin Investig* 1994;72:139–149

21 Guay AT, Perez JB, Velasquez E, Newton RA, Jacobson JP. Clinical experience with intraurethral alprostadil (MUSE) in the treatment of men with erectile dysfunction. A retrospective study. Medicated urethral system for erection. *Eur Urol* 2000;38: 671–676

22 Hellstrom WJ, Montague DK, Moncada I, et al. Implants, mechanical devices, and vascular surgery for erectile dysfunction. *J Sex Med* 2010;7:501–523

23 McLaren RH, Barrett DM. Patient and partner satisfaction with the AMS 700 penile prosthesis. *J Urol* 1992;147:62–65

24 Jarow JP. Risk factors for penile prosthetic infection. *J Urol* 1996;156:402–404

25 Wilson SK, Delk JR, 2nd. Inflatable penile implant infection: predisposing factors and treatment suggestions. *J Urol* 1995;153:659–661

26 Lotan Y, Roehrborn CG, McConnell JD, Hendin BN. Factors influencing the outcomes of penile prosthesis surgery at a teaching institution. *Urology* 2003;62:918–921

27 Montague DK. Chapter 27: Prosthetic surgery for erectile dysfunction. In: Wein AJ, Kavoussi LR, Novick AC, Partin AW, Peters CA, editors. *Campbell-Walsh Urology*. 10th ed. Vol. 1. Philadelphia, PA: Saunders; 2011. pp. 780–791

28 Hellstrom WJ. History, epidemiology, and clinical presentation of Peyronie's disease. *Int J Impot Res* 2003;15 (Suppl 5):S91–S92

29 Jordan GH, McCammon KA. Chapter 28: Peyronie's disease. In: Wein AJ, Kavoussi LR, Novick AC, Partin AW, Peters CA, editors. *Campbell-Walsh Urology*. 10th ed. Vol. 1. Philadelphia, PA: Saunders; 2011. pp. 792–809

30 Greenfield JM, Levine LA. Peyronie's disease: etiology, epidemiology and medical treatment. *Urol Clin North Am* 2005;32:469–478, vii

31 Ralph DJ, Schwartz G, Moore W, Pryor JP, Ebringer A, Bottazzo GF. The genetic and bacteriological aspects of Peyronie's disease. *J Urol* 1997;157:291–294
32 Dominguez-Malagon HR, Alfeiran-Ruiz A, Chavarria-Xicotencatl P, Duran-Hernandez MS. Clinical and cellular effects of colchicine in fibromatosis. *Cancer* 1992;69:2478–2483
33 Jack GS, Gonzalez-Cadavid N, Rajfer J. Conservative management options for Peyronie's disease. *Curr Urol Rep* 2005;6:454–460
34 Coughlin PW, Carson CC, 3rd, Paulson DF. Surgical correction of Peyronie's disease: the Nesbit procedure. *J Urol* 1984;131:282–285
35 Carson CC. Penile prosthesis implantation in the treatment of Peyronie's disease and erectile dysfunction. *Int J Impot Res* 2000;12 (Suppl 4):S122–S126

Answers to multiple choice questions

1 c
2 e
3 a
4 c
5 e

Section 4 Emergency urology

7 Genitourinary trauma

Adam Kern

The James Buchanan Brady Urological Institute and Department of Urology, The Johns Hopkins School of Medicine, Baltimore, MD, USA

KEY POINTS

- Traumatic injury is a leading cause of morbidity and mortality among young persons.
- Genitourinary evaluation should not delay initial trauma survey or hemodynamic stabilization.
- Acute onset hematuria following trauma is suspicious for genitourinary injury.
- Most renal injuries may be managed conservatively.
- The most important principle of the surgical repair of ureteral injury is formation of a tension-free anastomosis.
- Extraperitoneal bladder rupture is generally managed with prolonged bladder drainage.
- Intraperitoneal bladder rupture is generally managed operatively.

Traumatic injury is a leading cause of death among young persons in the United States. Rapid assessment and treatment of the trauma patient can significantly decrease morbidity and mortality. While major renal trauma tends to cause morbidity in the acute phase, lower urinary tract trauma also causes long-term morbidity that may severely impact a patient's life.

The initial management of trauma always first involves stabilization of the patient with the Acute Trauma Life Support resuscitation. Next, any available history should be gathered. Examples of useful historical information would be what type of instrument caused a penetrating injury, or the degree of deceleration or impact in a blunt trauma. Any possibility of retained foreign bodies such as bullets should be thoroughly addressed.

Hematuria

Hematuria may be caused by a wide range of genitourinary injuries and is suggestive of occult GU trauma. Microscopic hematuria of >5 RBC/high powered field (hpf) following a trauma is suggestive of GU tract injury. However, the degree of hematuria does not absolutely correlate with the severity of injury, and some major injuries may not cause immediate hematuria. Shock accompanying microscopic hematuria increases the likelihood of concomitant renal or vascular injury [1]. Voided or catheterized urine should be collected at the time of presentation to avoid dilution of red blood cells by resuscitation fluid.

Renal trauma

The kidney is the most common genitourinary organ injured by trauma. Injuries may be caused by either blunt trauma or penetrating mechanisms, and may be predisposed toward exacerbated bleeding by preexisting renal lesions. After initial stabilization, imaging to characterize renal trauma should be undertaken in any patient with penetrating injury to the flank or abdomen, significant blunt injury involving deceleration, blunt trauma accompanied by hematuria

Handbook of Urology, First edition. J. Kellogg Parsons, John B. Eifler and Misop Han. © 2014 by John Wiley & Sons, Ltd. Published 2014 by John Wiley & Sons, Ltd.

or shock, or any pediatric patient with microscopic hematuria. Imaging should only be performed on hemodynamically stable patients. Hemodynamically unstable patients in whom there exists a high likelihood of renal injury based on mechanism should be managed operatively without delay.

CT with IV contrast is the gold standard for the evaluation of renal injury. Hematomas and parenchymal lacerations can be visualized and collecting system or vascular injuries are identified on delayed series. An immediate nephrogenic delayed phase may be followed by a 10 minute delayed phase in order to identify extravasation from the collecting system. The cortical rim sign is a radiographic feature sometimes seen on CT after high-grade renal injury that is suggestive of parenchymal ischemia with continued perfusion of only the superficial cortex from peripheral collateral circulation. Benign forniceal rupture may also be present, especially after blunt trauma, and may be distinguished from renal vascular injury by the lack of perinephric hematoma, parenchymal laceration, and adequate visualization of the ureter. Hemodynamically unstable patients in whom obtaining a CT is not possible may also be assessed with an on-table intravenous pyelogram (IVP) 10 minutes following an IV push of 2 mL/kg of contrast [2].

Renal trauma is graded according to the American Association for the Surgery of Trauma (AAST) Renal Injury Scaling System. The odds of renal surgery increase by 15-fold for every increase in AAST grade. Grade I injuries are nonexpanding contusions or subcapsular hematomas without parenchymal laceration. Grade II injuries are nonexpanding perirenal hematomas or lacerations into the cortex with a depth of <1 cm, without urine extravasation. Grade III injuries are cortical lacerations >1 cm in depth without urine extravasation. Grade IV injuries are either nonvascular lacerations >1 cm in depth penetrating the collecting system, or vascular injuries involving the hilar or segmental vessels with contained thrombus. Grade V injuries involve complete shattering of the parenchyma or vascular injuries causing complete avulsion of the pedicle. If urine extravasation is seen, the presence of a parenchymal laceration must be determined. Urine extravasation without laceration is consistent with benign forniceal rupture, while urine extravasation with concomitant laceration is a minimum grade IV injury.

Management of most renal trauma is conservative. The only absolute indication for surgical exploration is hemodynamic instability with associated expanding retroperitoneal hematoma, usually in the setting of grade IV or grade V injury. Grade III and nonvascular grade IV injuries may be followed closely in the inpatient setting, while grade I and II injuries can usually be observed. Typical management of low-grade renal trauma consists of bed rest and Foley catheter drainage until gross hematuria resolves, if present. Serial hemoglobin values are also initially monitored for many grade III–IV injuries, and repeat imaging is undertaken selectively. Options for conservative intervention include selective arterioembolization and placement of percutaneous drains in urine and hematoma collections. Predictive features of failed nonoperative management include increasing AAST organ injury scale grade, penetrating or gunshot mechanism of injury, transfusion requirement, shock, and the entrance of a penetrating wound anterior to the anterior axillary line.

Initial operative management of renal trauma is indicated in grade V and vascular grade IV injuries and/or in the hemodynamically unstable patient. A significant number of these cases involve penetrating trauma. If a CT cannot be performed preoperatively, an intraoperative IVP at the time of repair of other non-urologic injuries may be used to determine whether renal exploration is necessary. The major goal of renal trauma exploration is control of bleeding. A midline transabdominal incision is used to expose both kidneys and to allow access to the renal hilum. Early vascular control proximal to the injury is associated with lower rates of total nephrectomy, especially when vascular control is obtained prior to opening Gerota's fascia [3]. Access to the renal vascular pedicle is achieved by incising the posterior parietal peritoneum, just over the aorta. The left renal vein is then identified and elevated, exposing the renal arteries. The renal blood supply may then be controlled, if necessary. Warm ischemia time should be minimized when possible. At this point the renal cortex may be inspected and defects repaired with suture. After hemostasis is achieved, methylene blue may be injected into the renal pelvis while occluding the ureter in order to identify extravasation of urine. After these defects are repaired, a drain or drains are placed. Suction drains may promote continued urine leakage—a Penrose drain placed in the dependent portion of the hematoma bed may alternatively be used. If these approaches fail, nephrectomy may be performed as a life-saving maneuver.

The most common complications of renal trauma are urinary extravasation, delayed retroperitoneal bleeding, and hypertension. Persistent urine extravasation lasting >3 days after initial repair may be managed by the placement of a ureteral stent and Foley catheter, and can be followed by serial ultrasound imaging. Delayed retroperitoneal bleeding is a life-threatening complication and is usually associated with penetrating trauma, which may lead to arteriovenous fistula formation. Selective arterioembolization is usually effective at repairing delayed bleeding after the source is radiographically identified. Hypertension is a rare and usually late complication of renal trauma, and may occur either as a result of persistent external compression of the cortex or may be a renin-mediated effect secondary to a persistently ischemic segment of parenchyma. Medical management is the first-line treatment of renal-trauma-associated hypertension, although partial nephrectomy may be required in refractory cases.

Ureteral trauma

The most common cause of ureteral injury in adults is iatrogenic, followed by penetrating injury to the abdomen or flank. Diagnosis may be difficult because hematuria and retroperitoneal hematomas are present in only two-thirds of the cases, and also because urinary extravasation from isolated ureteral injury is usually only seen on delayed series 10 minutes post-contrast or greater. Gunshot wounds are significantly more likely to cause ureteral injuries than are stab wounds. Since gunshot wounds are also commonly associated with other injuries, concomitant multiple organ injury should raise the index of suspicion for occult ureteral injury. Children are particularly susceptible to ureteral injuries at the ureteropelvic junction (UPJ) following deceleration injuries owing to spinal hyperextensibility.

While isolated ureteral injuries may cause hematuria, the absence of hematuria does not exclude a ureteral injury. Ureteral injuries may also present with flank pain or masses, ileus, or elevated serum creatinine. These injuries are classified based on both the location of injury (UPJ vs. abdominal ureter vs. distal pelvic ureter) and when the diagnosis is made. Delayed diagnoses are associated with greater rates of urinoma, renal loss, and mortality. While a single-shot IVP may be used in a trauma setting to diagnose ureteral injury, its reliability is poor and CT remains the gold standard. A periureteral pattern of contrast extravasation on CT with poor visualization of contrast within the ipsilateral distal ureter is suggestive of a ureteral injury. The diagnosis can also be made at the time of surgical exploration, either by inspecting the ureter along its length or by administering colored dye by IV, renal pelvic injection or retrograde ureteral injection, or an intraoperative fluoroscopic retrograde pyelogram with contrast may be performed.

Management of ureteral injuries depends on both the timing and location of injury. Immediate repair of recognized injuries is best. If temporization of an unstable patient is required, a percutaneous nephrostomy tube may be placed, allowing subsequent surgical repair while preventing urinoma formation. Examples of scenarios involving immediate recognition of injury and repair are ureteral perforation during endourologic procedures, intraoperative ureteral crush injuries, trauma patients where injuries are immediately recognized, or children who have large UPJ disruptions following deceleration injuries. Minor ureteral perforations and crush injuries can usually be managed with indwelling stents that remain in place 4–6 weeks after the injury. Healing is then reevaluated using retrograde pyelography. Larger ureteral injuries that are recognized at the time of presentation may be managed either by percutaneous nephrostomy tube placement or through ureteric exteriorization, where a ureteral catheter is placed and the distal end is brought to the skin. Either approach temporizes the injury and allows for subsequent definitive repair. UPJ distractions are treated simply with ureteral stent placement, ureteropyelostomy over a stent, or formal ureterocalycostomy, depending on the degree of injury. As in the other scenarios, percutaneous drainage proximal to the UPJ injury may also be helpful. Delayed recognition of ureteral injury is associated with ureteral stricture formation and is best managed initially by percutaneous drainage of any urinoma that is present, and percutaneous nephrostomy and/or ureteral stent placement, followed by elective repair.

The *sine qua non* of surgical ureteral repair is the tension-free anastomosis. This requires adequate debridement of devitalized tissue and sufficient mobilization of the ureteral segments to allow the creation of a watertight closure. Typically, the ureteral ends are spatulated to allow mucosal-to-mucosal contact and the defect is closed over a stent. The location and length of injury dictates the surgical approach required to allow adequate mobilization of the remaining ureteral segments.

Distal ureteral injuries are repaired with ureteroneocystostomy. Short defects may be directly reimplanted into the bladder with either refluxing or nonrefluxing anastomoses. Longer distal defects may also be corrected with ureteroneocystostomy, although mobilization of the bladder may be required to compensate for the lack of ureteral length. A psoas hitch can be performed if the bladder capacity and elasticity are normal: the contralateral superior vascular pedicle of the bladder is ligated and the bladder is then fixed to the ipsilateral psoas tendon. This usually mobilizes the bladder at least to the level of L5. This maneuver can also be combined with a downward nephropexy to gain additional mobilization. More extensive distal injuries can also be corrected with ureteroneocystostomy if a Boari flap is performed. Here the bladder is rotated cranially and a tubularized flap is formed. The ureteral stump is then reimplanted into the tubularized bladder segment. However, the Boari flap is contraindicated when the bladder capacity or elasticity is already compromised.

Mid-ureteral defects above the pelvic brim are best managed either by end-to-end anastomosis (ureteroureterostomy) or, in the case of large defects, transureteroureterostomy (TUU). End-to-end repair is also aided by combination with a downward nephropexy. Omental flaps may be used for additional coverage, particularly when other injuries to abdominal organs are present. If adequate ureteral length cannot be mobilized for end-to-end repair, then the ligated ureter is anastomosed to the contralateral ureter by TUU. The injured ureter is brought through the colonic mesentery cranial to the inferior mesenteric artery. It is then ligated end-to-side with the contralateral ureter using a spatulated repair.

Upper ureteral or UPJ injuries of short length can be managed by primary reanastomosis with the kidney (ureteropyelostomy) and ureteral stenting and/or percutaneous nephrostomy tube drainage. More extensive upper ureteral injuries are corrected by ureterocalycostomy, where the lower pole of the kidney is removed and the ureter anastomosed directly to the infundibulum.

In cases of extreme ureteral injury involving the entire length of the ureter or multiple segments, or when proximal and distal mobilization cannot be performed, ileal ureteral interposition or kidney autotransplantation may be performed. Ileal ureter interposition involves placement of an isoperistaltic segment of ileum across the ureteral defect. However, the morbidity of the necessary bowel segment excision and reanastomosis is justified only when other ureteral repair techniques will fail.

Bladder injury

Bladder injury is often associated with blunt trauma and particularly with pelvic fracture. Some series report up to 90% of bladder ruptures occurring with associated pelvic fracture. Conversely, the incidence of bladder rupture after pelvic fracture is between 6% and 10% [4] and more likely with fracture of the pubic arch or pubic symphyseal diastasis. Severe associated injuries are often seen when both pelvic fracture and bladder rupture are present, and mortality may occur in 12–22% of cases [5]. Broadly speaking, bladder injuries may be classified as resulting from blunt or penetrating trauma, and the nature of injury may be a simple contusion, or either extraperitoneal or intraperitoneal rupture. The symptoms of bladder injury are often nonspecific, although complete ruptures are accompanied by microscopic or gross hematuria 95% of the time [6]. The AAST five-point injury scale for bladder trauma classifies grade I lesions as either contusions or partial thickness lacerations. Grade II injuries involve extraperitoneal bladder wall lacerations <2 cm. Grade III injuries involve extraperitoneal lacerations >2 cm or intraperitoneal lacerations <2 cm. Grade IV injuries involve intraperitoneal lacerations >2 cm. Grade V injuries involve any laceration extending into the bladder neck or ureteral orifice.

Diagnosis of bladder rupture hinges on the observation of extravasation of urine. Early signs are nonspecific and can be heralded by fever, anuria, and peritonitis. A definitive diagnosis is made by cystography, either plain cystogram or CT cystogram. Complete filling of the bladder is mandatory to avoid making a false-negative diagnosis. Alternatively, bladder injury may be diagnosed intraoperatively by administration or instillation of colored dyes or visual cystoscopy.

Management is dependent on whether the rupture is intraperitoneal or extraperitoneal. Extraperitoneal defects can be managed conservatively with Foley catheter drainage of the bladder. However, open surgical repair may still be indicated when a bone fragment is projecting into the bladder, when an open pelvic fracture is present, when there is rectal perforation, or when there is suspicion of bladder neck injury. Classic dogma teaches that intraperitoneal ruptures must be repaired, especially considering that these defects may be larger than as suggested on cystogram. Anecdotally, intraperitoneal ruptures may be managed conservatively with percutaneous peritoneal drainage in very select patients where the degree of injury is objectively known to be small and the urine is thought to be sterile.

All open surgical repair techniques aim to achieve watertight closure of the bladder in several layers. When open cystotomy is performed to repair an intraperitoneal rupture, the remaining mucosa should be carefully examined, as concomitant extraperitoneal rupture may be present in up to 12% of patients [7]. After the bladder is inspected from the inside out, the detrusor is reapproximated and a large-bore Foley catheter is placed. A suprapubic drainage tube is utilized if Foley catheter placement is contraindicated by bladder neck or urethral injury. However, there is no inherent advantage to using a suprapubic tube over a Foley catheter unless a specific contraindication to the use of the Foley exists [8]. In some instances a drain is left near the bladder closure in the extravesical space. Typically the Foley will be left in place for a minimum of 7–10 days, and preferentially for 2 weeks before reexamination with repeat cystography.

Urethral injury

Traumatic urethral injury is significantly more common among men and, like bladder rupture, is more likely in the setting of pelvic fracture. Indeed, pelvic fractures are the most common cause of posterior urethral injuries, with posterior urethral injuries occurring in between 4% and 14% of pelvic fracture cases [9]. Injuries to the posterior urethra are also associated with bilateral pubic rami fractures and with diastasis of the sacroiliac joint. While the vast majority of these injuries occur in men, girls younger than 17 years of age have a significantly increased risk compared to older women [10]. Conversely, anterior urethral injuries are less common, comprising only 10% of all urethral injuries, [11] with the majority being associated with straddle injury.

Initial observations suggestive of urethral injury are blood at the urethral meatus, inability to void, dysuria, high-riding prostate, difficulty with urethral catheterization, and a butterfly deformity of the perineum. While blood at the meatus is present in up to 50% of urethral injuries, the degree of meatal bleeding does not correlate to the severity of the injury. The combination of meatal bleeding and urinary retention should be considered highly suspicious. If any of these signs are observed, Foley catheter placement without proper urologic evaluation is contraindicated.

Urethral injuries are best diagnosed by performing a retrograde urethrogram (RUG). A small Foley catheter or angiocath is introduced into the urethral meatus and a clamp or steady pressure is applied to occlude the urethra. Contrast is then instilled retrograde and the length of the urethra is visualized fluoroscopically. Injuries may be classified either according to the Colapinto scheme or the more recent AAST urethra injury scale. Pragmatically, urethral injuries can be classified as complete versus partial rupture, given that the accurate assessment of the exact degree of urethral injury is often difficult.

Immediate open surgical primary realignment of the posterior urethra is associated with increased incontinence and stricture formation, and is avoided unless the patient has a rectal or bladder neck injury [12]. Otherwise, the bladder is temporarily drained either by urethral realignment over a catheter or placement of a suprapubic tube and a delayed repair is subsequently performed. Evidence shows that primary endoscopic realignment allows healing without stricture ~50–65% of the time, whereas patients who are not realigned and solely undergo initial suprapubic tube placement develop urethral strictures requiring posterior urethroplasty up to 96% of the time [13]. This suggests that initial placement of a Foley catheter across the urethral defect portends a favorable ultimate outcome. In this setting, a catheter may be placed under controlled conditions by a urologist by gentle blind passage or with cystoscopy, or in extreme cases, by anterograde cystoscopy in the operating room through an open cystostomy. After 6 weeks, a pericatheter RUG is used to evaluate the defect prior to Foley removal. Unhealed injuries are treated first with delayed endoscopic techniques; however, the failure rate of delayed endoscopic repair is high. Longer strictures or unhealed defects refractory to endoscopic management require delayed open reconstruction.

Anterior urethral injuries may be accompanied by hematoma contained under Buck's fascia, causing an "eggplant deformity" of the penile shaft. If the Buck's fascia is ruptured, the hematoma extravasates outward until it is contained by Colles' fascia, leading to swelling of the scrotum and perineum. As opposed to posterior urethral injuries, anterior injuries are best served by immediate primary open repair or suprapubic tube placement followed by open repair. Catheter realignment and delayed repair have less favorable outcomes in anterior injuries than in posterior injuries [14].

Penile injury

Penile injuries are caused by a range of etiologies, including blunt and penetrating trauma, vigorous intercourse, and even self-mutilation. The flaccid penis is usually resistant to blunt trauma, while the erect penis is more liable to injury, and therefore penile fracture is usually associated with missed intromission during sexual intercourse. Penetrating injuries of the penis and external genitalia often accompany other vascular injuries of the spermatic cord, testis, bladder, and other genitourinary structures.

Although most commonly caused by missed intromission during vigorous intercourse, penile fracture has been described after trauma to the erect penis, rough masturbation, and even rolling over in bed [15]. Patients often hear a snapping or popping sound at the time of injury. Shortly thereafter a penile hematoma forms, causing the penile shaft to mimic an eggplant shape. Extreme fractures may also cause urethral tears or hematoma extravasation along the scrotum into the perineum. The diagnosis of penile fracture is primarily clinical. Although cavernosography, ultrasonography, and ultrasound can be used as adjuncts, the clinical picture is usually unambiguous. The only diagnostic study routinely suggested in addition to the clinical diagnosis is a RUG, which will rule out urethral injury. Penile fracture is an emergency and management is operative. A Foley catheter is placed to aid in avoiding iatrogenic urethral injury. Then a circumcising incision is used to deglove the affected area of the penis and allow repair of the underlying fascial layers. Care is taken not to inadvertently plicate the penile shaft and cause a chordee unless it is necessary to close a very large defect. Some surgeons have reported using graft materials to close large defects. The tunica albuginea is then closed with absorbable sutures. Finally, the repair may be tested intraoperatively by saline injection artificial erection.

Penile amputation is usually the result of self-mutilation. Reimplantation is attempted if adequate tissue is salvaged from the preserved penis. The severed penis should be wrapped in wet gauze and placed on ice until reimplantation. Up to 24 hours of cold ischemia time may pass before reimplantation. If reimplantation is not possible, it is usually then necessary to formalize the amputation and create a perineal urethrostomy.

Genital bites, burns, and skin loss

Genital bite injuries, like other cutaneous wounds, can be irrigated and debrided to remove foreign material and then closed primarily if the risk of contamination is low, antibiotics are given, and the injury is only a few hours old. Otherwise, the wound should be left open and allowed to granulate. Inspection of the underlying tissue should be performed prior to primary closure rule out violation of Buck's fascia or hematoma.

Burns to the external genitalia are often full thickness owing to the thin penile skin. Like other burns, burn eschar is resected and coverage with skin grafts is used where necessary. Attention to formation of circumferential bands of scar is particularly necessary in the setting of penile burns, but also has been reported following use of vacuum-assist constriction devices or during sadomasochistic sex play. Skin avulsion injuries caused by machinery may also mimic the genital skin loss caused by burns. In both instances, initial management is coverage of the area with wet gauze and/or silvadene, with surgical management of large areas of full-thickness skin loss. Foreskin or scrotal flaps may be used in distal or proximal injuries, respectively. Potent men should only have nonmeshed split-thickness skin grafts placed so as to avoid avulsion of the graft and subsequent graft contracture.

Scrotal skin loss is encountered either following injury or after intentional debridement, such as in treating Fournier's gangrene. When large amounts of scrotal skin are missing, the testicles may either be placed in surgically tunneled thigh pouches or may simply be wrapped in moist gauze dressings. Frequent dressing changes 2–3 times per day may be performed for several weeks until formal reconstruction is performed. Delayed primary closure is sometimes possible. Otherwise, meshed split-thickness skin grafts or plastic surgical consultation and the transposition of pedicled thigh flaps or free flaps are used to close the defect.

WHAT TO AVOID/PITFALLS

- Blind Foley catheter insertion should not be performed when a urethral injury is suspected until adequate diagnostic workup has been performed and an experienced professional is available to insert the catheter.
- Immediate primary open repair of posterior urethral injuries is not recommended because it usually leads to poorer outcomes than suprapubic tube drainage with delayed repair.
- Gerota's fascia should not be opened while repairing traumatic renal injury until proximal control of the vascular supply is achieved.
- Diagnostic CT and delay of operative management of suspected renal trauma is contraindicated in the setting of acute hemodynamic instability.

KEY WEB LINKS

http://www.aast.org/Default.aspx – AAST trauma guidelines

CASE STUDY

A 17-year-old male presents to the emergency room 3 hours following a rugby match. He reports sustaining a large collision with another player and the onset of right-sided flank pain and one episode of "pink urine". He is afebrile and hemodynamically stable. CT scan with IV contrast in the emergency room reveals a large right-sided perinephric fluid collection that does not enhance on delayed imaging and a 2.5 cm laceration of the right renal parenchyma.

Multiple choice questions

1 The first step in management of the patient should be:
 a Repeat CT scan in 1 hour
 b Placement of percutaneous drainage tube
 c Open surgical repair of parenchymal laceration
 d Advanced trauma life support (ATLS) trauma survey
 e Right total nephrectomy

2 According to the AAST renal trauma guidelines, this patient has what grade of renal injury?
 a Grade I
 b Grade II
 c Grade III
 d Grade IV
 e Grade V

3 Ultimate repair and salvage of the injured kidney is best achieved by:
 a Percutaneous drainage of perinephric fluid
 b Initial bed rest followed by expectant management
 c Placement of ipsilateral percutaneous nephrostomy tube
 d Placement of ipsilateral ureteral stent
 e Partial nephrectomy of injured renal segment

References

1 Miller KS, McAninch JW. Radiographic assessment of renal trauma: our 15-year experience. *J Urol.* 1995; 154(2 Pt 1):352–355.
2 Morey AF, McAninch JW, Tiller BK, Duckett CP, Carroll PR. Single shot intraoperative excretory urography for the immediate evaluation of renal trauma. *J Urol* 1999;161(4):1088–1092.
3 McAninch JW, Carroll PR. Renal trauma: kidney preservation through improved vascular control-a refined approach. *J. Trauma* 1982;22(4):285–290.
4 Hochberg E, Stone NN. Bladder rupture associated with pelvic fracture due to blunt trauma. *Urology* 1993;41(6):531–533.
5 Cass AS, Luxenberg M. Features of 164 bladder ruptures. *J Urol* 1987;138(4):743–745.
6 Cass AS. Urethral injury in the multiple-injured patient. *J. Trauma* 1984;24(10):901–906.
7 Carroll PR, McAninch JW. Major bladder trauma: mechanisms of injury and a unified method of diagnosis and repair. *J Urol* 1984;132(2):254–257.

8 Volpe MA, Pachter EM, Scalea TM, Macchia RJ, Mydlo JH. Is there a difference in outcome when treating traumatic intraperitoneal bladder rupture with or without a suprapubic tube? *J Urol* 1999;161(4):1103–1105.
9 Colapinto V, McCallum RW. Injury to the male posterior urethra in fractured pelvis: a new classification. *J Urol* 1977;118(4):575–580.
10 Hemal AK, Singh I, Chahal R, Gupta NP. Core through internal urethrotomy in the management of post-traumatic isolated bladder neck and prostatic urethral strictures in adults. A report of 4 cases. *Int Urol Nephrol* 1999;31(5):703–708.
11 Mitchell JP. Injuries to the urethra. *Br J Urol* 1968; 40(6):649–670.
12 Webster GD, Mathes GL, Selli C. Prostatomembranous urethral injuries: a review of the literature and a rational approach to their management. *J Urol* 1983;130(5): 898–902.
13 Elliott DS, Barrett DM. Long-term followup and evaluation of primary realignment of posterior urethral disruptions. *J Urol* 1997;157(3):814–816.
14 Husmann DA, Boone TB, Wilson WT. Management of low velocity gunshot wounds to the anterior urethra: the role of primary repair versus urinary diversion alone. *J Urol* 1993;150(1):70–72.
15 Karadeniz T, Topsakal M, Ariman A, Erton H, Basak D. Penile fracture: differential diagnosis, management and outcome. *Br J Urol* 1996;77(2):279–281.

Answers to multiple choice questions

1 d The first step in the management of all trauma patients is ATLS trauma survey to identify any acute or occult life-threatening injury and to achieve hemodynamic stabilization. Diagnostic genitourinary survey should not be performed at the expense of initial stabilization of the patient. If major renal trauma leading to hemodynamic instability is suspected, diagnostic workup is bypassed and operative management is indicated.
2 c The patient has a grade III renal injury: a cortical laceration >1 cm in depth without urine extravasation.
3 b Most grade III injuries may be managed conservatively with bed rest. Once hematuria resolves and hemoglobin is stable, the patient may be observed as an outpatient. Care should be taken to avoid further trauma for at least 4–6 weeks while the renal parenchyma heals. Retroperitoneal hematoma and renin-induced hypertension are rare late complications.

8 Testicular torsion and trauma

Adam Kern

The James Buchanan Brady Urological Institute and Department of Urology, The Johns Hopkins School of Medicine, Baltimore, MD, USA

KEY POINTS

- The *acute scrotum* is a constellation of symptoms consisting of the acute onset of tenderness and/or swelling of the scrotum and its contents. The acute scrotum is a urological emergency.
- Testicular torsion, testicular trauma, torsion of the testicular appendages, epididymitis, orchitis, and incarcerated hernia may all cause acute scrotum.
- Testicular torsion must be recognized promptly as outcome is associated with time to intervention.
- Although color Doppler ultrasound is extremely useful in identifying testicular ischemia, surgical intervention should never be delayed when testicular ischemia is highly suspected.
- A portion of testicular injury patients may be managed nonoperatively if adequate testicular blood supply can be documented.

Testicular torsion is a common entity that all urologic practitioners will encounter, and is one of the classic urologic emergencies that must be promptly recognized. It is also one of the most common and serious urologic emergencies of children and adolescents. The constellation of symptoms of new onset of tenderness and swelling of the scrotum and associated structures is termed *acute scrotum*. Acute scrotum may be caused by several processes, of which testicular torsion is one. While other diagnoses may mimic the symptoms of acute testicular torsion, a high index of suspicion for torsion should always be held. Surgical management of testicular torsion generally yields satisfactory outcomes and may preserve testicular viability, although any significant delay in treatment will reduce the efficacy of intervention considerably. The use of high-definition color Doppler scrotal ultrasound has become commonplace in contemporary practice. However, in indeterminate cases, when the suspicion for acute testicular torsion is high, scrotal exploration is indicated.

General evaluation

A focused urological examination is the starting point for the workup of the acute scrotum, including a history of the nature and duration of the pain and any associated symptoms. Generally, the causes of acute scrotal pain may be delineated into several broad categories, including testicular torsion, testicular trauma, torsion of the appendices, epididymitis, malignancy, and other miscellaneous conditions including scrotal erythema, infectious orchitis, and discomfort due to hernia, hydrocele, and varicocele. Rarely Henoch–Schönlein purpura, an acute vasculitis, may also manifest in the pediatric patient as acute scrotal pain. A history of recent trauma and acute pain of <6 hours duration should be especially noted. Although severe

Handbook of Urology, First edition. J. Kellogg Parsons, John B. Eifler and Misop Han.
Published 2014 by John Wiley & Sons, Ltd.

pain, nausea, and vomiting are often encountered in testicular torsion and may be useful in making a diagnosis, they are not a prerequisite.

Epididymitis

Among adults, epididymitis is the most common cause of acute scrotal pain in the absence of obvious trauma. In pediatric populations, review of patients undergoing surgical exploration demonstrates that torsion of the testicular appendices is the most common finding upon exploration. One large retrospective trial of boys younger than 17 years who presented with signs of acute scrotum and underwent surgical exploration demonstrated that 45% had an appendix testis torsion, followed by spermatic cord torsion (26%), epididymitis (10%), incarcerated hernias (8%), and other conditions (11%) [1]. Epididymitis is most prevalent in infancy and around puberty [2], while appendix testis torsion is more common after infancy. Epididymitis may be either inflammatory or infectious. Epididymitis may be differentiated from torsion on examination, as the former will sometimes provoke extratesticular tenderness by careful palpation. Urinalysis and urine culture may reveal infectious epididymitis and should be part of the general workup. Fever and leukocytosis are also consistent with acute epididymitis. A color Doppler ultrasound will usually reveal a hyperemic epididymis and assist in making the diagnosis. Importantly, ultrasound will normally rule out acute testicular torsion by demonstrating testicular blood flow. Treatment with NSAID and rest will often resolve noninfectious pediatric epididymitis, although careful follow-up is necessary to ensure resolution. Infectious epididymitis should be treated with appropriate antibiotics.

Malignancy, erythema, and infectious orchitis

Germ cell and other testicular tumors may cause testis pain. However, solid or cystic intratesticular masses should be readily identified on ultrasound. Blood flow to the ipsilateral testis should be confirmed using Doppler techniques. If a suspicious intratesticular mass is identified, tumor markers including alpha-fetoprotein, beta-human chorionic gonadotropin (hCG), and serum lactate dehydrogenase (LDH) should be sent. (The workup of testicular masses is reviewed elsewhere in this text.) Scrotal erythema may also be associated with acute scrotal tenderness. New onset scrotal erythema can be associated with cellulitis, and rarely Fournier's gangrene. Once testicular involvement is excluded, appropriate treatment of any infection is initiated. In boys and adolescents who have not received immunizations or who are otherwise immunosuppressed, one should also consider infectious orchitis secondary to mumps virus infection. The presence of parotitis and fever usually accompany mumps virus infection.

Testicular torsion: predisposing factors

Testicular torsion is associated with several predisposing factors. The bell-clapper deformity is the most commonly encountered anatomic variant that leads to torsion. Children with bell-clapper deformity have incomplete fusion of the tunica vaginalis along the epididymis. This causes incomplete anchoring of the testis to a fixed point within the scrotum and allows the testis and epididymis to be mobile. These children are thought to suffer from testicular torsion at higher rates after acute trauma than their age-matched peers, in addition to having elevated rates of spontaneous torsion. Cryptorchid or undescended testes are also at higher risk for torsion before orchiopexy is performed. It is for this reason that the testicle should be well anchored within the scrotum at the time of orchiopexy.

Testicular torsion: types

Testicular torsion may be broadly classified into three categories: (1) acute intravaginal spermatic cord torsion, (2) intermittent intravaginal spermatic cord torsion, and (3) extravaginal spermatic cord torsion. These three types differ in their chronicity and etiology and also in the typical age at presentation.

Acute intravaginal spermatic cord torsion—which is associated with bell-clapper deformity—most commonly occurs in pubertal boys with a mean age at presentation of 13 years [3], although it may present frequently in boys ranging in age from 12 to 16 years and in young adults. Notably, this age range overlaps with that of peak incidence for appendix testis torsion. Torsion of the appendices is most common between the ages 9 and 13 years. Acute intravaginal spermatic cord torsion most commonly involves a single testicle with acute onset of ipsilateral pain of <6 hours duration with no prior known episodes. Athletic activity and/or trauma is thought to be associated with acute intravaginal torsion, although neither is a prerequisite, and indeed children may present with no known inciting factor.

Intermittent intravaginal spermatic cord torsion—or more colloquially known simply as "intermittent torsion"—also typically presents at ages similar to primary acute spermatic cord torsion. However, these boys will have spontaneous resolution of symptoms and very often will recall similar prior episodes. These patients may also carry diagnoses of epididymitis or orchitis from previous encounters where pain spontaneously resolved. Evidence suggests that the frequency of intermittent torsion events correlates with the per-incident risk of persistent torsion [4]. Diagnosis of intermittent torsion may be obscured by spontaneous resolution of symptoms by the time the urologist has had opportunity to evaluate the patient. Therefore, a careful history is integral to making the diagnosis.

Extravaginal spermatic cord torsion is more commonly associated with presentation during the pre- or perinatal period. These children often do not have a bell-clapper deformity. Rather, they are so young that there has not yet been an opportunity for the tunica vaginalis to fuse with the dartos fascia and become fixed within the scrotum. This allows the testis, tunica vaginalis, and epididymis the freedom to rotate *en bloc*. These boys may also present with asynchronous bilateral torsion [5]. Often the extravaginal torsion will occur before birth, resulting in a nonviable unilateral testis, although there are reports of asynchronous bilateral torsion taking place where the second testicle becomes affected after birth. There is still debate whether the added risk of contralateral extravaginal torsion following a prenatal unilateral torsion warrants preemptive surgical management in the neonatal period. As with adolescent intravaginal spermatic cord torsion, if an acute torsion is identified and testicular salvage is possible, urgent surgical exploration is indicated.

Testicular torsion: presentation

The presentation of acute testicular torsion almost always involves the acute onset of scrotal pain of duration <6 hours. Scrotal edema and swelling may also be present. A significant proportion of boys will experience nausea and vomiting. Acute testicular pain in an adolescent in the presence of nausea and vomiting is very suggestive of testicular torsion and prompt workup should not be delayed. The ipsilateral cremasteric reflex may also be absent when complete persistent torsion of the spermatic cord has taken place. While the absence of the reflex is concerning, torsion may still occur along with an intact cremasteric reflex. Intermittent torsion may also spare the cremasteric reflex. Many practitioners also use Prehn's sign to diagnose acute torsion and to differentiate it from epididymitis. Prehn's sign is the relief of testicular pain upon elevation of the affected testicle within the scrotum.

A positive Prehn's sign elicits pain relief upon elevation of the testicle and is suggestive of epididymitis. A negative Prehn's sign is consistent with an ischemic testicle, which may actually become more painful when manipulated. The observation of Prehn's sign has been largely supplanted by color Doppler ultrasound.

Ultrasound is the tool of choice for rapid diagnostic evaluation of acute testicular torsion. It is affordable, readily available, and has a low false-positive rate. Doppler ultrasound is used to visualize the blood flow to the testicle within the spermatic cord. The absence of flow on color Doppler is highly suggestive of acute torsion and necessitates appropriate surgical intervention. After the advent of color Doppler, this technique became widely used throughout pediatric urology. However, recently, some investigators have suggested that the sensitivity of color Doppler ultrasound may be lower than expected, approaching the order of 60% in some hands [6]. In this case, persistent blood flow is seen to a testicle which may subsequently be intraoperatively identified as being ischemic. False negative by ultrasound may be caused by persistent collateral or arterial blood flow or by operator error. Some groups have theorized that a thick spermatic cord may allow for the persistence of blood flow as seen on ultrasound, while the testicle itself remains clinically ischemic. For these reasons, some investigators have taken to direct ultrasound visualization of the spermatic cord as part of the diagnostic workup. High-resolution ultrasonography of the cord itself is performed to determine morphology and directly visualize torsion. Initial data suggest that this technique is highly sensitive to acute torsion, especially when taken in combination with traditional color Doppler ultrasonography of the vascular supply [7, 8]. However, prospective correlation of this technique with the definitive finding of torsion at surgery is ongoing. Direct high-resolution imaging of the spermatic cord may also be pragmatically limited outside of large centers due to the availability of appropriate equipment and personnel.

Urinalysis should always be performed as part of the workup for acute scrotum. The presence of pyuria more commonly indicates epididymitis, but it may be observed along with torsion as well. Radionuclide scanning has also been used to diagnose acute testicular torsion, although this modality is largely of historical interest since the advent of widely available color Doppler ultrasound.

There is no role for nonsurgical management of acute testicular torsion. While manual detorsion may be attempted at the bedside, even if successful, this technique does not address any anatomic anomaly that may put the patient at risk for future torsion. Furthermore, its success is hindered by lack of *a priori* knowledge of the direction of torsion, making it difficult to know in which direction to rotate the affected testicle. Finally, this maneuver may subject the patient to undue additional discomfort and anxiety. We recommend that a single attempt at manual detorsion be made in selected cases, but that this should not delay operative intervention in the patient with refractory symptoms. Even when manual detorsion is successful, the patient should still be counseled to undergo elective orchiopexy.

Testicular torsion: surgical management

The time to intervention after torsion has a direct impact on testicular salvage rates. The risk of orchiectomy after <6 hours since the onset of symptoms is on the order of 5% [9]. The risk of orchiectomy climbs to 20% after 6 hours and doubles to 40% after 12 hours. At 24 hours, it is 80%. These data underscore the importance of prompt intervention.

Surgical management of testicular torsion has four principal goals: (1) rapid identification and confirmation of torsion, (2) reestablishment of testicular perfusion, (3) assessment of testicular viability, and (4) prevention of future recurrence. A transverse hemiscrotal or midline (median raphe) incision is made and the affected testicle is delivered first. It should be immediately inspected and decompressed (in a clockwise direction, similar to opening a book). Initial subjective assessment of its color and viability can then be made, as well as intraoperative ultrasound to establish reestablishment of flow. Once the affected testicle is decompressed, it should be wrapped in sponges soaked in warm saline, and attention should be turned to the contralateral testicle. The contralateral testicle should be fixed in place to the scrotum with three-point orchidopexy using nonabsorbable, monofilament sutures placed through the tunica albuginea. After fixation of the contralateral testis, attention may be turned back to the symptomatic side. If the testicle appears viable, bilateral orchidopexy is completed.

Torsion of the testicular appendices

The testicular appendages are remnants of obliterated Mullerian and Wolffian structures. The appendix testis derives from primordial female Mullerian tissues, whereas the appendix epididymis derives from male Wolffian precursors. Torsion of the appendages is the most common torsion in prepubertal boys. (Extravaginal testicular torsion predominates in the perinatal period, while intravaginal torsion is most common in the pubertal phase.) The classic finding of torsion of the appendages is the "blue dot sign," seen at the superior pole of the testis where necrotic tissues may be seen through the thin transilluminated scrotal skin. The presenting signs of appendix torsion can be nonspecific and often mimic that of acute testicular torsion, but with a more protracted course. The epididymis may also appear hyperemic on examination or ultrasound. If testicular torsion may be absolutely ruled out on the basis of examination and Doppler ultrasound, then management of the appendix torsion may be conservative; however, definitive exclusion of testicular torsion is difficult. Surgical exploration often is indicated to rule out testicular torsion. A torsed appendix may be removed at the time of surgery, although a torsed appendix is not in and of itself an indication for preemptive orchidopexy.

Testicular trauma

Acute scrotum may also be due to trauma. Many traumas are secondary to athletic activity, although a significant proportion will also occur as a result of accident or assault. There are two broad categories: blunt and penetrating. Testicular trauma may have sequelae not just on fertility but on endocrine function and self-image as well.

Testicular injuries are graded according to the American Academy for the Surgery of Trauma (AAST) scale from I to V [10]. Grade I lesions are simple contusions; grade II involve laceration of the tunica albuginea; grade III involve <50% parenchymal loss; grade IV involve ≥50% parenchymal loss; and grade V lesions describe total testicular destruction. There is some evidence that AAST injury scale assessment may be accurately used to determine the appropriateness of conservative versus surgical management [11]. In all cases where conservative management is considered, a scrotal ultrasound should demonstrate lack of testicular rupture and adequate testicular blood flow.

Testicular trauma may be grouped into four broad categories: (1) intratesticular hematoma without rupture, (2) testicular fracture, (3) traumatic testicular torsion, and (4) testicular dislocation. Intratesticular hematoma appears as a heterogeneous lesion on ultrasound and is associated with acute onset of pain. On examination, a noncomplex testicular hematoma or contusion may be difficult to distinguish from a more ominous rupture because both present with pain and subjective changes on ultrasound. In suspicious cases, unless the diagnosis of contusion can be made unequivocally by ultrasound, diagnostic surgical exploration should be performed to rule out a rupture or fracture. Testicular fracture, on the other hand, is more likely to cause a hematocele because of displacement of testicular contents outside of the tunica vaginalis. A hematocele visible on ultrasound should be viewed with suspicion. Fractured or ruptured testes require prompt surgical intervention in order to preserve viability. The testicular contents should be replaced and the tunica then closed. Traumatic testicular torsion should be managed similar to persistent intravaginal spermatic cord torsion, as above. Finally, testicular dislocation may present with pain and an empty hemiscrotum on examination. Diagnostic imaging may be required to ascertain the position of the testicle. The mechanism of these injuries is usually high-energy impacts. After the patient is stabilized, every attempt should be made to salvage the displaced testicle. This may require an inguinal surgical approach to allow for adequate mobilization of tissues. The affected gonads should be carefully inspected for evidence of fracture or devitalization prior to orchidopexy.

Nonoperative management of the testicular trauma patient may be considered when the patient is hemodynamically stable with no evidence of expanding hematoma or hematocele. Pain control should be adequate and both testicles should be visualized in orthotopic position with adequate blood flow. Neither testicle should have significant intraparenchymal heterogeneity on ultrasound. These patients will have injuries classified as AAST grade I–II. Serial monitoring of these patients is advisable to ensure that a hematoma does not form and compromise testicular vascularity or global hemodynamic stability.

WHAT TO AVOID

- Acute testicular torsion may present without all of the characteristic subjective findings. The clinician must have a low index of suspicion.
- The false-negative rate on color Doppler ultrasound may approach 40% depending on conditions. Some ischemic testicles may demonstrate flow on ultrasonography.
- A case of recurrent presumptive epididymitis may actually be intermittent testicular torsion. Examination should be performed when acute pain is present.
- Surgical exploration is diagnostic, whereas delay of surgical intervention on a torsioned testicle is known to correlate with poorer outcomes. If in doubt, go explore in the operating room (OR).

KEY WEB LINKS

AAST trauma guidelines
http://www.trauma.org/index.php/main/articles/C16/

Radiological Society of North America review on scrotal ultrasound
http://radiology.rsna.org/content/227/1/18.abstract

CASE STUDY

A 13-year-old boy is admitted to the pediatric emergency room 4 hours after the acute onset of right-sided scrotal pain. The child was born at 36 weeks with normal prenatal ultrasounds. He demonstrates age-appropriate secondary sexual characteristics on examination. Earlier in the day, he was playing soccer at school when a ball impacted him in the groin. Several minutes later he developed significant scrotal pain radiating to his right inguinal canal. He was able to void urine spontaneously afterward and no hematuria was seen.

On admission he is afebrile and hemodynamically stable, and he vomits twice while being examined. He is reluctant to allow his genitalia to be examined because of pain. His mother states that he had similar sharp pain on several prior occasions, although he was never nauseous during prior episodes. At birth he was noted to have a contralateral left-sided "retractile" testis which never necessitated orchidopexy, and the left testicle is now palpated in an orthotopic position in the scrotum.

Multiple choice questions

1 The first step in management of the patient should be:

- a Manual detorsioning of the testicle
- b IV pain medication
- c Urinalysis
- d Scrotal color Doppler ultrasound
- e High-resolution ultrasound of the spermatic cord

2 The optimal window of time to intervene after the onset of symptoms is:

- a <2 hours
- b <4 hours
- c <6 hours
- d <12 hours
- e <24 hours

3 Which feature puts the patient most at risk for metachronous contralateral testicular torsion?

- a History of trauma
- b Preterm delivery
- c Retractile testis
- d Any incidence of unilateral testicular torsion, regardless of etiology
- e Prior episodes of scrotal pain

References

1 Mäkelä E, Lahdes-Vasama T, Rajakorpi H, Wikström S. A 19-year review of paediatric patients with acute scrotum. *Scand J Surg* 2007;96(1):62–66.

2 Sidler D, Brown RA, Millar AJ, Rode H, Cywes S. A 25-year review of the acute scrotum in children. *S Afr Med J* 1997;87(12):1696–1698.

3 Anderson PA, Giacomantonio JM. The acutely painful scrotum in children: review of 113 consecutive cases. *Can Med Assoc J* 1985;132(10):1153–1155.

4 Hayn MH, Herz DB, Bellinger MF, Schneck FX. Intermittent torsion of the spermatic cord portends an increased risk of acute testicular infarction. *J Urol* 2008; 180(4 Suppl):1729–1732.

5 Baglaj M, Carachi R. Neonatal bilateral testicular torsion: a plea for emergency exploration. *J Urol* 2007;177(6):2296–2299.

6 Bentley DF, Ricchiuti DJ, Nasrallah PF, McMahon DR. Spermatic cord torsion with preserved testis perfusion: initial anatomical observations. *J Urol* 2004;172 (6 Pt 1):2373–2376.

7 Kalfa N, Veyrac C, Baud C, Couture A, Averous M, Galifer RB. Ultrasonography of the spermatic cord in children with testicular torsion: impact on the surgical strategy. *J Urol* 2004;172(4 Pt 2):1692–1695.

8 Kalfa N, Veyrac C, Lopez M, et al. Multicenter assessment of ultrasound of the spermatic cord in children with acute scrotum. *J Urol* 2007;177(1):297–301.

9 Visser AJ, Heyns CF. Testicular function after torsion of the spermatic cord. *BJU Int* 2003;92(3):200–203.

10 Moore EE, Malangoni MA, Cogbill TH, et al. Organ injury scaling VII: cervical vascular, peripheral vascular, adrenal, penis, testis, and scrotum. *J Trauma* 1996;41(3):523–524.

11 Mohr AM, Pham AM, Lavery RF, Sifri Z, Bargman V, Livingston DH. Management of trauma to the male external genitalia: the usefulness of American Association for the Surgery of Trauma organ injury scales. *J Urol* 2003;170(6 Pt 1):2311–2315.

Answers to multiple choice questions

1 The first step in management of the patient should be scrotal color Doppler ultrasound. The imperative in the management of testicular torsion is rapid

confirmation of the diagnosis. Manual detorsioning of the testicle may then be attempted, if appropriate. Urinalysis should be performed in all patients presenting with an acute scrotum, but this should not delay prompt evaluation of testicular vascularization. High-resolution ultrasound of the spermatic cord is a promising technique but is not a substitute for visualization of testicular blood flow.

2 The optimal time to correct a testicular torsion is within the first 6 hours.
3 Any incidence of unilateral testicular torsion puts the patient at elevated risk for contralateral metachronous torsion, regardless of the etiology of the first event. This is thought to be due to the frequently bilateral presence of the bell-clapper deformity. Any retractile testis is itself at a higher risk for torsion.

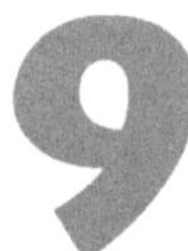

Acute gross hematuria: etiology and management

Kenneth S. Tseng

The James Buchanan Brady Urological Institute and Department of Urology, The Johns Hopkins School of Medicine, Baltimore, MD, USA

KEY POINTS

- A significant proportion of patients who develop gross hematuria while on anticoagulation or aspirin therapy will still have an underlying abnormality.
- Most hematuria will resolve spontaneously. The objective of conservative management strategies should be to maintain hemodynamic stability and adequate drainage of the bladder until the bleeding resolves.
- Persistent, severe hemorrhagic cystitis requiring multiple transfusions may require intravesical instillation of silver nitrate, aluminum, or formalin.
- Hyperbaric oxygen treatment can be used with success in refractory cases of hematuria, although resolution of symptoms may require up to 60 treatments.
- Selective embolization of the internal iliac arteries may obviate the need for more invasive surgical intervention, although it comes at the risk of gluteal claudication or bladder necrosis.

CASE STUDY

An 80-year-old gentleman with a history of prostate cancer s/p radiation therapy presented to the urology clinic for a single episode of gross hematuria. Upon endoscopic evaluation, he was found to have a urethral stricture which was dilated. After dilation of the stricture, the bladder had pale urothelium with diffuse telangiectasias and neovascularity. Two days later, the patient presented to the emergency department (ED) unable to pass urine. He reported dark merlot colored urine 12 hours earlier with quarter-sized clots passing per urethra. A 24F 3-way catheter was placed and manually irrigated until the clots were fully evacuated. A complete blood count (CBC) in the ED revealed a hemoglobin level of 6 g/dL. He was admitted, transfused with four units of packed red blood cells and placed on continuous bladder irrigation (CBI). Urine cytology showed no signs of atypia or malignancy. Over the subsequent 2 days, he required frequent manual irrigation due to clot obstruction, and required another four units of packed red blood cells. The patient was taken to the operating room, where clot was evacuated and intravesical silver nitrate was instilled after a cystogram showed no vesicoureteral reflux. After the procedure, the patient's CBI was weaned to off and he was clear for 2 days. However, his urine became bloody again, and another dose of intravesical silver nitrate was instilled without success. He was taken back to the OR, and intravesical formalin was instilled in his bladder for 30 minutes. Postoperatively, his hematuria resolved, the CBI was discontinued, and his urine was seen to remain clear. He was discharged to home.

Handbook of Urology, First edition. J. Kellogg Parsons, John B. Eifler and Misop Han.
Published 2014 by John Wiley & Sons, Ltd.

Acute onset of gross hematuria accounts for many outpatient and inpatient urology consultations. The majority of cases are self-limited. However, the possibility that this symptom is a harbinger of insidious disease mandates that work-up be performed in certain populations. In cases where hematuria does not resolve on its own and is refractory to conservative treatment, urologists have several treatment options that vary in efficacy, safety, and morbidity.

The most common causes of gross hematuria include neoplastic, infectious, traumatic, or iatrogenic processes. Neoplasms arising anywhere along the urinary tract can lead to bleeding; prostate cancer, bladder cancer, upper urinary tract transitional cell carcinoma, and renal tumors are the most common. Infectious processes include cystitis and prostatitis. Menses can sometimes be misinterpreted as hematuria. The initial presenting symptoms for a stone in the kidney, ureter, or bladder may be gross hematuria. Postradiation cystitis (Figure 9.1) and cyclophosphamide-induced hemorrhagic cystitis are often the most refractory of all the etiologies. Iatrogenic causes include traumatic urethral catheterization or removal of a Foley catheter without deflating the balloon. Urinary tract instrumentation may also cause clinically significant hematuria.

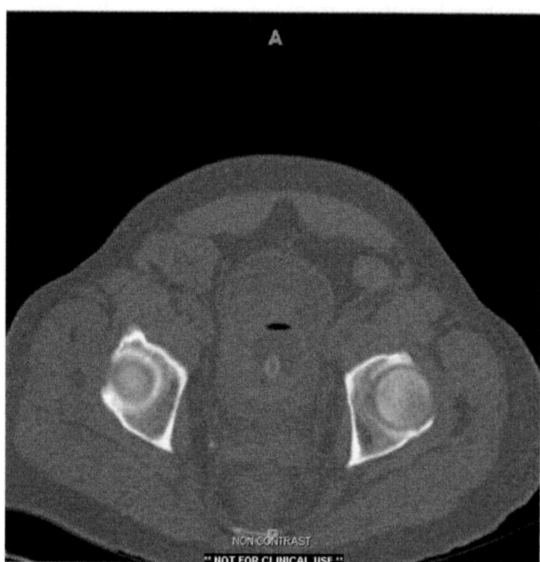

Figure 9.1 CT of the pelvis shows bladder with radiation cystitis and blood clot surrounding Foley catheter balloon.

The initial work-up of gross hematuria should include a thorough history and physical examination. The history should include the onset, timing, and duration of bleeding. Prior need for blood transfusions, episodes of clot retention, or hospitalizations for hematuria may inform the physician about the severity of hematuria. A past medical history that includes a personal history of malignancy in the urinary tract, other malignancies requiring chemotherapy or pelvic radiation, a history of stones, or lower urinary tract symptoms may provide clues to the etiology of the current episode. Although a history of bleeding at other body sites can explain a predisposition for hematuria, up to 80% of patients who develop hematuria while on anticoagulation still have a significant urologic abnormality [1].

Physical examination should include examination of catheterized urine in patients with a catheter, and voided urine in those who do not. Examination of the genitalia should focus on anatomic abnormalities of the meatus that may have made catheterization difficult in men, or the presence of menstruation in women. An abdominal examination should be performed to evaluate for a palpable bladder indicating clot retention, or abdominal masses indicative of large renal tumors. Costovertebral angle tenderness may be a sign of pyelonephritis, or hydronephrosis from a ureteral stone. A digital rectal examination can identify palpable prostate adenocarcinoma, a boggy prostate suggestive of prostatitis, or an enlarged gland.

The goal of diagnostic studies is to evaluate for upper and lower tract abnormalities associated with hematuria. A urinalysis and urine culture should be sent whenever the cause of the hematuria is not immediately obvious from the history and physical examination to evaluate for infection or signs of renal disease. A CBC with differential, PT, and PTT should be considered in a patient whose hematuria is considered significant enough to cause hemodynamic instability, or in patients on anticoagulation or antiplatelet medications. Urine cytology should be performed to evaluate for urothelial malignancy, especially in patients over 40 or those with a history of smoking [2]. Flexible cystoscopy can be performed in the outpatient setting to further evaluate for bladder tumor, mucosal abnormalities, or foreign bodies. CT urogram can also be performed electively, with a dry phase to evaluate for stone disease, an arterial phase to evaluate for enhancing renal masses, and an excretory phase to evaluate for upper tract filling defects that may be indicative of transitional cell carcinoma. If the initial work-up for gross hematuria is normal, repeat urinalysis, urine cytology, and blood pressure should be checked every 6 months until 3 years after the initial episode [3].

For patients who are acutely bleeding, the initial management strategy should aim to ensure adequate bladder drainage and hemodynamic stability. Patients who meet these criteria should be encouraged to maintain adequate oral hydration. Any coagulopathies should be reversed, and consideration should be given to stopping anticoagulants (NSAIDs, heparin, warfarin, or clopidogrel) when possible. Men who are passing large clots may be at risk for clot retention, and manual irrigation of their bladder should be performed until there is no longer any residual clot. If the bleeding is thought to be from the bladder neck or from urethral injury, such as after traumatic urethral catheterization, a large-caliber (22/24F) urethral catheter can be left indwelling to tamponade the bleeding. Placing the catheter on light traction can further place pressure on the bladder neck and prostate, although extended periods of traction may theoretically cause ischemia.

In all patients who present with clot retention and appear to be actively bleeding after manual irrigation and evacuation of all clot burdens, continuous bladder irrigation (CBI) should be considered to maintain dilute concentrations of urine to prevent further clot retention. The CBI can be titrated to a light color of effluent while the bleeding has time to resolve on its own.

A word of caution regarding CBI: for patients with organized bladder clots refractory to manual irrigation, CBI runs the risk of outflow obstruction and bladder perforation. Untrained nurses managing CBI should be instructed to clamp the inflow port for suprapubic pain or low urine output and to contact the urologist.

Etiologies

Hemorrhagic cystitis can be one of the most difficult urologic conditions to treat. It is caused by bladder inflammation, often from prior pelvic radiation or chemotherapy (especially cyclophosphamide or ifosfamide). Infections (bacterial or viral) may also be associated with hemorrhagic cystitis in immunocompromised hosts. Approximately 23% of patients with gross hematuria are found to have evidence of urologic malignancy on initial evaluation. Furthermore, out of the 8% of patients who do not have any discernible cause of hematuria after initial evaluation, 18% are later found to have urologic malignancy [3].

Patients with hemorrhagic cystitis should undergo cystoscopy to evaluate the cause of the bleeding, evacuate organized clot refractory to catheter irrigation, and if possible, to control bleeding with fulguration. Urine culture and cytology should be obtained. If hematuria from an upper tract etiology is suspected, a CT urogram would be indicated for patients with normal renal function.

Treatment of refractory hematuria

Refractory bleeding from a renal source, such as an angiomyolipoma, should be treated with embolization. If embolization is unsuccessful, partial or total nephrectomy should be considered.

Bleeding from the prostate can be treated medically with aminocaproic acid (Amicar), androgen deprivation, or 5α-reductase inhibitors. Finasteride has been shown in noncontrolled case series to be effective in up to 77% of patients who receive treatment for refractory hematuria from benign prostatic hypertrophy [4]. It is thought to work by decreasing expression of vascular endothelial growth factor (VEGF) in the prostate and limiting angiogenesis [5]. A transurethral procedure can be performed to cauterize bleeding venous sinuses, or to resect gland overgrowth. Palliative radiation therapy is also an option.

Bladder bleeding occasionally responds to medical treatment with aminocaproic acid or, in cases where the bleeding is from distinct areas, transurethral cauterization. More often, though, refractory hematuria from the bladder is due to a diffuse abnormality of the mucosa, as occurs in hemorrhagic or radiation cystitis, and requires intravesical therapy or hyperbaric oxygen treatments. Nephrostomy tubes can be used to divert urine and urokinase away from the bladder [6]. Selective embolization of internal iliac arteries can be attempted prior to more invasive surgical interventions [7]. Lastly, cystectomy or urinary diversion is also an option in severe cases that do not respond to any of the above treatments.

Aminocaproic acid (Amicar)

Mechanism of action: inhibits conversion of plasminogen to plasmin, an enzyme that lyses fibrin clots; at higher doses, direct inhibition of plasmin activity
Contraindications: disseminated intravascular coagulation (DIC); risk of thrombosis; hypersensitivity to aminocaproic acid
Precautions: cardiac, hepatic, or renal insufficiency; renal or ureteral bleeding
Dose: 5 g IV diluted in 250 mL of D5W or NS infused intravesically over 1 hour, followed by 1 g/hour (50 mL/hour) continuous infusion for 8 hours or until bleeding is controlled; 5 g PO once, followed by 1 g PO qhour for 8 hours or until bleeding is controlled; 0.1% intravesical instillation
Adverse effects: rhabdomyolysis, hypotension [8–11]

Sodium pentosan polysulfate (Elmiron)

Mechanism of action: reinforce glycosaminoglycan layer of bladder
Contraindications: allergy to pentosan polysulfate
Precautions: risk of hemorrhage; hepatic insufficiency; splenic disorders
Dose: 100 mg PO TID either 1 hour before or 2 hours after meals
Adverse effects: alopecia, rectal hemorrhage
Note: may require chronic treatment for several weeks before results are seen [12–15]

Conjugated estrogens

Mechanism of action: stabilization of vascular fragility
Contraindications: arterial thromboembolic disease, breast cancer, DVT/PE, liver dysfunction, pregnancy, thrombophilia
Precautions: hypertension, hereditary angioedema, asthma, diabetes, epilepsy, lupus
Dose: 5 mg PO daily (± an initial dose of 1 mg/kg IV BID for 2 days)
Adverse effects: hypercoagulability [16–19]

Hyperbaric oxygen

Mechanism of action: increased angiogenesis in bladders with endarteritis secondary to radiation-induced tissue hypoxia; vasoconstriction
Contraindications: use of cisplatin or doxorubicin; severe pulmonary disease such as pneumothorax or oxygen-dependent COPD; active viral infections
Dose: 14–60 daily sessions with 100% oxygen inhalation at 0.3 MPa, 90 minutes per session
Adverse effects: sinus barotrauma, oxygen toxicity
Note: successful in up to 70–90% of cases [20–24]

Intravesical formalin

Mechanism of action: precipitates proteins on mucosa surface; coagulation of telangiectasias and small capillaries
Contraindications: small volume bladder
Dose: instill 1% formalin (equivalent to 0.37% formaldehyde) intravesically under gravity for 10 minutes; the endoscopic placement of cotton pledgets soaked with higher concentrations of formalin has also been described
Adverse effects: reflux leading to pyonephrosis and fatal sepsis; vesicovaginal fistula; contracted bladder
Notes: all clots must be evacuated prior to instillation; must be performed under general or spinal anesthesia due to discomfort; a cystogram is required to rule out ureteral reflux; Fogarty catheters can be used to occlude the ureteral orifices if reflux is present; formalin can scar or fibrose the bladder, occasionally leaving the bladder completely defunctionalized, which can be troublesome in younger patients [25–32]

Intravesical 1% alum

Mechanism of action: precipitates proteins on cell surface and in interstitial spaces, leading to clotting of capillaries
Dose: 50 g alum dissolved in 5 L sterile water; bladder irrigated at a rate of 200–300 mL/hour
Precautions: renal insufficiency, children
Adverse effects: suprapubic pain, low-grade fever, encephalopathy
Notes: prothrombin time correlates with serum aluminum levels and can be used as a surrogate measure for aluminum toxicity; alum irrigation can precipitate and block the catheter outflow [33–37]

Intravesical silver nitrate

Mechanism of action: precipitates protein, leading to clotting of surface capillaries

Contraindications: bladder perforation, vesicoureteral reflux

Dose: instill 0.5–1% in sterile water intravesically for 10–20 minutes, placing the catheter on light traction to avoid silver nitrate contact with the urethra; after draining the catheter, irrigate the bladder copiously with normal saline

Adverse effects: methemoglobinemia; sensation of burning of skin

Notes: similar to formalin, all clots must be evacuated prior to instillation; at concentrations >0.5%, must be performed under general or spinal anesthesia due to discomfort; a cystogram is required to rule out ureteral reflux; Fogarty catheters can be used to occlude the ureteral orifices if reflux is present; silver nitrate can cause scarring of the bladder [35, 38–40]

WHAT TO AVOID/KEY PITFALLS

- Patients who develop gross hematuria while on anticoagulant therapy are still at risk for an underlying anatomic abnormality and should be evaluated endoscopically.
- Vesicoureteral reflux is a contraindication to intravesical instillation of formalin and silver nitrate, but not alum.
- Aminocaproic acid can be used for treating prostatic or bladder bleeding, but should be avoided in hematuria from the upper urinary tract because of concern that clots in the upper tract can lead to ureteral obstruction.
- Intravesical alum treatments can be absorbed systemically and may be toxic in patients with renal insufficiency.
- Because of scarring that can occur with intravesical instillations of formalin and silver nitrate, alternate therapies should be considered for younger patients.

KEY WEB LINK

http://kidney.niddk.nih.gov/kudiseases/pubs/hematuria/

Multiple choice questions

1 A 60-year-old man develops severe hemorrhagic cystitis after receiving cyclophosphamide as part of his chemotherapy regimen for Hodgkin lymphoma. He is started on CBI and transfused with several units of blood for symptomatic anemia. His bleeding persists despite a single intravesical instillation of 2% formalin. The next step is

a Intravesical instillation with 1% aluminum
b Bilateral percutaneous nephrostomy tubes
c Administration of sodium 2-mercaptoethane sulfonate (Mesna)
d Administration of sodium pentosan polysulfate (Elmiron)
e Hyperbaric oxygen treatment

2 The following should be done prior to instillation of intravesical formalin *except*

a Cystogram to rule out vesicoureteral reflux
b Renal ultrasound to rule out hydronephrosis
c Positioning of patient in reverse Trendelenburg to minimize vesicoureteral reflux
d Administration of general anesthesia
e Evacuation of all clots

References

1 Avidor Y NA, Matzkin H. Clinical significance of gross hematuria and its evaluation in patients receiving anticoagulant and aspirin treatment. *Urology* 2000;55(1):22–24.
2 Grossfeld GD, Litwin MS, Wolf JS, Jr., et al. Evaluation of asymptomatic microscopic hematuria in adults: the American Urological Association best practice policy—part II: patient evaluation, cytology, voided markers, imaging, cystoscopy, nephrology evaluation, and follow-up. *Urology* 2001;57(4):604–610.
3 Sutton JM. Evaluation of hematuria in adults. *JAMA* 1990;263(18):2475–2480.
4 Kearney MC, Bingham JB, Bergland R, Meade-D'Alisera P, Puchner PJ. Clinical predictors in the use of finasteride for control of gross hematuria due to benign prostatic hyperplasia. *J Urol* 2002;167(6):2489–2491.
5 Pareek G, Shevchuk M, Armenakas NA, et al. The effect of finasteride on the expression of vascular endothelial growth factor and microvessel density: a possible mechanism for decreased prostatic bleeding in treated patients. *J Urol* 2003;169(1):20–23.
6 Sneiders A, Pryor JL. Percutaneous nephrostomy drainage in the treatment of severe hemorrhagic cystitis. *J Urol* 1993;150(3):966–967.
7 Liguori G, Amodeo A, Mucelli FP, et al. Intractable haematuria: long-term results after selective embolization of the internal iliac arteries. *BJU Int* 2010;106(4):500–503.
8 *PDR Physicians' Desk Reference*. 42nd ed. Oradell, NJ: Medical Economics Company; 1988.
9 *CPS Compendium of Pharmaceuticals and Specialties*. 22nd ed. Ottawa, Canada: Canadian Pharmaceutical Association; 1987.
10 Product Information: Amicar. Lederle, Canada.
11 *PDR Physicians' Desk Reference*. 48th ed. Montvale, NJ: Anon Medical Economics Data; 1994.

12 Ortho-McNeil Pharmaceutical I. Product information: ELMIRON(R) oral capsules, pentosan polysulfate sodium oral capsules. Raritan, NJ 2006.
13 Parsons CL. Successful management of radiation cystitis with sodium pentosanpolysulfate. *J Urology* 1986;111:603.
14 Sandhu SS, Goldstraw M, Woodhouse CR. The management of haemorrhagic cystitis with sodium pentosan polysulphate. *BJU Int* 2004;94(6):845–847.
15 Hampson SJ, Woodhouse CR. Sodium pentosanpolysulphate in the management of haemorrhagic cystitis: experience with 14 patients. *Eur Urol* 1994;25(1):40–42.
16 Liu YK, Harty JI, Steinbock GS, Holt HA, Jr., Goldstein DH, Amin M. Treatment of radiation or cyclophosphamide induced hemorrhagic cystitis using conjugated estrogen. *J Urol* 1990;144(1):41–43.
17 Miller J, Burfield GD, Moretti KL. Oral conjugated estrogen therapy for treatment of hemorrhagic cystitis. *J Urol* 1994;151(5):1348–1350.
18 Ordemann R, Naumann R, Geissler G, Bornhauser M, Schuler U, Ehninger G. Encouraging results in the treatment of haemorrhagic cystitis with estrogen—report of 10 cases and review of the literature. *Bone Marrow Transplant* 2000;25(9):981–985.
19 FDA WPIp. Product Information: PREMARIN(R) oral tablets, conjugated estrogens oral tablets. Philadelphia, PA.
20 Corman JM, McClure D, Pritchett R, Kozlowski P, Hampson NB. Treatment of radiation induced hemorrhagic cystitis with hyperbaric oxygen. *J Urol* 2003;169(6):2200–2202.
21 Bevers RFM, Bakker DJ, Kurth KH. Hyperbaric oxygen treatment for haemorrhagic radiation cystitis. *Lancet* 1995;346:803–805.
22 Crew JP, Jephcott CR, Reynard JM. Radiation-induced haemorrhagic cystitis. *Eur Urol* 2001;40(2):111–123.
23 Mathews R, Rajan N, Josefson L, Camporesi E, Makhuli Z. Hyperbaric oxygen therapy for radiation induced hemorrhagic cystitis. *J Urol* 1999;161(2): 435–437.
24 Del Pizzo JJCB, Jacobs SC, Sklar GN. Treatment of radiation induced hemorrhagic cystitis with hyperbaric oxygen: long-term follow-up. *J Urol* 1998;160(3 Pt 1): 731–733.
25 Shah BC, Albert DJ. Intravesical instillation of formalin for the management of intractable hematuria. *J Urol* 1973;110:519–520.
26 Ferrie BG, Rundle JS, Kirk D, Paterson PJ, Scott R. Intravesical formalin in intractable haematuria. *J Urol* (Paris) 1985;91(1):33–35.
27 Vicente J, Rios G, Caffaratti J. Intravesical formalin for the treatment of massive hemorrhagic cystitis: retrospective review of 25 cases. *Eur Urol* 1990;18(3):204–206.
28 Dewan AK, Mohan GM, Ravi R. Intravesical formalin for hemorrhagic cystitis following irradiation of cancer of the cervix. *Int J Gynaecol Obstet* 1993;42(2):131–135.
29 Fair WR. Formalin in the treatment of massive bladder hemorrhage. Techniques, results, and complications. *Urology* 1974;3(5):573–576.
30 Lowe BA, Stamey TA. Endoscopic topical placement of formalin soaked pledgets to control localized hemorrhage due to radiation cystitis. *J Urol* 1997;158(2):528–529.
31 Lojanapiwat B, Sripralakrit S, Soonthornphan S, Wudhikarn S. Intravesical formalin instillation with a modified technique for controlling haemorrhage secondary to radiation cystitis. *Asian J Surg* 2002;25(3):232–235.
32 Donahue LA, Frank IN. Intravesical formalin for hemorrhagic cystitis: analysis of therapy. *J Urol* 1989;141(4):809–812.
33 Arrizabalaga M, Extramiana J, Parra JL, Ramos C, Diaz-Gonzales R, Leiva O. Treatment of massive hematuria with aluminous salts. *Br J Urol* 1987;60:223–226.
34 Goswami AK, Mahajan RK, Nath R, Sharma SK. How safe is 1% alum irrigation in controlling intractable vesical hemorrhage? *J Urol* 1993;149(2):264–267.
35 Rastinehad AR, Ost MC, VanderBrink BA, Siegel DN, Kavoussi LR. Persistent prostatic hematuria. *Nat Clin Pract Urol* 2008;5(3):159–165.
36 Ostroff EB, Chenault OW. Alum irrigation for the control of massive bladder hemorrhage *J Urol* 1982;128: 929–930.
37 Kanwar VS, Jenkins JJ, 3rd, Mandrell BN, Furman WL. Aluminum toxicity following intravesical alum irrigation for hemorrhagic cystitis. *Med Pediatr Oncol* 1996;27(1):64–67.
38 deVries CR, Freiha FS. Hemorrhagic cystitis: a review. *J Urol* 1990;143(1):1–9.
39 Raghavaiah NV, Soloway MS. Anuria following silver nitrate irrigation for intractable bladder hemorrhage. *J Urol* 1977;118(4):681–682.
40 Jerkins GR, Noe HN, Hill DE. An unusual complication of silver nitrate treatment of hemorrhagic cystitis: case report. *J Urol* 1986;136(2):456–458.

Answers to multiple choice questions

1 b In patients with severe hemorrhagic cystitis requiring repeated transfusions of packed red blood cells, bilateral nephrostomy tubes are used to divert urine (and urokinase) away from the bladder in order to increase the likelihood of tamponade and clotting. Having the urine diverted also allows more aggressive intravesical therapy [6].

2 b

10 Priapism

Debasish Sundi and Trinity J. Bivalacqua

The James Buchanan Brady Urological Institute and Department of Urology, The Johns Hopkins School of Medicine, Baltimore, MD, USA

KEY POINTS

- Ischemic priapism requires emergent diagnosis and treatment.
- High-flow priapism may be treated electively.
- Check prior to aspiration/injection: consent, antibiotics, telemetry monitor.
- As an adjunct to surgical shunts, corporal tunneling maneuvers are highly effective in evacuating blood clots.

Presentation and diagnosis

General principles

Obtain a complete blood count with differential, coagulation profile, sickle cell prep and hemoglobin electrophoresis. Toxicology screening should be performed when suspicion is triggered by the history.

Ischemic priapism

A man with ischemic priapism may describe a past medical history of sickle cell disease or other blood dyscrasia. The lifetime prevalence of priapism in sickle cell disease is 29–42%, and two-thirds of men with sickle-cell-disease-associated ischemic priapism will have experienced prior stuttering episodes [1]. For adult priapism overall, sickle cell disease is the underlying etiology in 23% of cases. There may be a history of erectile dysfunction with recent intracavernosal injection with combinations of phentolamine, papaverine, and alprostadil (referred to as "bimix" or "trimix" injections), recreational drugs, or centrally acting drugs for the treatment of depression or psychosis. Ischemic priapism is typically progressively painful with time, and the shaft is usually fully rigid and tender to palpation. The corporal blood will appear very dark, and the corporal blood gas will have, typically, $pO_2 < 30$ mm Hg, $pCO_2 > 60$ mm Hg, and $pH < 7.25$ [2]. Color duplex ultrasound (CDU) may be used as an adjunct test, and it will show no flow in the cavernosal arteries [3]. CDU can be performed in a frog-legged or lithotomy position; the perineum and corpora should be scanned in their entirety. CDU is not essential to diagnose ischemic priapism and must not delay initiation of timely treatment.

Stuttering priapism

A man with stuttering priapism will most often have an associated history of sickle cell disease, with painful priapism episodes that may have started as early as his childhood or teenage years [1, 2]. The priapism episodes may have been the sequelae of routine morning erections or specific stressors such as dehydration, fever, or cold ambient temperatures. A man with stuttering priapism who presents with ischemic priapism (>4 hours) is likely to have had an episode of ischemic priapism in the past as well (approximately

Handbook of Urology, First edition. J. Kellogg Parsons, John B. Eifler and Misop Han.
Published 2014 by John Wiley & Sons, Ltd.

one-third). The symptoms, physical examination, corporal blood gas, and CDU in stuttering priapism that has lasted >4 hours and ischemic priapism are, by definition, identical.

High-flow priapism

The patient with high-flow priapism will most often have a history of penile or perineal trauma, such as during intercourse, saddle or sports injuries to the perineum, or pelvic fractures [1]. The trauma may be related to needle puncture such as with intracavernosal injection therapy for erectile dysfunction. Other causes of high-flow priapism that should be elucidated on history relate to malignant infiltration of the corpora causing an arteriocorporal fistula (primaries may be locally infiltrative such as prostate or bladder or distant metastatic lesions such as lymphoma). An increasingly recognized category of high-flow priapism is the subset related to surgical shunt procedures to treat ischemic priapism. A patient with symptomatic high-flow priapism may present in delayed fashion (such as the morning after or several days after) the traumatic event. The penis may only be partially erect, and is typically not painful, nor tender to palpation. CDU is sufficient to confirm the diagnosis [3]. It will demonstrate normal to high flow in the cavernous arteries and may even show an arteriolar–sinusoidal fistula. The corporal blood gas will have, typically, a normal arterial profile with $pO_2 > 90$ mm Hg, $pCO_2 < 40$ mm HG, and pH near 7.40 [2]. Though arteriography can also confirm the diagnosis of high-flow priapism, this technique should only be used when performed in conjunction with arterial embolization as an elective treatment for this condition.

Treatment

Ischemic priapism (low flow)

Ischemic priapism is a penile compartment syndrome with progressive time-dependent tissue hypoxia, acidosis, necrosis, and fibrosis of the corpora cavernosa. These irreversible cellular changes begin at the 4-hour time point [4]. It is the result of blood that, during erection, had engorged the corporal bodies, but which can no longer exit the sinusoidal spaces. As an ultimate result, arterial flow in the cavernous arteries stops. In sickle cell disease, the pathophysiology of vascular occlusion may be brought on by low oxygen tension that causes HbS polymerization and RBC sickling/clumping and hemolysis. Release hemoglobin and free radicals also quench NO, thus impairing NO-mediated vasodilation.

Treatment for ischemic priapism must be initiated in a timely manner. The chance of spontaneous erections (with or without phosphodiesterase-type 5 (PDE-5) inhibitors) has been reported to be 100% in men with priapism reversed within 12 hours, 78% within 12–24 hours, 44% in 24–36 hours, and 0% after a priapism duration >36 hours [1].

The initial treatment of ischemic priapism should involve penile aspiration and injection. Steps:

1 Consent—make the patient aware that erectile dysfunction is an additional consequence of penile aspiration and injection, along with pain, bleeding, infection, failure to detumesce, and the cardiogenic sequelae of systemic distribution of injected alpha-agonists (hypertension, reflex bradycardia, arrhythmias, myocardial infarction, stroke).

2 All patients and particularly those with cardiovascular risk factors should have continuous cardiac monitoring and frequent serial blood pressure measurements during injection therapy.

3 Systemic pre-procedure antibiotics, such as with cefazolin 2 g or clindamycin 600 mg intravenous.

4 Sterile prep and drape.

5 Administer local anesthesia. A penile block with lidocaine or bupivacaine is sufficient, though an additional subdermal wheal at the site of injection is also acceptable.

6 Insert a 21- or 18-gauge butterfly (scalp–vein) needle connected to long tubing into the right or left corporal body near the base of the penis, but taking care to avoid the urethra. Lateral punctures at the 9–10 o'clock and/or 2–3 o'clock positions are acceptable. Larger gauge needles may facilitate effective aspiration of static corporal blood.

7 Aspirate the dark (old) blood until the returned blood is bright red (evidence of oxygenated blood). The first aspirate may be sent for a confirmatory corporal blood gas at this time if the history and physical examination +/– CDU were diagnostic for ischemic priapism already.

8 Irrigation with normal saline has no demonstrated benefit. We advise against this since saline injection causes the corpora to regain rigidity and may

dilute the injected alpha-agonist, and is therefore counterproductive.

9 If necessary, injection and aspiration may be done through an additional second puncture (keeping the first needle in place) in the contralateral corporal body.

10 If detumescence is nil or unsatisfactory with aspiration alone, inject dilute phenylephrine into the corpora through the existing 21-gauge needle. Typically, phenylephrine should be diluted with normal saline into a 200 mcg/mL concentration, and be injected in 0.5 to 1 mL doses in 5–10 minute intervals for a maximum total dose of 1000 mcg. For children or patients who are elderly or with significant cardiovascular disease, use a 100 mcg/mL concentration. If at the maximal phenylephrine dose or after 1 hour, the penis does not detumesce, aspiration and injection should be deemed a failure and one should proceed to a surgical shunt procedure.

Aspiration alone is sufficient to resolve the priapism up to 36% of the time. Aspiration with injection of an alpha-agonist has a higher success rate, up to 81% [2]. In the setting of sickle cell disease, note that systemic strategies such as oxygenation, opioid analgesics, alkaline intravenous rehydration, and exchange transfusion are not primary treatments for priapism, but can be used as an adjunct to aspiration/injection and shunting—either during or after.

When aspiration and injection fail to resolve the priapism, the next step is a shunt procedure performed in the operating room [4]. Distal shunts are attempted first, and if those fail, proximal shunts are performed. A Winter's shunt involves using a biopsy needle (such as a "TruCut") to remove cores of the distal corpora percutaneously through the glans [5]. Ebbehoj shunts involve using an 11- or 15-blade to make multiple stab incisions into the distal corpora through the glans, with or without a 90 degree outward turn of the blade to increase the size of the corporal puncture. A T-shunt (Lue shunt) involves a single vertical stab incision through the glans into the tip of each corporal body with a 10-blade, and with subsequent rotation of the blade of the knife outward 90 degrees to achieve a bigger corporal puncture. In one modification, the corpora are then tunneled proximally to the crura with 20F dilating sheaths or 20F bougies in order to evacuate the old ischemic blood [6]. The glans incisions are closed with 4-0 chromic simple interrupted sutures. These aforementioned shunt procedures (Figure 10.1) are technically feasible at the bedside using local anesthesia, though for comfort and convenience regional or general anesthesia in the operating room may facilitate the procedure.

The Al-Ghorab shunt involves a single transverse or two vertical incisions in the dorsum of the glans to expose the tips of the corpora, which are then grasped with Kocher clamps and excised. The snake maneuver (Burnett shunt) involves dilation of the corporal bodies to the crura with 9 mm Hegar dilators to facilitate milking out of the old blood and establishing a more robust shunt (Figure 10.2) [7].

Proximal shunts include Quackle's corporoglanular shunt, which may be performed bilaterally or unilaterally through a scrotal or perineal incision; the Grayhack shunt that involves anastomosis of the saphenous vein to one of the corpora (often complicated by venous thrombus and embolism); and the Barry shunt that involves anastomosis of the penile deep dorsal vein to a window in one of the corpora (which has not been very effective in practice) [5]. The Grayhack and Barry shunts are historical shunts that are seldom used in current practice. The successful execution of a shunt procedure may result in a non-tender penile erection with arterial-profile corporal blood gases—this represents iatrogenic conversion of ischemic priapism into a non-ischemic, or high-flow priapism state. This type of post-shunt high-flow priapism is *not* treated with arterial embolization.

Stuttering priapism (recurrent)

Stuttering priapism is a recurrent form of ischemic priapism. When a stuttering episode lasts beyond 4 hours it should be treated as an ischemic priapism event.

Several strategies could be employed in the non-urgent setting to prevent stuttering ischemic episodes. Some advocate the use of chronic androgen deprivation, though this may have untoward side effects (loss of energy, low libido, depression, gynecomastia, decreased muscle mass) [8]. Androgen deprivation must not be used in males who have not yet completed full masculinization and skeletal linear growth. Some properly instructed patients perform self-injection with intracavernosal phenylephrine to manage stuttering

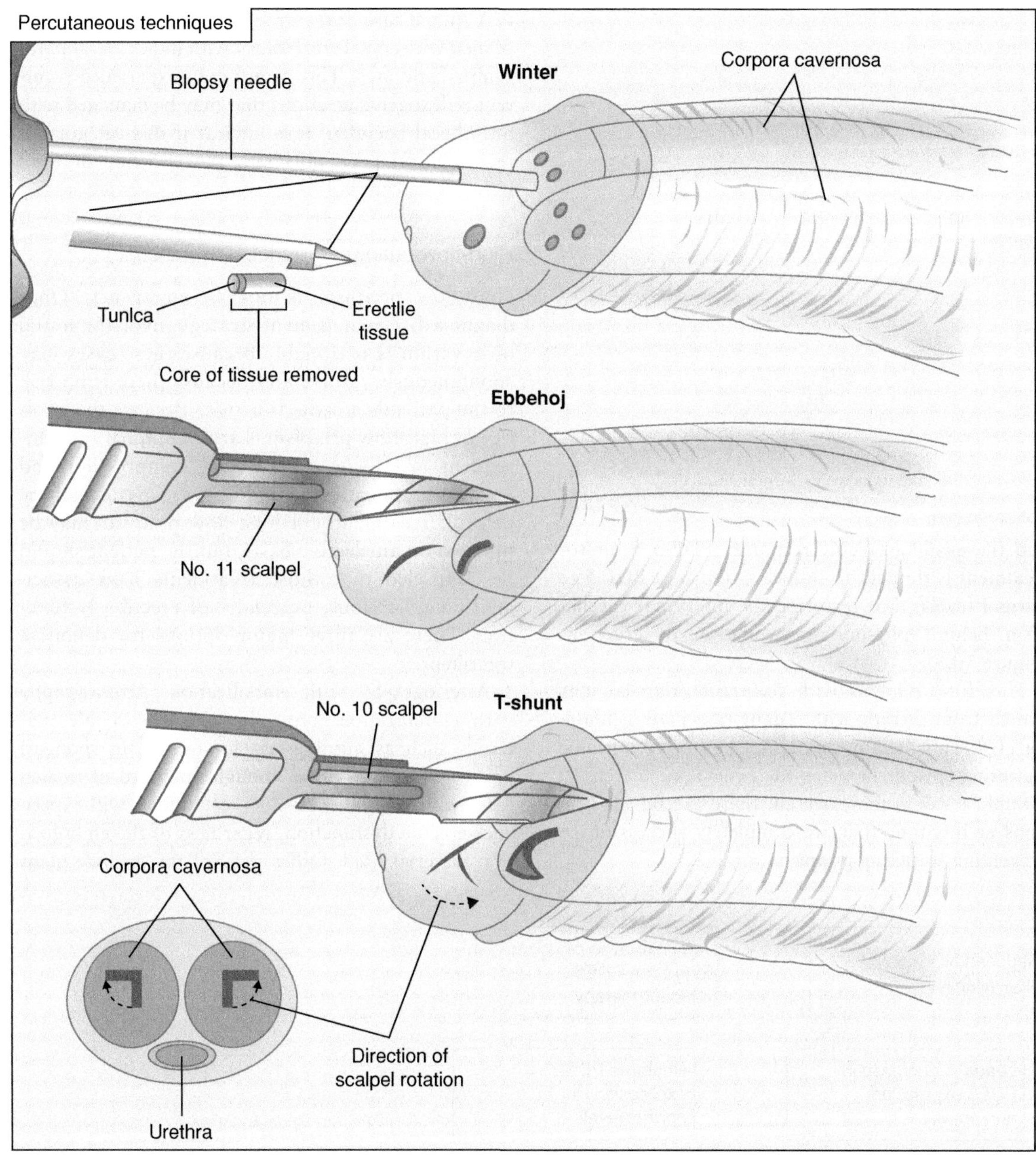

Figure 10.1 Distal percutaneous shunts [6].

events; this technique may be difficult to perform and carries the inherent cardiovascular risks of systemic alpha-agonism. A third strategy is the administration of a daily PDE-5 inhibitor—an initially counterintuitive approach that is mechanism based [9].

The molecular pathology of stuttering and ischemic priapism may be related to a paucity of local NO, and downregulated PDE-5. When a stimulus for erection causes a surge in cGMP, the low levels of PDE-5 cannot sufficiently regulate cGMP

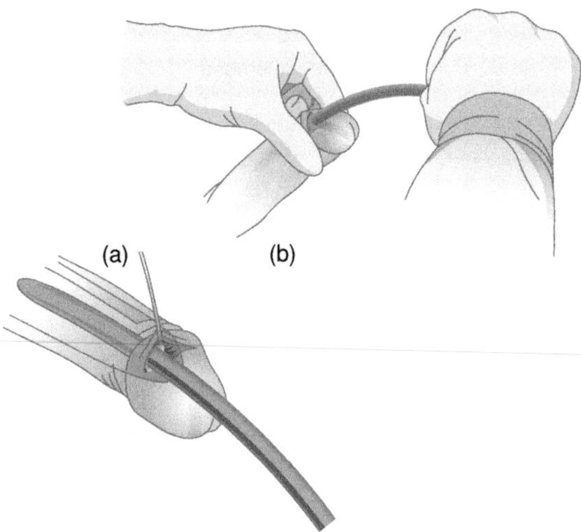

Figure 10.2 Snake maneuver (Burnett shunt) [7].

and the ensuing erectile response. PDE-5 inhibitor treatment is thought to induce a return of PDE-5 to normal levels, thus restoring the molecular mechanism behind physiologic regulation of erections (Figure 10.3).

Therefore, patients with recurrent priapism may benefit from therapy with a daily oral PDE-5 inhibitor [10]. This therapy should not be started during a stuttering episode or when the penis is tumescent. It should be noted that, overall, there are no medications at this time that are completely successful for preventing stuttering priapism.

A special case of recurrent priapism is in the group of men with spinal cord injury with intact sacral parasympathetic arcs. This group may experience recurrent reflexogenic erections that may be managed with intrathecal baclofen. It is unclear if this category of recurrent priapism falls into the ischemic or non-ischemic category.

High-flow priapism (arterial, non-ischemic)

High-flow priapism is not an emergency. Once diagnosed, a management strategy involving initial observation is reasonable because these cases may spontaneously resolve and because there is no risk to the patient's erectile function. Because the etiology of high-flow priapism is arterial injury and consequent arteriocorporal fistula, compression and ice-pack application to induce vasospasm may be helpful. Treatments for high-flow priapism may be pursued on an elective basis, but the patient should be counseled that those treatments have associated complications, especially of erectile dysfunction. There are three major options for definitive treatment.

1 Arteriography with embolization. Arteriography with embolization (typically with absorbable materials such as autologous clot or gelatin sponges) has a 90% success rate, though one-third of treated cases will recur, and 15–20% of patients will experience erectile dysfunction, regardless of the embolization material used. Other risks of this include glans

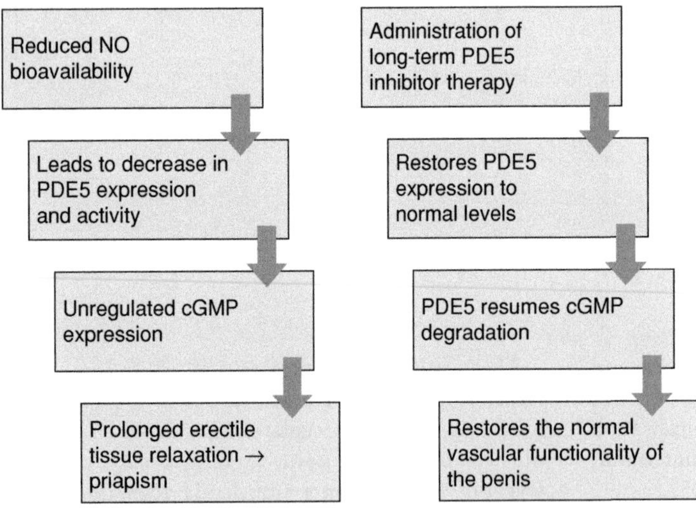

Figure 10.3 Molecular basis of daily PDE-5 inhibitor treatment for prevention of stuttering priapism [9].

necrosis and penile gangrene, gluteal ischemia, and perineal abscess [1, 5].

2 Conservative management. Over time (months to years) the arteriocorporal fistula may mature into a distinct lesion with a pseudocapsule. This can be ligated and excised via an open surgical approach [1].

3 Androgen deprivation. A very small case series demonstrated that 2–6 months of androgen deprivation therapy can potentially successfully treat high-flow priapism [11]. The postulated mechanism is that the resulting hypogonadism suppresses nocturnal erections, thus allowing arteriocorporal fistula to heal rather than repeatedly disrupt.

Implantable penile prostheses

The long-term functional consequence of untreated or unsuccessfully treated ischemic priapism is necrosis and fibrosis of the corpora cavernosa, which in turn results in irreversible erectile dysfunction. A man with erectile dysfunction secondary to priapism may elect to have a surgical placement of a penile prosthesis to restore sexual function. Penile prostheses come in two types. Malleable (two-piece) prostheses are flexible rods implanted into each corporal body that may be bent into an erect position for intercourse. Inflatable (three-piece) prostheses consist of cylindrical balloons that fill with fluid and become rigid when an erection is desired. A fluid-containing reservoir is placed into the space of Retzius adjacent to the bladder, and a pump that allows the man to inflate and deflate the balloon cylinders is placed in a subdartos scrotal pouch. Both types of prostheses can be implanted through a single, small vertical penoscrotal incision.

The main intraoperative complication of prosthesis placement is perforation of the urethra during dilation of the corporal bodies. If this occurs, standard management involves aborting the prosthesis placement, placing a urethral catheter to allow the urethra to heal, and delayed prosthesis placement in several weeks. The primary postoperative complications of penile prosthesis implantation are device infection and distal erosion. Infection may be manifested by purulent drainage, systemic signs and symptoms of infection, or sometimes marked tenderness of the penile shaft. Almost all penile prosthesis infections present within 12 months of implantation. Device infection is treated with urgent explantation and antimicrobial therapy. A new prosthesis may be implanted in several weeks. The rate of device infection is 2% overall, 5% for diabetics, and 10% in the setting of reimplantation for mechanical failure of the original device [12]. The risk of infection has been shown in multiple studies to be lower when the prosthetic cylinders are coated with an antibiotic such as rifampin/minocycline (InhibiZone™) [13].

Recall that rates of spontaneous erectile function (with or without the use of on-demand PDE-5 inhibitors) approach 0% for ischemic priapism episodes >36 hours. For this subgroup of extended ischemic priapism patients (who may have failed aspiration/injection and shunts), some authors have advocated immediate placement of a penile prosthesis [14]. The main benefit of this strategy is that it is thought to prevent the penile shortening that accompanies corporal fibrosis after ischemic priapism events. However, the main risk of this strategy is a higher risk of device infection (6%) and a high revision rate (24%), which some surgeons and patients will find unacceptable.

WHAT TO AVOID/PITFALLS

1 Inadequate history and physical examination can lead to misdiagnosis of priapism (e.g., end-stage ischemic priapism without pain masquerading as stuttering priapism, or inflated penile prosthesis in obtunded patients confused for priapism).

2 Aspiration/injection beyond 1 hour or 1000 mcg phenylephrine unlikely to cause detumescence; therefore make preparations for surgical shunt at that point.

3 Surgical shunts are best attempted in the operating room; bedside procedures are likely to be less effective and cause significant patient discomfort.

KEY WEB LINKS

AUA Clinical Practice Guidelines on Priapism
http://www.auanet.org/content/clinical-practice-guidelines/clinical-guidelines.cfm?sub=priapism

Clinical Trial of Sildenafil for Stuttering Priapism
http://clinicaltrials.gov/ct2/show/NCT00940901

CASE STUDY

A 19-year old African-American man presents to the emergency room complaining of a persistent penile erection that began with intercourse the evening prior. He has been fully rigid for 14 hours, and for the past 8 hours he has also experienced significant pain. His past medical history is notable for sickle cell trait. Throughout his teenage years, he confirms that he has had prolonged erections for several hours despite orgasm and the cessation of intercourse and sexual stimulation—these episodes have become slightly more frequent over time, although they have all resolved by the time he wakes in the morning.

Multiple choice questions

1 What is the most likely diagnosis?
- a Ischemic priapism
- b High-flow priapism
- c Physiologic erection in a young man
- d Stuttering priapism

2 What is this man's chance of spontaneous erections given his duration of symptoms at presentation?
- a 0%
- b 44%
- c 78%
- d 100%

3 After discussion with his urologist, the patient is interested in a medical therapy that will prevent a repeat episode of ischemic priapism. Which option is best for him?
- a Phenylephrine self-injection PRN
- b Oral ephedrine PRN
- c Oral terbutaline PRN
- d Daily sildenafil

References

1 Broderick GA, Kadioglu A, Bivalacqua TJ, Ghanem H, Nehra A, Shamloul R. Priapism: pathogenesis, epidemiology, and management. *J Sex Med* 2010;7(1 Pt 2):476–500.

2 Montague DK, Jarow J, Broderick GA, et al. American urological association guideline on the management of priapism. *J Urol* 2003;170(4 Pt 1):1318–1324.

3 Bella AJ, Lue TF. Colour duplex ultrasound and simplified corporoglanular shunting procedures with and without tunnelling in contemporary management of priapism. *Can Urol Assoc J* 2009;3(4):312–313.

4 Burnett AL, Bivalacqua TJ. Priapism: new concepts in medical and surgical management. *Urol Clin North Am*; 2011;38(2):185–194.

5 Bochinski DJ, Deng DY, Lue TF. The treatment of priapism–when and how? *Int J Impot Res* 2003; 15(Suppl 5):S86–S90.

6 Lue TF, Pescatori ES. Surgical techniques: distal cavernosum–glans shunts for ischemic priapism. *J Sex Med.* 2006;3:749–752. doi: 10.1111/j.1743–6109.2006.00281.x

7 Burnett AL, Pierorazio PM. Corporal "snake" maneuver: corporoglanular shunt surgical modification for ischemic priapism. *J Sex Med.* 2009;6:1171–1176. doi: 10.1111/j.1743-6109.2008.01176.x

8 Burnett AL. Castration for treating recurrent priapism: can we do better? *J Androl* 2012;33(3):291.

9 Levey HR, Kutlu O, Bivalacqua TJ. Medical management of ischemic stuttering priapism: a contemporary review of the literature. *Asian J Androl.* 2012;14(1): 156–163. doi: 10.1038/aja.2011.114. Epub 2011 Nov 7.

10 Pierorazio PM, Bivalacqua TJ, Burnett AL. Daily phosphodiesterase type 5 inhibitor therapy as rescue for recurrent ischemic priapism after failed androgen ablation. *J Androl* 2011;32(4):371–374.

11 Mwamukonda KB, Chi T, Shindel AW, Lue TF. Androgen blockade for the treatment of high-flow priapism. *J Sex Med* 2010;7(7):2532–2537.

12 Abouassaly R, Angermeier KW, Montague DK. Risk of infection with an antibiotic coated penile prosthesis at device replacement for mechanical failure. *J Urol* 2006;176(6 Pt 1):2471–2473.

13 Carson CC. Efficacy of antibiotic impregnation of inflatable penile prostheses in decreasing infection in original implants. *J Urol.* 2004;171(4):1611–1614.

14 Ralph DJ, Garaffa G, Muneer A, et al. The immediate insertion of a penile prosthesis for acute ischaemic priapism. *Eur Urol* 2009;56(6):1033–1038.

Answers to multiple choice questions

1 a This man describes a history of stuttering priapism, which makes him more susceptible to the current episode of ischemic priapism (>4 hours duration). High-flow priapism is unlikely since there is no history or evidence of saddle/sexual trauma and the likelihood of a malignancy-induced arteriovenous fistula at this age is overall low. High-flow priapism

also does not present with pain. Though sickle cell disease is commonly associated with stuttering and ischemic priapism, men with sickle cell trait can present similarly.

The decision to treat him at the bedside with corporal aspiration and phenylephrine injection is made. Informed consent is obtained, he receives antibiotics, and after sterile prep, drape, and anesthetic penile block, his erection is successfully detumesced with aspiration and a single injection of 200 mcg phenylephrine. His continuous cardiac rhythm strip and blood pressures remain normal. The first corporal aspirate blood gas result demonstrates ischemia.

2 c The chance of spontaneous erections (with or without PDE-5 inhibitors) has been reported to be 100% in men with priapism reversed within 12 hours, 78% within 12–24 hours, 44% in 24–36 hours, and 0% after a priapism duration >36 hours.

3 a Though daily sildenafil is used in clinical trials as a potential therapy to restore normal PDE-5 levels in men with stuttering priapism, the only current effective treatment for recurrent ischemic priapism prior to emergent urologic treatments is penile self-injections with phenylephrine. This is generally well tolerated though the patient should be counseled about the potential cardiovascular side effects of systemic phenylephrine absorption.

11 Urinary fistulae

Adam Kern

The James Buchanan Brady Urological Institute and Department of Urology, The Johns Hopkins School of Medicine, Baltimore, MD, USA

KEY POINTS

- Fistulae most commonly result from surgical injury, but may occur any time processes that lead to local tissue degradation are present.
- The tenets of management of fistulae are prevention, early intervention, and optimization of wound healing.
- Vesicovaginal fistulae (VVF) are the most common lower urinary tract fistulae.
- Most VVF encountered in industrialized countries occur as a result of injury accrued during abdominal or pelvic surgery.
- The optimal method of fistula repair depends both on patient factors and surgeon familiarity.

A fistula represents an abnormal connection or communication between two epithelial-lined hollow viscera or between the viscera and the skin. Fistulae may be formed by a variety of congenital processes, infection, malignancy, or may be caused by iatrogenic injury. Owing to the fact that the urinary tract is composed of epithelial-lined hollow viscera, fistulae may form between almost any genitourinary structure and other organs, given the proper conditions. The range of clinical presentations of fistulae is widely variable and depends in part on the physiologic impact of the fistula on the genitourinary function. In turn, the ideal treatments for fistulae depend on the exact location, etiology, and acuity of the fistula. Because many fistulae form in the setting of poor wound healing, both the prevention and correction of fistulae depend on addressing comorbid conditions that may have contributed to fistula formation, including malnutrition, malignancy, infection, poorly controlled diabetes, and ischemia.

The hallmarks of management of urinary tract fistula are prevention, early intervention to control urinary leakage, and optimization of nutritional and other factors to promote wound healing. Because of the discomfort and inconvenience associated with urinary fistulae, immediate control of urine leakage at the time of diagnosis, at least through supportive measures such as application of absorbent pads and meticulous skin hygiene, may significantly alleviate patient suffering. These maneuvers may also arrest further fistulous maturation and progression and prevent serious infectious complications.

Vesicovaginal fistulae

Vesicovaginal fistulae (VVF) are the most common acquired fistulae of the urinary tract [1]. The first records of surgical repair of VVF in the Western world date to the 1660s, but it was not until John Mettaur's successful closure of a VVF in 1838 that a durable technique of repair was reported in the United States. The famous North American surgeon James Marion Sims modernized the repair of VVF and became the

Handbook of Urology, First edition. J. Kellogg Parsons, John B. Eifler and Misop Han.
Published 2014 by John Wiley & Sons, Ltd.

father of the nascent field of urogynecology after the publication of a successful series of transvaginal VVF repairs using silver wire in 1852 [2]. However, Sims remained a controversial figure owing to his use of slaves as his surgical subjects amid unresolved questions about their willing participation and informed consent [3, 4]. Thirty years later Trendelenburg published the first series on transabdominal repair of VVF, and Martius described the labial fat pad interpositional flap in 1928.

The etiology of VVF differs greatly between those commonly encountered in the developing world versus those in industrialized nations. VVF seen in the United States are overwhelmingly the result of iatrogenic injury during pelvic surgery, frequently hysterectomy [5]. Abdominal hysterectomy seems to carry the highest risk, with the rate of VVF formation following the procedure estimated to be between 0.5% and 1% [6, 7]. The aggregate prevalence of VVF following hysterectomy in all approaches is estimated between 0.1% and 0.2% [8]. Post-hysterectomy VVF almost always result from occult cystotomy near the bladder cuff [9]. Obstetric trauma is an uncommon cause of VVF in the developed world. In contrast, lack of adequate perinatal care is a major public health problem in developing nations and obstructed labor remains a significant cause of VVF in these settings. Because these fistulae form as a result of prolonged abruption of the fetal head against the anterior vaginal wall, obstetric fistulae tend to be larger and are located distally in the vagina. Obstetric fistulae are also associated with other injuries to the lower urinary tract that may occur as a result of labor, such as urethral damage, urinary sphincter dysfunction, and neurologic deficit. In Sub-Saharan Africa, the rate of VVF after vaginal delivery is estimated to be as high as 10.3 per 100,000 deliveries [10].

Most urinary fistulae seen in developed countries initially present with symptoms of frequent or constant urinary drainage 1–2 weeks after a pelvic or abdominal surgical procedure or instrumentation. The degree of urinary leakage may be highly variable and ranges from constant dribbling to intermittent leakage which is dependent on bladder fullness and patient position. Exceptions to the above are fistulae stemming from radiation injury, which usually present after a delay of many years. Pain is an uncommon finding with VVF.

The initial evaluation of VVF focuses on ruling out other causes of urinary leakage, such as stress or urge incontinence, and on proving the existence of a fistulous tract. Physical examination, including pelvic examination with speculum, is critical in determining fistula location and size. Special note should be taken of the location of the fistula within the vagina to determine the feasibility of transvaginal repair. A starting point when looking for iatrogenic fistulae is to look at the vaginal cuff, where most fistulae are located. The quality of the tissue surrounding the fistula should also be noted in order to inform the timing of repair. The urethra should also be inspected, and a urinalysis and urine culture should be obtained.

Some fistulae are difficult to identify and in these instances additional diagnostic maneuvers are helpful. Occult or complex fistulae can be evaluated with cystoscopy. Cystoscopic examination can identify intravesical signs of inflammation, scarring, or malignancy. Furthermore, a pediatric catheter may be passed through the fistula from the vaginal aspect and visualized within the bladder, giving the surgeon a more accurate understanding of the geometry of the tract. This technique also identifies the proximity to the trigone, which will allow planning for ureteroneocystostomy, if needed at the time of reconstruction. A "double dye" test may also be performed to identify the position of a VVF. In this test, the vagina is packed with several pieces of moist white gauze that will stain with leaking dye from the fistula tract. Alternatively, a tampon may be used. The bladder is then instilled with a dye and another agent is given either IV or PO to color the urine filtered by the kidneys. Different regimes using carmine dyes or phenazopyridine and methylene blue have been described. In one routine, a red carmine dye is instilled into the bladder and indigo carmine is administered IV. The vaginal packing is then examined. A red-colored stain on the packing from the mid-vaginal or upper-forniceal packing is suggestive of VVF. A blue stain is suspicious for a ureterovaginal fistula, whereas red staining only at the distal packing near the vaginal opening is consistent with urethral leakage. In an alternative system, methylene blue is instilled into the bladder and oral phenazopyridine is administered. An orange stain suggests a ureterovaginal fistula, whereas blue staining indicates either VVF or urethral leakage.

Radiographic evaluation is also used in conjunction with cystoscopy and physical examination to identify and characterize VVF. Because concomitant ureteral injury is seen in 10–15% of cases of VVF [11], imaging of the upper tracts is an important component of the VVF workup. IVP or CT urogram is usually capable of identifying ureterovaginal fistulae. Endoscopic retrograde pyelography is also employed when CT urography is nondiagnostic or when the VVF is known to be in very close proximity to the ureter. Imaging of the bladder is best undertaken by performing a voiding cystourethrogram (VCUG). This study has the ability to evaluate for multiple fistulae, and to identify small fistulae where leakage is only provoked by detrusor contraction during the voiding phase. Evaluation with VCUG gives the additional benefit of assessing bladder capacity, which will aid preoperative planning. Cross-sectional imaging is often of less value in the workup unless malignancy or other pelvic pathology is present. Likewise, urodynamic studies are not routinely needed unless the history and physical examination suggest coexistent stress incontinence or detrusor instability.

Catheter drainage of the bladder is the initial management of VVF. Almost all patients will benefit from immediate catheter drainage early after injury is recognized because urinary leakage will be diminished and further maturation of the tract may be slowed. Very small fistulae may resolve with catheter drainage alone, as total urine diversion away from the tract will allow it to heal. Patients will also significantly benefit from the symptomatic relief of total urinary incontinence. An initial strategy is a trial of 4–6 weeks of catheter drainage with subsequent reevaluation of the patency of the tract. However, if urinary leakage does not stop after insertion of the catheter, the fistula is likely too large to ever heal with this conservative approach. Providers should also proactively manage bothersome secondary complications of chronic Foley catheter use such as bladder spasm to maximize patient comfort. Adjuvant usage of fulguration of the fistula tract may be combined with catheter drainage for small fistulae. The epithelium lining the tract is fulgurated with a Bugbee electrode or similar device, allowing healing and eventual reapproximation along the tract. However, this strategy can backfire if high electrocautery currents are used, as surrounding tissue becomes devitalized and the size of the fistula may actually increase. Careful selection only of small fistulae and application of meticulous technique are essential to the success of this procedure.

Larger or more complex fistulae are managed surgically. Contemporary understanding of the timing of fistula repair has evolved since the early 1900s. Traditionally, surgical repair was delayed many months. The rationale was that this allowed maximal resolution of surrounding inflammation and maturation of the tract that would aid visual identification at the time of surgery. However, this approach left patients having to deal with bothersome problems of incontinence for long periods of time, and ultimately has not been shown to significantly increase surgical success rates in modern series. Indeed, early repair of VVF has success rates that approach 90–100% in a variety of transabdominal or transvaginal modalities. The timing of surgical repair is a decision customized for each patient, based on the anticipated surgical strategy and adequate resolution of local edema and necrosis.

Likewise, the choice of surgical approach is also customized to each individual situation and based both on clinical factors and surgeon familiarity. Controversy exists as to the superiority of transabdominal versus transvaginal approaches. Highly complex fistulae may be most amenable to transabdominal repair given the maximal exposure and ability to employ omental interpositional flaps. However, the vast majority of fistulae may not require such extensive dissection and are best treated with less-invasive transvaginal techniques that minimize perioperative patient morbidity and speed recovery time. Factors to consider are whether repair of the tract will require ureteral reimplantation or bladder augmentation, desire to minimize the possibility of vaginal shortening, the location of the tract, and the general quality of surrounding tissues. Most transvaginal techniques only require patients to be hospitalized for 1–2 nights and are often associated with less overall catheter time. The primary risk of transvaginal repair is insufficient closure of the fistula or vaginal foreshortening or stenosis. In either general approach, certain surgical tenets should be adhered to, namely adequate debridement of devitalized tissues, watertight closure in multiple layers using a tension-free repair and complete postoperative urinary catheter drainage to allow the defect to heal.

The transvaginal repair technique usually involves placing the patient in lithotomy position and obtaining exposure with either a weighted speculum or a Brantley Scott (a.k.a. Lone Star) retractor. The distal aspect of the fistula is then isolated and mobilized and then closed by the creation and folding of vaginal flaps. Inverting sutures are placed into the tract in multiple layers before positioning the vaginal flap over the defect. Optionally, an additional soft tissue flap such as a vascularized Martius fat pad may be rotated over the defect to provide additional coverage.

A partial colpocleisis (a.k.a. Latzko procedure) is one popular option for transvaginal repair of fistulae located right at the cuff of the vagina. In the Latzko repair, a portion of the vaginal epithelium is denuded from the cuff across an area that traverses both the anterior and the posterior vagina. The denuded area is then plicated onto itself over the vaginal cuff in layers, encompassing the area of the fistula, and the mucosa is then closed over the top of the repair. Latzko repair is an attractive option when a minimal transvaginal approach is desired and the location of the fistula is known and the size of the defect is small. However, the potential risk of the technique is that plication of the cuff will lead to shortening of the vaginal canal and negatively impact sexual function.

The traditional open abdominal repair begins by bivalving the bladder along the midline to approach the fistula from above. The proximal tract is then isolated and mobilized, and then closed. A careful examination of the bladder and ureters is also done at this time to identify any other occult fistulae or other injury. Bladder flaps are then formed and used to close the fistula in layers, and omental flaps may also be applied for maximal coverage. The bladder is then closed in layers.

Ureterovaginal fistulae

Ureterovaginal fistulae, similarly to VVF, are most often caused by injury during pelvic or abdominal surgery. Ureteral injuries during abdominal hysterectomy or other major gynecologic surgery are especially common in the distal one-third of the ureter, and it is these injuries that can lead to ureterovaginal fistula formation. Additionally, other factors such as prior radiation exposure diminish the quality of surrounding tissues and predispose toward ureteral fistulae. While ureterovaginal fistulae often present with continuous dribbling of urine similar to VVF, patients with ureteral fistulae may also develop ipsilateral ureteral obstruction, and hydroureteronephrosis or even flank pain may be apparent.

The evaluation and diagnosis of ureterovaginal fistulae is similar to that undertaken of the upper tracts during the workup of VVF. Intravenous pyelography, CT urogram, or retrograde pyelography can identify extravasation from the ureter and localize the level of the defect. Retrograde pyelography may also be therapeutic, as a ureteral stent can be placed at the time of the study to at least temporize the injury. Cystoscopy performed at the same time as retrograde pyelography allows visual inspection of the trigone for occult injury. Finally, a filling cystogram, or ideally a VCUG, assists with the estimation of bladder capacity for surgical planning and identifies any vesicoureteral reflux that may be present. Cross-sectional imaging is useful as a diagnostic adjunct when the patient displays clinical signs of complex UTI or pyelonephritis. CT can identify perinephric and periureteral collections and also identify radiographic signs of renal parenchymal compromise consistent with pyelonephritis. A notable difference between ureterovaginal fistulae and VVF is that in the former, patients will still report normal voiding habits because the contralateral kidney continues to fill the bladder with urine. This stands in contradistinction to VVF, which usually prevents the bladder from filling to large volumes. A careful history may elicit these signs and guide early diagnostic workup. The "double dye" test can also be used to differentiate VVF from ureteral fistulae.

As with VVF, the initial management of ureteral fistulae is diversion of urine away from the fistulous tract. This is most easily achieved by placing a ureteral stent across the defect. Percutaneous nephrostomy tubes can also be placed for maximal urinary drainage. Small defects may resolve with conservative management alone if the urine is diverted from the tract for a period of 4–8 weeks [12]. If conservative management is insufficient, open surgical repair is required. Because the majority of ureterovaginal fistulae occur at the most distal portion of the ureter, repair usually involves ureteroneocystostomy and ureteral reimplantation. It is not necessary to excise the distal ureteral stump distal to the defect unless significant vesicoureteral reflux is present. If a defect involves a large portion of the ureter or other pathology is involved, it may be necessary to excise a portion of the ureter and mobilize tissues to effect a repair similar to the approach in trauma. If short lengths of additional ureter are required to allow reimplantation, a psoas hitch or Boari flap may be employed. Alternatively, the rare large distal ureterovaginal fistula may require reconstruction with transureteroureterostomy, ileal ureter formation, or renal autotransplantation.

Urethrovaginal fistulae

Urethrovaginal fistulae, like other genitourinary fistulae involving the vagina, are most commonly seen in the setting of surgical trauma, particularly vaginal or urethral reconstructive surgeries. However, many urethrovaginal fistulae may be initially asymptomatic if located distally because continent control is maintained over the portion of urethra where the fistula branches. Vague symptoms such as dyspareunia or sporadic incontinence can be the presenting signs. The diagnosis is made by VCUG and cystoscopy. Complex urethrovesicovaginal fistulae are sometimes seen in instances of obstructed labor resulting in wide areas of tissue necrosis.

Conservative management of urethrovaginal fistulae is possible if symptoms are minimal and there is no significant ongoing local necrotic or inflammatory process. When operative intervention is required, techniques similar to those employed in VVF and urethral trauma repair are utilized. The fistula is isolated and mobilized and local flaps are then reflected over the defect. Additional vascularized adjuvant interpositional flaps or grafts similar to those used in VVF repair may be optionally used. Several weeks of postoperative Foley catheter drainage ensure adequate healing of the repair.

Uroenteric fistulae

Enterovesical fistulas usually result from complications of bowel disease including inflammatory bowel disease, Crohn's disease, diverticulitis, and malignancy. Diverticulitis was the most common cause of enterovesical fistula in some small contemporary series [13]. However, enterovesical fistulae secondary to trauma or urologic instrumentation may also occur.

Many enterovesical fistulae are clinically silent, but when symptomatic, they most often manifest with urinary symptoms, including pneumaturia (air in the urine), fecaluria (fecal material in the urine), and recurrent urinary infections. The fistula can then be confirmed with either visual or radiographic means. A charcoal test may be used where the patient ingests activated charcoal and the urine is analyzed for the presence of charcoal in the voided urine. A potentially easier, cheaper, and more effective test is the "poppy seed test," where the patient ingests poppy seeds and the urine is studied to see if any seeds are present in the voided specimen. One group reported a 100% diagnostic success rate using the poppy seed test, at a cost 100× lower than competing modalities [14]. Cystoscopy also has a high success rate in identifying uroenteric fistulae and allows for simultaneous biopsy if malignancy or other pathology is suspected. Radiographic workup can be performed using a combination of barium enemas, VCUG, or CT. Any air or contrast tracking between the urinary and digestive viscera is indicative of a fistula.

Conservative treatment of enterovesical fistulae can be initially attempted, given that many of these fistulae are clinically silent. Symptomatic fistulae that are shown to be small and noncomplex on examination may respond to prolonged bowel rest facilitated by parenteral nutrition supplementation. Any underlying contributing factors such as malignancy or inflammatory disease should also be addressed at this time. Refractory cases can be repaired surgically, although these procedures are often extensive and benefit from a team approach between genitourinary and gastrointestinal surgeons. Fecal and/or urinary diversion may be required along with intra-abdominal reconstruction using transposition of omental flaps.

WHAT TO AVOID/PITFALLS

- New onset incontinence should not be automatically attributed to a urinary fistula even in the setting of recent surgery. Appropriate workup for detrusor instability, urinary sphincter deficiency, etc. is still required.
- Prevention is the best strategy for managing iatrogenic fistulae.
- Up to 12% of iatrogenic VVF have an associated ureteral injury.
- Often the best modality of surgical management of urinary fistulae is dependent on surgeon comfort and familiarity.
- Most large fistulae will not heal unless local wound care and nutritional status are optimized.

GUIDELINES AND WEB LINKS

1 *Living With Obstetric Fistula.* G Esegbona.BMJ 2011;342:d2881
2 www.endfistula.org
3 http://www.isofs.org/wp-content/uploads/2011/04/report_2010_000_full_report_LR.pdf

CASE STUDY

A 48-year-old woman undergoes a laparoscopic abdominal hysterectomy and develops vaginal leakage of urine 7 days after surgery. She has no prior history of abdominal or pelvic radiation.

Multiple choice questions

1 The first step in management of the patient should be:
- a Reexploration of the surgical bed
- b Placement of percutaneous nephrostomy tubes
- c Optimization of nutritional status
- d VCUG
- e Foley catheter placement

2 Two weeks later the patient continues to complain of urinary leakage. The best first diagnostic test to perform is:
- a Retrograde urethrogram
- b Double dye test
- c Cystoscopy
- d VCUG
- e Pelvic CT scan

3 A ureterovaginal fistula is identified 2–3 cm above the bladder. Endoscopic attempts to pass a ureteral stent in both retrograde and antegrade fashions fail. The best next step is:
- a Percutaneous nephrostomy placement
- b Ureteroneocystostomy with psoas hitch
- c Transureteroureterostomy
- d Ileal ureter
- e Renal autotransplantation

References

1 Gerber GS, Schoenberg HW. Female urinary tract fistulas. *J Urol* 1993;149(2):229–236.
2 Sims JM. On the treatment of vesico-vaginal fistula. 1852. *Int Urogynecol J Pelvic Floor Dysfunct* 1998;9(4):236–248.
3 Sartin JS. J. Marion Sims, the father of gynecology: hero or villain? *South Med J* 2004;97(5):500–505.
4 Spettel S, White MD. The portrayal of J. Marion Sims' controversial surgical legacy. *J Urol* 2011;185(6): 2424–2427. doi:10.1016/j.juro.2011.01.077
5 Tancer ML. Observations on prevention and management of vesicovaginal fistula after total hysterectomy. *Surg Gynecol Obstet* 1992;175(6):501–506.
6 Eilber KS, Kavaler E, Rodríguez LV, Rosenblum N, Raz S. Ten-year experience with transvaginal vesicovaginal fistula repair using tissue interposition. *J Urol* 2003;169(3):1033–1036. doi:10.1097/01.ju.0000049723.57485.e7
7 Keettel WC, Sehring FG, deProsse CA, Scott JR. (1978). Surgical management of urethrovaginal and vesicovaginal fistulas. *Am J Obstet Gynecol* 1978;131(4):425–431.
8 Harris WJ. Early complications of abdominal and vaginal hysterectomy. *Obstet Gynecol Surv* 1995;50(11): 795–805.
9 Kursh ED, Morse RM, Resnick MI, Persky L. Prevention of the development of a vesicovaginal fistula. *Surg Gynecol Obstet* 1988;166(5):409–412.
10 Vangeenderhuysen C, Prual A, Ould el Joud D. Obstetric fistulae: incidence estimates for sub-Saharan Africa. *Int J Gynaecol Obstet* 2001;73(1):65–66.
11 Goodwin WE, Scardino PT. Vesicovaginal and ureterovaginal fistulas: a summary of 25 years of experience. *J Urol* 1980;123(3):370–374.
12 Selzman AA, Spirnak JP, Kursh ED. The changing management of ureterovaginal fistulas. *J Urol* 1995;153 (3 Pt 1):626–628.
13 Najjar SF, Jamal MK, Savas JF, Miller TA. The spectrum of colovesical fistula and diagnostic paradigm. *Am J Surg* 2004;188(5):617–621. doi:10.1016/j.amjsurg.2004.08.016
14 Kwon EO, Armenakas NA, Scharf SC, Panagopoulos G, Fracchia JA. The poppy seed test for colovesical fistula: big bang, little bucks! *J Urol* 2008;179(4):1425–1427. doi:10.1016/j.juro.2007.11.085

Answers to multiple choice questions

1 c Optimization of nutritional status to promote wound healing is a cardinal principle of the management of urinary fistulae and should be started in the early phase of care. A VCUG is highly useful in the diagnostic workup, as it can potentially identify and localize vesicovaginal, ureterovaginal, and vesicoureteral fistulae and also characterize bladder capacity and identify other occult bladder injury and vesicoureteral reflux. However, the first step in management after a clinical diagnosis of incontinent urinary fistula is made is Foley catheter placement. The Foley catheter will keep the patient dry and also may lead to spontaneous closure of small fistulae. Immediate reexploration or percutaneous urinary diversion is not indicated.

2 a A retrograde urethrogram is unlikely to identify the source of leakage given the history. Cystoscopy, VCUG, and CT scan are all useful adjuncts in the advanced diagnostic workup. An easy and rapid initial test that can be performed in the office is the double dye test. Methylene blue dye solution is instilled into the bladder and the patient is given a dose of oral phenazopyridine. Extravasation of blue dye onto the vaginal packing suggests a VVF, whereas leakage of orange dye indicates a ureterovaginal fistula.

3 b Planning for surgical repair of ureterovaginal fistulae involves considerations similar to repair of traumatic injury. The type of ureteral reconstruction is dependent on the location and size of the ureteral defect. Ureterovaginal fistulae 2–3 cm above the bladder can be corrected by ureteral reimplantation. It is not necessary to resect the distal ureteral stump unless vesicoureteral reflux is present.

12 Urethral stricture disease

Debasish Sundi and Arthur L. Burnett

The James Buchanan Brady Urological Institute and Department of Urology, The Johns Hopkins School of Medicine, Baltimore MD, USA

KEY POINTS

- Urethral strictures are most commonly traumatic in etiology.
- Direct vision internal urethrotomy (DVIU) is not a durable treatment for urethral strictures.
- The extent of urethral strictures can be assessed preoperatively by retrograde urethrogram (RUG) or voiding cystourethrogram (VCUG)–RUG when there is also an indwelling suprapubic (SP) tube.
- Strictures ≤2 cm are amenable to scar excision, urethral spatulation, and primary anastomosis.
- Strictures >2 cm typically require additional tissue mobilization or substitution urethroplasty with buccal graft or non–hair-bearing skin flap.

Etiology and pathogenesis

In a large single-surgeon series, 53% of urethral strictures were secondary to trauma [1]. The most common type of injury is a saddle trauma event. Forty percent of cases had no known cause and are inclusive of iatrogenic, infectious, and inflammatory conditions such as urethral instrumentation, chlamydia, gonorrhea, and lichen sclerosus–balanitis xerotica obliterans (LS–BXO). A history of hypospadias was found in 7% of strictures. Another cause of strictures is radiation (e.g., pelvic external beam or brachytherapy for prostate cancer) [2].

Iatrogenic strictures have become less common with the development of smaller caliber cystoscopes and more less frequent indications for cystoscopy in boys [3]. Urethritis-related strictures (secondary to gonorrhea and chlamydia) have also become less common over time [4]. Reiter's syndrome remains a rare cause of urethral stricture disease. LS–BXO is an idiopathic inflammatory process of the glans penis that may cause meatal stenosis. This is commonly associated with diffuse urethral stricture disease. The exact relationship is unknown but one hypothesis is that distal urethral obstruction from meatal stenosis causes high pressure voiding and urine intravasation into the paraurethral glands of Littre, which could result in chronic peri-urethral injury and inflammation.

The primary insult (trauma, infection, and ischemia) ultimately leads to an inflammation response and subsequent fibrosis of the urethra and its investing spongy tissue, the corpus spongiosum. The length of this fibrosis determines the appropriate treatment.

Diagnosis

The predominant symptom of a significant urethral stricture is progressive obstructive voiding. Less commonly, the patient presents with irritative voiding symptoms, prostatitis, epididymitis, or painful ejaculation. The patient with a urethral stricture may even be in urinary retention and attempts at urethral catheterization will likely be unsuccessful. The next step is urethroscopy

Handbook of Urology, First edition. J. Kellogg Parsons, John B. Eifler and Misop Han.
Published 2014 by John Wiley & Sons, Ltd.

(such as with a flexible cystoscope) to visualize the stricture. Though it may be tempting to use serial dilators to widen the stricture in order to pass a catheter over a wire, this practice is discouraged for two reasons. First, it may ultimately result in more extensive urethral scar. Second, it will disrupt the anatomy of the stricture, making diagnostic urethrography difficult to interpret. Therefore, the preferred method for bladder drainage in the setting of urinary retention secondary to a stricture is the placement of a suprapubic tube.

The study of choice to delineate the length of a urethral stricture is a retrograde urethrogram (RUG). This is a fluoroscopic study with the patient in a relatively steep lateral oblique position and his penis on gentle stretch. Radiopaque contrast is injected retrograde into the urethra via either an angiocath or a 12F Foley catheter inserted into the tip of the penis with 1–2 mL inflated in the balloon to prevent the catheter from slipping out. If a suprapubic tube is present, contrast can also be instilled into the bladder; the patient is asked to void during the RUG. This antegrade voiding cystourethrogram (VCUG) in concert with the RUG is a combined VCUG–RUG; it is sometimes referred to an "up-and-down" study. Alternatively, if a mature suprapubic tract is present, then a flexible cystoscope can be placed antegrade into the bladder neck to the proximal-most aspect of the stricture. This is an alternative to the VCUG–RUG to study the stricture length in simultaneous antegrade and retrograde fashion.

Ultrasound is a less-commonly used alternative or adjunct technique to study urethral stricture length [5]. Some authors propose that ultrasound is preferred since it may also assess the extent of spongiofibrosis and stricture depth. If narrowing of the urethra is suspected to be a malignancy based on the history and urethroscopy, transurethral biopsy in indicated, and MRI may be considered as an additional imaging modality.

Conservative treatments and temporizing measures

There are three conservative treatment options for urethral stricture disease. (1) Urethral dilation with or without subsequent self-catheterization (periodic urethral "calibration"). (2) DVIU with or without subsequent periodic self-catheterization. (3) The placement of an endoprosthesis (UroLume® stent) across the stricture. Dilation may be achieved in serial fashion using filiforms and followers, fascial (Amplatz®) dilators over a stiff guidewire, sounds, or urethral balloon-dilating catheters. The idea is to stretch the scar but not injure and rip it (as evidenced by postdilation bleeding). Traumatic stricture dilation will likely lead to rapid scar recurrence, leading perhaps to a worse stricture than before the dilation.

DVIU (endoscopic cold knife or laser) is often used to treat strictures. The patient should be counseled that this maneuver can cause longer, denser strictures subsequently and may require periodic self-catheterization (urethral calibration) on a tapering schedule for several weeks after the procedure. This technique is less durable and may have to be repeated over time (as often as once every several months). Overall reported success rates of DVIU vary widely from 20% to 74%. Other data are more sobering, with published 5-year stricture-free rates as low as 5–7%. In a 15-year retrospective study of 76 patients who underwent DVIU, the stricture-free rate was only 8% (median time to recurrence 7 months, mean overall follow-up 18 months) [6]. Subsequent DVIU operations were associated with even lower success rates.

A third option is the placement of a UroLume® stent for strictures in the bulbar urethra [7]. This option is seldom employed due to many stent-related complications that may require a lifetime of endoscopic maintenance procedures. If the stent is placed or migrates distal to the bulbar urethra, the patient may experience significant pain during sitting or intercourse. Overlapping stents placed for longer strictures may migrate away from each other and lead to the need to place a third, intervening stent across the gap. The stents often epithelialize and may obstruct when this process is hypertrophic. The stent is also a nidus for (potentially obstructing) stones and is a risk factor for urinary tract infection. Another risk, especially if the stent is placed over the external rhabdosphincter, is incontinence that may require implantation of an artificial urinary sphincter (AUS). If stent-associated complications are significant, unfortunately the UroLume® is often exceedingly difficult to remove using endoscopic methods. However, successful open removal and concomitant urethroplasty through a perineal approach has been described [8]. The UroLume® is contraindicated in patients with pelvic fracture urethral distraction injuries and for recurrent strictures in an area of prior urethroplasty with skin flap substitution. These stents are also less successful in the setting of deep spongiofibrosis, often associated with saddle perineal trauma.

Definitive management

The most successful treatment for urethral stricture disease is stricture excision and urethroplasty [3]. The entire scar must be excised. Defects of ≤2 cm are typically repaired by spatulation of the proximal and distal urethral ends and primary anastomosis. Defects >2 cm may also be closed primarily if the tissue is compliant enough or with additional mobilization of the proximal urethra. The problems associated with primary anastomotic urethroplasty with larger defects include excessive tension on the anastomosis, foreshortening of the penis, and creation of a penile chordee. Traditionally, when the urethral defect after stricture excision is >2 cm, the technique of choice is substitution urethroplasty, using either a graft or flap interposed between the proximal and distal urethral segments. A graft or flap may be applied to the ventral, dorsal, or lateral urethra. The most commonly used graft is derived from the buccal mucosa. Other grafts include split- and full-thickness skin grafts, bladder epithelium, and rectal mucosa. Skin flaps may be transposed on a vascular pedicle to bridge the urethral defect. It is essential that the skin flap be derived from a patch of hairless skin. Hair-bearing skin grafts can cause voiding irritation, recurrent infections, voiding obstruction, and serve as a nidus for stones. A variation of the skin flap, for very long anterior urethral strictures, is the Quartey flap [9]. This involves harvesting an island of penile and preputial skin derived from the axial blood supply of the superficial external pudendal artery. It may be used as a patch or a rolled tube for urethral substitution.

Urethroplasty is typically performed with a perineal approach, with the patient positioned in high or exaggerated dorsal lithotomy [4]. It is beneficial to minimize time in this position, pad the lower extremities with care, and use sequential compression devices; because prolonged dorsal lithotomy carries risks of rhabdomyolysis and compartment syndrome [10]. Complex or very long urethral strictures that are not amenable to repair with a single operation may be treated by a strategy of staged urethroplasty. In the first stage, a urethrostomy is created at the perineum or ventral penile shaft. In the second stage, the urethroplasty is completed by urethral tubularization distal to the prior urethrostomy. In one retrospective study of 38 men who underwent first-stage urethroplasty, the success rate (requiring no further procedures) was 84%, and only 24% was elected to proceed with the second stage, indicating that a perineal or penile urethrostomy results in satisfactory voiding function and quality of life in most cases [11].

Postoperatively, patients are maintained on culture-specific or prophylactic antibiotics until the urethral catheter is removed. Patient status after graft substitution urethroplasty will require 48–72 hours of bed rest to allow graft imbibition and therefore also require venous thrombus prophylaxis with subcutaneous heparin injections in addition to compression stockings and pneumatic compression boots. About 2–3 weeks after the urethroplasty, a RUG and/or VCUG is performed with the urethral catheter *in situ*. If this peri-catheter RUG demonstrates a widely patent urethra with no extravasation at the site or urethroplasty, the urethral catheter may be removed. If a suprapubic tube is in place, this is capped and removed a few days later if the patient has no subsequent voiding difficulty. Scheduled follow-up with RUGs at 3 and 12 months postoperatively may be appropriate, with further interventions such as a urinary flow rate undertaken as needed if symptoms develop.

In a single-surgeon series of 495 patients who had undergone urethroplasty, a multivariate analysis showed that smoking, prior DVIU, and prior urethroplasty were predictors of failure (defined as urine flow rate <15 cm/s or the need for subsequent DVIU or revision urethroplasty) [1]. The studied population included anterior or posterior urethroplasties performed by a primary anastomotic approach or with graft or flap substitution. In this series, the 5-year rate of stricture-free survival was 79%. Consistent with this finding, a prior study of 51 patients who had undergone anastomotic urethroplasty for posttraumatic urethral stricture found that the 1-year rate of a satisfactory result was 90% in men who had not undergone prior urethral manipulation such as endoscopic realignment, DVIU, or urethroplasty, but only 60% in those men who did have prior urethral manipulation [12]. In this series, the 5-year rate of stricture-free survival was 55%.

As discussed previously, urethral strictures may also be sequelae of radiation therapy. The incidence of urethral strictures in men who have undergone either pelvic external beam radiation therapy or brachytherapy for prostate cancer is approximately

2% [13]. Urethroplasty is a feasible treatment option for radiation-induced strictures as well. In a multi-institutional retrospective study of 30 men who underwent urethroplasty for radiation-induced strictures, the stricture-free rate was 73% at a 21-month median follow-up, with the main side effect being new-onset urinary incontinence, which effected 50% of men [2].

A major side effect of urethroplasty is erectile dysfunction. This has been prospectively studied at one center. In a single-surgeon series analyzing 52 men, erectile dysfunction (defined as a 5 point or greater decrease in the international index of erectile function (IIEF)) occurred in 38% of men, with a slightly higher rate in men undergoing bulbar versus penile urethroplasty [14]. By a mean of 190 days, IIEF scores returned to baseline in 90% of the men who experienced postoperative erectile dysfunction. Interestingly, the subgroup that did not experience a statistically significant decrease in IIEF was the group of men undergoing substitution urethroplasty for bulbar strictures. However, it should be noted that many men with urethral stricture disease have significant erectile dysfunction even before urethroplasty, which may be related to prior trauma and pelvic fractures. In a small series of men with posterior urethral strictures secondary to pelvic fractures, the rate of preoperative erectile dysfunction (negative nocturnal "Rigiscan" tumescence test) was 72%. Cavernosal arterial duplex ultrasonography of these men was abnormal in 28%, indicating a probable neurogenic etiology in 72% of the men with preoperative erectile dysfunction [15]. Some authors recommend that men with arteriogenic erectile dysfunction should undergo arteriography and penile revascularization prior to urethroplasty in order to avoid urethral ischemia, necrosis, and recurrent stricture [15].

WHAT TO AVOID/PITFALLS

- Strictures or dilations that result in tearing/bleeding rather than gentle stretching may cause even more severe recurrent strictures.
- During urethroplasty, the lower extremities must be well-padded, carefully positioned, and periodically lowered during long surgeries, to avoid rhabdomyolysis and compartment syndrome.
- Patients undergoing urethroplasty must be counseled regarding the risk of erectile dysfunction.

KEY WEB LINKS

AUA Foundation urethral stricture
http://www.urologyhealth.org/urology/index.cfm?article=66

CASE STUDY

A 34-year-old man presents to the clinic with several months of progressive lower urinary tract symptoms (LUTS), the most prominent of which is decreased force of stream. His stream has lately become only a dribble, even with straining. He additionally feels—that is, having more of the sense—that he cannot empty his bladder completely. He has a history of appendectomy and is otherwise healthy. He takes no medications. He has been sexually active for most of the past decade (multiple partners), using condoms a majority of the time and is now in a monogamous relationship. He denies a history of urinary tract infection. He is physically active and has completed several triathlons. His vitals are normal, his physical and genitourinary examinations are unremarkable, and a urinalysis is normal.

Multiple choice questions

1 What is the most likely etiology and condition for this man's obstructive LUTS?
- a Benign prostatic hypertrophy
- b Urethral stricture secondary to remote perineal trauma
- c Urethral stricture secondary to history of sexually transmitted urethritis
- d Early-onset prostate cancer
- e Hypertonic bladder neck

2 The treatment with the lowest retreatment rate is
- a Urethroplasty with excision of scar and primary anastomosis
- b Urethroplasty with excision of scar and buccal mucosal graft interposition
- c Direct vision internal urethrostomy (DVIU)
- d Endoscopic placement of a UroLume® urethral stent
- e There are no significant differences in retreatment rates among the above options

References

1 Breyer BN, McAninch JW, Whitson JM, et al. Multivariate analysis of risk factors for long-term urethroplasty outcome. *J Urol* 2010;183(2):613–617.

2 Meeks JJ, Brandes SB, Morey AF, et al. Urethroplasty for radiotherapy induced bulbomembranous strictures: a multi-institutional experience. *J Urol* 2011;185(5):1761–1765.
3 Jordan G. Surgery of the penis and urethra. In: Wein AJ, Kavouss LR, Novick AC, Partin AW, Peters CA, editors. *Campbell-Walsh Urology*. 9th ed. Philadelphia, PA: Elsevier Inc.; 2007. pp. 956–1000.
4 Jordan GH, Virasoro R, Eltahawy EA. Reconstruction and management of posterior urethral and straddle injuries of the urethra. *Urol Clin North Am* 2006;33(1): 97–109, vii.
5 Gupta N, Dubey D, Mandhani A, Srivastava A, Kapoor R, Kumar A. Urethral stricture assessment: a prospective study evaluating urethral ultrasonography and conventional radiological studies. *BJU Int* 2006;98(1):149–153.
6 Santucci R, Eisenberg L. Urethrotomy has a much lower success rate than previously reported. *J Urol*; 2010;183(5):1859–1862.
7 Wilson TS, Lemack GE, Dmochowski RR. UroLume stents: lessons learned. *J Urol* 2002 ;167(6):2477–2480.
8 Parsons JK, Wright EJ. Extraction of UroLume endoprostheses with one-stage urethral reconstruction. *Urology* 2004;64(3):582–584.
9 Quartey JK. One-stage penile/preputial cutaneous island flap urethroplasty for urethral stricture: a preliminary report. *J Urol* 1983;129(2):284–287.
10 Anusionwu I, Wright E. Compartment syndrome after positioning in lithotomy: what a urologist needs to know. *BJU Int* 2011;108(4)477–478.
11 Elliott SP, Eisenberg ML, McAninch JW. First-stage urethroplasty: utility in the modern era. *Urology* 2008;71(5):889–892.
12 Culty T, Boccon-Gibod L. Anastomotic urethroplasty for posttraumatic urethral stricture: previous urethral manipulation has a negative impact on the final outcome. *J Urol* 2007;177(4):1374–1377.
13 Elliott SP, Meng MV, Elkin EP, McAninch JW, Duchane J, Carroll PR. Incidence of urethral stricture after primary treatment for prostate cancer: data from CaPSURE. *J Urol* 2007;178(2):529–534; discussion 534.
14 Erickson BA, Granieri MA, Meeks JJ, Cashy JP, Gonzalez CM. Prospective analysis of erectile dysfunction after anterior urethroplasty: incidence and recovery of function. *J Urol* 2010;183(2):657–661.
15 Shenfeld OZ, Kiselgorf D, Gofrit ON, et al. The incidence and causes of erectile dysfunction after pelvic fractures associated with posterior urethral disruption. *J Urol*. 2003;169(6):2173–2176.

Answers to multiple choice questions

1 b The majority of urethral strictures are secondary to perineal trauma (straddle injury), which may be remote in the patient's history. They occur most frequently in the bulbar urethra. Sexually transmitted infections are a less common cause of urethral stricture. In this age group, benign prostatic hyperplasia (BPH) and prostate cancer are rare in incidence.

Flexible urethroscopy demonstrates an 8F stricture in the bulbar urethra, preventing passage of the scope into the bladder. A bladder scan ultrasound shows a 150 mL post-void residual, and because the symptoms are subacute, a suprapubic tube is not placed. The next day, the patient undergoes retrograde urethrography. The RUG is shown below.

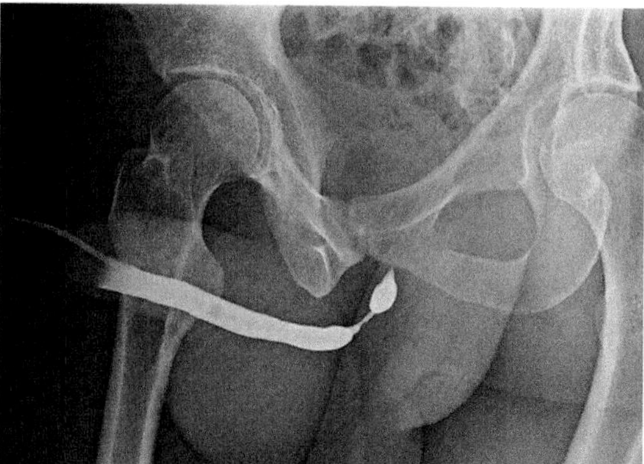

Courtesy of Dr. Arthur Burnett, The Johns Hopkins School of Medicine.

2 a Strictures recur after DVIU. The stricture-free rates from 5 to 15 years after DVIU are less than 10%, and the median time to recurrence is between 6 and 12 months. In contrast, the 5-year stricture-free rate after urethroplasty (any technique) is about 80%. Factors that reduce the stricture-free rates over time include prior urethral instrumentation/manipulation such as DVIU, exposure to local radiation therapy, revision urethroplasty, substitution with graft or flap instead of primary anastomosis, and smoking history.

Section 5 Urine storage and emptying

13 Neurourology

Ifeanyichukwu Anusionwu

The James Buchanan Brady Urological Institute and Department of Urology, The Johns Hopkins School of Medicine, Baltimore, MD, USA

KEY POINTS

- Lesions above the brainstem initially lead to detrusor areflexia associated with "cerebral shock," then later to detrusor overactivity with coordinated synergistic smooth and external sphincter; bladder sensation is usually normal or somewhat impaired.
- A complete lesion of the spinal cord above level T6 leads to autonomic hyperreflexia, detrusor overactivity, and smooth sphincter dyssynergia.
- Complete lesions between spinal cord level T6 to S2 lead to spinal shock initially and then smooth sphincter synergy with striated sphincter dyssynergy; bladder sensation is usually impaired and involuntary detrusor contraction is present.
- Lesions below spinal cord level S2 lead to decreased bladder compliance, an open smooth sphincter, and a resting striated sphincter tone that is not under voluntary control.
- Patients with Shy–Drager syndrome typically have an open bladder neck due to smooth and striated sphincter deficiency.
- Goals of treatment for neurogenic voiding dysfunction include preservation of renal function, facilitation of low pressure storing and adequate low pressure voiding, continence, and a socially acceptable independent function.

CASE STUDY

The patient is a 30-year-old female with a history of progressive multiple sclerosis diagnosed at the age of 20 years. Over the past 5 years, she noted worsening urge incontinence. She rarely has sensation of a need to void, and voids only twice daily. Between these voids, she has several episodes of urge incontinence. She is mobile with a walker although she can walk short distances without a walker; she is concerned that her limited mobility also contributes to inability to make it to the bathroom on time. She recently underwent a renal and bladder ultrasound, which showed no hydronephrosis, and a postvoid residual of 300 cc without any sensation of incomplete emptying. Her serum creatinine on laboratory testing 4 months before was 0.8. She does not report frequent urinary tract infections, and has roughly one or fewer episodes of cystitis yearly. Past medical history is notable for multiple sclerosis with optic neuritis and left-hand ataxia. She is right-handed and has adequate right-hand dexterity. Past surgical history is notable for remote history of gastric bypass surgery and abdominoplasty and recent ventral hernia repair. Medications include dalfampridine, baclofen, duloxetine, clonazepam, esomprazole, methadone, carbamazepine, pregabalin, diphenhydramine, natalizumab infusion, cyclobenzaprine, and methylphenidate. Physical examination was unremarkable. It was recommended that she undergo urodynamics testing to better characterize her voiding dysfunction. After this evaluation, possible management with anticholinergic medication in conjunction with self-catheterization will be discussed, with hopes that her manual dexterity will permit self-catheterization. In the mean time, she will practice timed voiding every 3 hours. She was also counseled about the importance of surveillance renal ultrasonography and serum creatinine testing at least yearly to detect any developing impairment of renal function.

Handbook of Urology, First edition. J. Kellogg Parsons, John B. Eifler and Misop Han.
Published 2014 by John Wiley & Sons, Ltd.

Normal micturition

The viscoelastic properties of the bladder allow it to fill at low pressure during normal physiologic conditions. This property of the bladder wall is called accommodation, and depends on its composition of smooth muscle, collagen, and elastin [1]. When this property is impaired, the bladder is said to be non-compliant. Patients who have a detrusor leak point pressure (detrusor pressure at which leakage occurs) of >40 cm H_2O are at increased risk for upper tract damage.

Neural control of micturition is organized in the pontine micturition center (PMC) and sacral micturition center. There is normally a negative inhibition from higher brain centers to PMC, and micturition requires release of this negative inhibition. The sacral micturition center receives parasympathetic and somatic inputs which are integrated there, and together with thoracolumbar sympathetic components, regulate micturition [1]. The first event to occur during micturition is relaxation of the striated sphincter. After this, there is a rise in detrusor pressure. The urethral pressure also falls until a point is reached when the detrusor pressure is equal to the urethral pressure. At this point, the bladder neck and urethra open and urine outflow occurs [1].

Continence depends on a number of factors: (1) a bladder which maintains low pressure over a range of filling volumes, and is free from intermittent pressure rises from involuntary detrusor contractions; (2) a sphincter mechanism which remains closed during filling but opens during voiding; and (3) intact neural network to the bladder and outlet [1].

Etiology of urinary incontinence

Bladder compliance: Several factors, neurogenic and non-neurogenic, may alter bladder compliance. These include radiation cystitis, tuberculous cystitis, bladder outlet obstruction, spina bifida, and radical pelvic surgery such as abdominoperineal resection or radical hysterectomy.

Detrusor overactivity: This, likewise, may be due to neurogenic or non-neurogenic causes. Neurogenic detrusor overactivity, formerly known as detrusor hyperreflexia, is often due to lesions above the PMC such as cerebrovascular accident, Parkinson's disease, brain tumor, and traumatic brain injury. Non-neurogenic detrusor overactivity, formerly known as detrusor instability, may be caused by bladder tumors or carcinoma *in situ*, bladder stones, and bladder outlet obstruction.

Impaired sphincter function: The sphincteric mechanism of men and women is fundamentally different. The male sphincteric mechanism consists of two elements: first, the bladder neck mechanism and second, the urethral sphincteric mechanism, located just distal to the prostatic apex, which contains the external sphincter muscle. In contrast, in the female, the bladder neck mechanism is quite weak and often incompetent [1]. Thus, the urethral sphincter, located in the proximal two-thirds of the urethra, is primarily responsible for maintaining and women are at higher risk for stress incontinence than men.

Impaired sphincter function may be due to (1) intrinsic sphincter deficiency (ISD) or (2) a poor support mechanism of the urethra, which leads to hypermobility. Although ISD and hypermobility are on a spectrum, there is likely at least a small component of ISD in most cases of impaired sphincter function [1]. It is widely accepted that a Valsalva leak point pressure (the intravesical pressure at which leakage occurs due to increased abdominal pressure) <60 cm H_2O is consistent with ISD while a Valsalva leak point pressure >90 cm H_2O is consistent with absence of ISD and thus the presence of hypermobility [1]. According to De Lancey's hammock theory, during increases in abdominal pressure, the urethra is normally compressed by a hammock of muscle and connective tissue. In patients with poor support, there is instead, rotational descent of the bladder neck with increased abdominal pressure and stress incontinence ensues [2].

Labor and vaginal delivery have long been known to be major risk factors for impaired sphincter function in women; the mechanism for this may include pudendal nerve injury, damage to pelvic floor connective tissue or its vasculature, and direct injury to the structures of the urinary tract. Women with severe perineal tears at the time of delivery or larger neonatal birth weight are at higher risk for sphincteric damage [3–6].

Other risk factors for impaired sphincter function include prior urethral surgery (e.g., sling procedure or urethral diverticulectomy which can predispose to periurethral fibrosis), radiation therapy, and denervation of the external sphincter.

Neurologic conditions leading to lower urinary tract dysfunction

Cerebrovascular accident: This event is initially associated with "cerebral shock" which is characterized by urinary retention due to detrusor areflexia. Once this phase resolves within a few weeks or months, overactive bladder usually manifests and persists long term.

Traumatic brain injury: This event may be associated with initial detrusor areflexia. If injury is above PMC, overactive bladder then develops. In cases where injury is in the brainstem below the PMC, detrusor-striated sphincter dyssynergia may develop.

Normal pressure hydrocephalus: This condition may be associated with incontinence due to bladder overactivity. The sphincter is usually synergic.

Cerebral palsy: This condition often has no associated voiding dysfunction, but may occasionally be associated detrusor overactivity with synergic sphincter.

Parkinson's disease: This disorder is often associated with voiding dysfunction of the following patterns: detrusor overactivity, smooth sphincter synergia, and striated sphincter bradykinesia (the striated sphincter is slow to relax at the beginning of voluntary voiding). Pseudodyssynergia (voluntary contraction of the striated sphincter to inhibit leakage during involuntary detrusor contraction) may also be present. Both pseudodyssynergia and striated sphincter bradykinesia may be confused with true dyssynergia on urodynamics.

Shy–Drager syndrome (also known as multiple system atrophy): This disorder consists of Parkinsonism, cerebellar dysfunction, pyramidal cortical dysfunction, and autonomic dysfunction (including orthostatic hypotension, urinary, and erectile dysfunction). Anhidrosis may also be present. Unlike Parkinson's disease in which urinary symptoms present several years *after* diagnosis, patients with multiple system atrophy often have urinary symptoms *before or at the time of* diagnosis. The features of the voiding dysfunction often include bladder overactivity, poor compliance, smooth and striated sphincter deficiency with an open bladder neck, difficulty in initiating voluntary voiding, and impaired detrusor contractility. The sphincter abnormalities in these patients make prostatectomy or other outlet procedures risky.

Multiple sclerosis: Urinary manifestations of this disease include detrusor overactivity, striated sphincter dyssynergia, and impaired detrusor contractility. The smooth sphincter is usually synergic and pseudodyssynergia may be present.

Spinal cord injury: Spinal shock is usually present for the first 6–12 weeks after complete suprasacral spinal cord injury and slightly less for incomplete suprasacral cord injuries. It is characterized by an areflexic bladder and a competent bladder neck. Both autonomic and somatic activities are suppressed [1].

After resolution of spinal shock, patients with suprasacral spinal cord injury have detrusor overactivity, smooth sphincter synergy, and striated sphincter dyssynergia. The striated sphincter dyssynergia puts these patients at risk for impaired renal function. Thus management should be directed at preservation of renal function as the main priority before attainment of continence. Patients with cord lesion above T6 may also have smooth sphincter dyssynergy. Patients with sacral spinal cord injury usually have detrusor areflexia, normal bladder compliance, competent nonrelaxing smooth sphincter, and a striated sphincter that has some fixed tone but is not under voluntary control [1].

Autonomic hyperreflexia occurs in patients with spinal cord injury above T6–T8 and involves an excessive sympathetic response to stimulation below the level of the lesion. This may be expressed as hypertension, reflex bradycardia, diaphoresis, and flushing of the face and skin above the level of the lesion. Inciting stimuli include genitourinary tract instrumentation (i.e., cystoscopy) or bladder distention and will abate once the stimulus is removed. Treatment is immediate removal of the inciting stimulus and alpha- or beta-adrenergic blockade. Oral nifedipine may be used for prophylaxis prior to instrumentation; alternatively, genitourinary tract interventions may be performed under spinal anesthesia in at-risk patients.

Care of the spinal cord injury patient: Patients should follow up yearly for the first 10 years after injury. If stable and doing well, follow-up can be extended to once every 2 years. During follow-up visits, evaluation of upper and lower tract functions, urodynamics, and cystoscopy (if patient has an indwelling catheter) are recommended. At cystoscopy, the bladder should be evaluated for tumors or stones. Patients with spinal cord injury—particularly those with an indwelling catheter, recurrent urinary tract infection, or bladder stones—are at increased risk for bladder cancer compared to the general population (squamous cell carcinoma) [1].

Bacteriuria, which is prevalent in spinal cord injury patients, should not be treated unless symptomatic. Prophylactic antibiotics should only be given to patients with recurrent urinary tract infections without a defined cause, particularly those with reflux or dilated upper tracts.

In patients who develop vesicoureteral reflux, management should be directed at correcting the bladder dysfunction that led to the reflux rather than correcting the reflux itself. Treatments directed at decreasing intravesical pressure include anticholinergic agents, sphincterotomy, and augmentation cystoplasty.

Myelomeningocele: Findings in these patients include an areflexic bladder and an open bladder neck. The bladder fills until it reaches a point where it overcomes the fixed resting pressure of the external sphincter, at which point urine leakage occurs.

Tabes dorsalis and pernicious anemia: Both of these disorders can lead to loss of bladder sensation and attendant large distended bladder.

Poliomyelitis: This disorder can lead to impaired motor function with attendant detrusor areflexia and urinary retention.

Herpesvirus: Herpes zoster virus may infect the sacral dorsal root ganglia leading to detrusor areflexia which may last 1–2 months. The dysfunction usually resolves spontaneously. Occasionally, detrusor overactivity and urinary incontinence may also be seen. With genital herpesvirus infection, urinary retention may develop within the first week after appearance of genital lesions.

Pelvic surgery: This voiding dysfunction occurs most frequently after abdominoperineal resection, abdominal hysterectomy, and proctocolectomy. The dysfunction is characterized by impaired bladder contractility, poor bladder compliance, and residual fixed striated sphincter tone. Thus, they present with obstruction, incontinence, or both. Most patients will have spontaneous improvement or resolution of their symptoms within 12 months and are therefore best managed with self-catheterization.

Management of neurogenic bladder disorders

Some of the goals of treatment for neurogenic lower urinary tract disorders include preserving renal function, avoiding urinary tract infections, facilitating low pressure urine storage and emptying, achieving continence, promoting independence in management of lower urinary tract function, and allowing for a socially acceptable function. In selecting the most appropriate treatment for a patient, several factors should be considered, including the patient's ability to perform necessary tasks (e.g., manual dexterity and mental capacity), social/home support system, patient's lifestyle (e.g., vocation and activity level), and patient's personal desires (e.g., desire to use only reversible treatments and desire to be catheter free).

For patients with bladder overactivity, behavioral modifications may be attempted, and if unsuccessful, pharmacologic management with anticholinergic medications is instituted. In patients who fail anticholinergic medications, intravesical botulinum toxin injection is an option.

For patients with myelomeningocele who have an areflexic bladder with an open bladder neck, treatment involves increasing the resistance of the bladder outlet (e.g., sling or injection of urethral bulking agents) combined with clean intermittent catheterization.

For patients with spinal cord injury where there is both a storage (detrusor overactivity and/or poor compliance) and an emptying (detrusor sphincter dysynergia) defect, management is usually twofold: the most popular strategy involves decreasing detrusor pressure and/or overactivity with anticholinergic medication in addition to instituting clean intermittent catheterization to adequately empty the bladder. Alternatively, sphincterotomy or sphincteric botulinum toxin injection can be used to decrease sphincter tone, and then incontinence can be managed with collecting device such as condom catheter.

Some recent management strategies for neurogenic lower urinary tract dysfunction have been described. Sacral deafferentation and anterior root stimulation have been reported to be associated with decreased incontinence and urinary tract infection [7].

Urinary diversion is a treatment of last resort which can be used to manage patients with neurogenic lower urinary tract dysfunction. Various types of diversion may be used, but again, consideration should be given to the above-described patient-specific factors; for example, if manual dexterity is limited, an ileal conduit may be more appropriate than a catheterizable pouch.

WHAT TO AVOID

- Avoid confusing pseudodyssynergia (voluntary contraction of the striated sphincter to inhibit leakage during involuntary detrusor contraction) or striated sphincter bradykinesia (delayed or slow relaxation of sphincter at the beginning of voluntary void) with true dyssynergia on urodynamics.
- Avoid immediate surgical or irreversible intervention in patients with voiding dysfunction after radical pelvic surgery, as most patients will have spontaneous improvement or resolution of their symptoms within 12 months; they may be managed with self-catheterization.
- In managing patients with neurogenic voiding dysfunction, avoid prescribing managements that involve tasks that will be challenging or impossible for the patient to perform; it is critical to assess manual dexterity, mental capacity, and support systems in place for the patient before constructing a management plan.
- Avoid treating asymptomatic bacteriuria in patients managed with long-term catheterization.

KEY WEB LINK

American Urological Association (AUA)/Society of Urodynamics, Female Pelvic Medicine & Urogenital Reconstruction (SUFU) Guideline (2012)
http://www.auanet.org/content/media/adult_urodynamics_guideline.pdf.

Multiple choice questions

1 A 35-year-old man sustains complete transection of T8 spinal cord level during a motor vehicle collision. Six months after the injury, the most likely finding on urodynamic testing is

a Detrusor areflexia
b Striated sphincter dyssynergy
c Smooth sphincter dyssynergy
d Low voiding pressure

2 All of the following findings may be seen after cerebrovascular accident except:

a Detrusor overactivity
b Pseudodyssynergy
c Smooth sphincter dyssynergy
d Detrusor areflexia

References

1 Campbell MF, Wein AJ, Kavoussi LR, et al. Urology. In: Wein AJ, Kavouss LR, Novick AC, Partin AW, Peters CA, editors. *Campbell-Walsh Urology*. 9th ed. Philadelphia, PA: Saunders Elsevier; 2007
2 DeLancey JO. Structural support of the urethra as it relates to stress urinary incontinence: the hammock hypothesis. *Am J Obstet Gynecol* 1994;170:1713.
3 Snooks SJ, Swash M, Henry MM, et al. Risk factors in childbirth causing damage to the pelvic floor innervation. *Int J Colorectal Dis* 1986;1:20.
4 Handa VL, Harris TA, Ostergard DR. Protecting the pelvic floor: obstetric management to prevent incontinence and pelvic organ prolapse. *Obstet Gynecol* 1996;88:470.
5 Brown S, Lumley J. Maternal health after childbirth: results of an Australian population based survey. *Br J Obstet Gynaecol* 1998;105:156.
6 Rortveit G, Daltveit AK, Hannestad YS, et al. Vaginal delivery parameters and urinary incontinence: the Norwegian EPINCONT study. *Am J Obstet Gynecol* 2003;189:1268.
7 Kutzenberger J, Domurath B, Sauerwein D. Spastic bladder and spinal cord injury: seventeen years of experience with sacral deafferentation and implantation of an anterior root stimulator. *Artif Organs* 2005;29:239.

Answers to multiple choice questions

1 b Spinal shock and associated detrusor areflexia in most cases are resolved by 6–12 weeks. Patients with complete spinal cord transection between T6 and S2 usually have smooth sphincter synergy, but striated sphincter dyssynergy and high voiding pressure.

2 c After cerebrovascular accident, both the smooth and striated sphincters are usually synergic.

14 Urogynecology

Ifeanyichukwu Anusionwu

The James Buchanan Brady Urological Institute and Department of Urology, The Johns Hopkins School of Medicine, Baltimore, MD, USA

KEY POINTS

- The Q-tip test may be used to evaluate for urethral hypermobility. It involves placing a Q-tip in the urethra and measuring the angle of deflection as the patient performs a Valsalva maneuver; an angle more than 30 degrees is consistent with hypermobility.
- Occult stress incontinence is stress incontinence masked by obstruction or kinking of the urethra by severe pelvic organ prolapse. It may be unmasked if the patient is asked to perform a Valsalva maneuver after the anterior vaginal wall is supported with a half speculum.
- In developed countries, the most common etiology for a vesicovaginal fistula (VVF) is iatrogenic bladder injury during pelvic surgery; in developing countries, the most common etiology is obstetric complication, particularly obstructed labor.
- In contrast to a post pelvic surgery, a VVF due to obstructed labor tends to be larger, more distal in the vagina, and involves a larger area of bladder and proximal urethra.
- The classic presenting signs of a urethral diverticulum are the "3 Ds": dysuria, dyspareunia, and dribbling.

CASE STUDY 1

The patient is a 73-year-old gravida 2, para 2 with a history of fecal soiling, urinary incontinence, and vaginal bulge. Urine leakage was with exertion and urge, and she reported a visible and palpable protrusion from the vagina with exertion. She required splinting (digital manipulation of the rectum) for defecation and noted discomfort with intercourse. Past medical history was notable for hyperlipidemia, hypertension, obstructive sleep apnea, and chronic low back pain. She had undergone prior hysterectomy as well as anterior and posterior colporrhaphy 1 year prior. She was moderately active, married, and never smoked. On physical examination, external genitalia and urethral meatus were normal and the bladder was nonpalpable. On pelvic examination, cervix and uterus were absent, and POPQ score was as following: Ba: 0, Bp: −1, C: −2, D: −2, TVL: +9. Urinalysis was within normal limits. She was diagnosed with stress incontinence, urge incontinence, POP, and defecatory dysfunction. She underwent an uncomplicated robotic-assisted laparoscopic abdominal sacral colpopexy, midurethral sling, and resection rectopexy. Postoperatively, she continued to have urgency with occasional episodes of urge incontinence. She denied sensation of incomplete bladder emptying, and was practicing timed voiding every 4 hours. Stress incontinence and vaginal bulge were resolved. An anticholinergic medication was started, and sacral neuromodulation was discussed as a second line management strategy if she failed anticholinergic therapy.

Handbook of Urology, First edition. J. Kellogg Parsons, John B. Eifler and Misop Han. © 2014 by John Wiley & Sons, Ltd. Published 2014 by John Wiley & Sons, Ltd.

CASE STUDY 2

The patient is a 20-year-old gravida 0, para 0 who presented with an enlarging anterior vaginal wall mass. She first noted this mass ~5–6 years prior, and it gradually enlarged over time. She admitted to dyspareunia, dribbling, discharge, and spraying of urinary stream, but denied dysuria. She had no past medical or surgical history. Physical examination was notable for a protuberant, ~1 cm, mass of the anterior vaginal wall, just proximal to the urethral meatus. There was no discharge on palpation, but the mass was tender. She underwent MRI of the pelvis, which showed this high signal intensity mass on T2 images originating from the urethra, thought to be consistent with a urethral diverticulum. She underwent an uncomplicated urethral diverticulectomy with an unremarkable postoperative course.

Classification of urinary incontinence

Urinary incontinence is the involuntary loss of urine severe enough to pose a social or hygienic problem [1]. There are three primary types of incontinence. **Stress incontinence** is the involuntary leakage of urine with exertion or abdominal pressure; it may be precipitated by activities such as coughing or sneezing. Urodynamic stress incontinence refers to the leakage of urine in the absence of detrusor contraction but synchronous with increased abdominal pressure. **Urgency incontinence** refers to involuntary urine loss subsequent to strong desire to void or urgency. Urodynamic testing will reveal involuntary detrusor contraction with urine leakage. **Mixed urinary incontinence** refers to the presence of both stress incontinence and urgency incontinence. Two other, less common types of incontinence include **continuous incontinence** (continuous leakage of urine caused by anatomic disruption of the lower urinary tract, such as by a fistula or ectopic ureter) and **overflow incontinence** (urine leakage in the setting of urinary retention).

There are several other related diagnoses. **Overactive bladder** refers to urgency with or without urgency incontinence, frequency, and nocturia. The minimal necessary symptom for diagnosis of overactive bladder is urgency. **Mixed urinary symptoms** refer to the presence of both stress incontinence and symptoms of overactive bladder without urgency incontinence. **Situational urinary incontinence** is associated with specific situations, including sexual intercourse or laughing.

Evaluation

A thorough history of the present illness should be obtained as to whether the incontinence is associated with urge, exertion, or both. The severity of the incontinence should be ascertained using number of pads used daily, with or without formal pad weight testing to estimate the volume of leakage. The presence of other associated voiding complaints should be determined (e.g., incomplete emptying, frequency, nocturia, weak stream) and the voiding pattern should be recorded on a voiding diary. Complete past medical and surgical history should be obtained, with particular interest in history of neurologic disorders, obstetric history, and prior pelvic surgery or genitourinary tract procedures. Medication use should be assessed, specifically querying for diuretics and adrenergic antagonists. The effect of the incontinence on quality of life should be assessed. Questionnaires such as Incontinence Impact Questionnaire (IIQ) and Urogenital Distress Inventory-6 short form (UDI-6) are useful.

A general physical examination including a general assessment for performance status and debilitation, an abdominal examination, and a neurologic examination should be performed. Pelvic examination includes assessment of: (1) the external genitalia; (2) the urethral meatus for location, lesions, prolapse, and hypermobility; (3) the vagina for lesions, prolapse, and occult stress incontinence, which can be unmasked if the patient is asked to strain while supporting the anterior vaginal wall with a half speculum; (4) the cervix and uterus for size, position, tenderness, and mobility; (5) the adnexa for masses or tenderness; and (6) the rectum for tone and masses.

The Q-tip test involves placing a Q-tip in the urethra and measuring the angle of deflection as the patient performs a Valsalva maneuver. An angle >30 degrees is consistent with hypermobility.

Urinalysis and ascertainment of post void residual are indicated. Routine performance of cystoscopy is not absolutely indicated in all cases, but is often indicated in patients with hematuria, storage symptoms, or complex histories, such as pelvic radiation, prior prolapse, or previous incontinence surgery [1]. Likewise, routine urodynamics is not recommended, but is indicated in patients with neurologic disease, obstructive voiding symptoms, mixed incontinence, or failed prior pelvic floor surgery [1].

Management

First line management of women with stress or mixed incontinence is pelvic floor muscle training [2]. For patients who fail this initial step, midurethral sling surgery may be offered. Autologous rectus fascial sling and open colposuspension are alternatives to midurethral sling [2].

First line treatment for women with urge or mixed incontinence is bladder training [2]. If bladder training is ineffective, anticholinergic medication should be offered. For patients who fail these initial management steps, sacral nerve stimulation may be performed. Intravesical botulinum toxin injection is also an alternative.

Pelvic floor anatomy and support

Bony structures

The pelvis is made up of pubis, ischium, ilium, and sacrum.

Musculature

The levator ani muscles are made up of three components: (1) the puborectalis and pubourethralis muscles which run from the pubis and wrap around the rectum and urethra in a U shape, (2) the pubococcygeus which runs from pubis to coccyx, and (3) the iliococcygeus which runs from arcus tendineus levator ani to the coccyx. The opening in the levator ani through which the urethra and vagina run is called the urogenital hiatus. Innervation to the levator ani, striated urethral sphincter, and striated anal sphincter comes from pudendal nerve.

Fascia and ligaments

The arcus tendineus fascia pelvis (ATFP) is a fibrous fascial band that runs from pubis to ischial spine bilaterally.

Arcus tendineus levator ani is a fibrous part of the obturator fascia that runs from the pubis to the ischial spine. Its origin on the pubis is lateral to that of ATFP, and it forms the origin of part of the levator ani musculature.

Pubourethral ligament attach the anterior midurethra to the pubic bone.

Sacrospinous ligament runs from ischial spine to the sacrum.

Uterosacral ligaments attach the cervix to sacral segments S2–S4.

Cardinal ligaments attach the cervix to the pelvic sidewall.

The endopelvic fascia is the superior fascial covering of the levator ani muscle while the pubocervical fascia is the inferior fascial covering for the levator ani. Pubocervical fascia attaches the vagina and cervix to the ATFP and also runs in the space between the vagina and bladder. Pubocervical fascia and endopelvic fascia both fuse at the ATFP.

Perineal body is a condensation of fibrous tissue in the midline of the perineum between the vagina and anus.

Pelvic organ prolapse

Pelvic organ prolapse (POP) is the descent of pelvic organs (bladder, rectum, or uterus) resulting in an external bulge of the vaginal wall. **A cystocele (anterior vaginal wall prolapse)** may be associated with incompetent urethral sphincter in some patients. It is also possible for a cystocele to mask underlying stress incontinence by kinking the urethra—this condition is called *occult* or *latent* stress incontinence and usually becomes evident only once the prolapse is treated. A **rectocele (posterior vaginal wall prolapse)** may lead to fecal impaction and need for manual reduction of the prolapse (i.e., by placing the fingers in the vaginal vault and pressing against the prolapse) in order to defecate. There is also increased prevalence of fecal incontinence in patients with POP.

Anterior compartment prolapse is most common, while apical prolapse is least common.

Risk factors for POP include older age, history of hysterectomy, prior pelvic surgery, increased parity, Hispanic or Caucasian race, smoking, estrogen deficiency, and genetic predisposition.

Evaluation

The pelvic examination should be performed both in lithotomy and in standing position (with one foot on a stool and legs apart). The pelvic floor is assessed for sensation and motor strength by placing a finger in the vagina and asking the patient to contract pelvic floor muscles. Retracting the posterior vaginal wall with half of a Graves speculum facilitates evaluation of the anterior compartment support. Likewise, the anterior vaginal wall can be retracted during evaluation of the posterior compartment, and both anterior and posterior compartments can be retracted with two half speculums to facilitate evaluation of the apical compartment.

POP is characterized using the pelvic organ prolapse quantification (POPQ). This scoring system measures the location of six vaginal points during Valsalva with reference to the hymen. Vaginal points are measured in centimeters above (negative value) or below (positive value) the hymen. Stage 0 denotes absence of prolapse. Stage I denotes a leading edge of the prolapse that is more than 1 cm above the hymen. Stage II denotes a leading edge of the prolapse that is within 1 cm above or below the hymen. Stage III denotes a leading edge that is more than 1 cm below the hymen but less than TVL-2 (total vaginal length minus 2 cm) below the hymen. Stage IV denotes a leading edge that is more than TVL-2 below the hymen [1]. The genital hiatus (gh), perineal body (pb), and total vaginal length (TVL) are also measured as part of the POPQ score. The perineal body measures the distance between the vagina and the rectum, while the genital hiatus is the size of the vaginal opening. The TVL is measured after reducing the prolapse.

The bulbocavernosus reflex, which reflects the function of the sacral nerve roots S2, S3, and S4, can be tested by squeezing the clitoris and observing for anal and pelvic floor contraction. This reflex is present in 70% of females.

Management

Initial management of POP can focus on lifestyle modifications (weight loss and smoking cessation), pelvic floor muscle training, and vaginal pessary [3]. Alternatively, a multitude of surgical techniques have been described. In a recent Cochrane review [4], native tissue repair of anterior compartment defect was associated with more failures than polypropylene mesh overlay and transobturator armed mesh. However, there was no difference in subjective symptoms and, in those treated with mesh, there was a 10% prevalence of mesh exposure. A prior review reported that abdominal sacral colpopexy was superior to vaginal sacrospinous colpopexy with regard to recurrence for management of vault prolapse [5]. Posterior wall defects may be managed transvaginally or transanally. Posterior colporrhaphy, which is a transvaginal plication of the rectovaginal tissue, may be performed with or without graft interposition. Transvaginal repair of rectoceles has been associated with lower recurrence rates than transanal repair [5]. Vaginal mesh kits and laparoscopic/robotic rectopexy are also being used for posterior compartment defects.

Urinary tract fistulae

Fistulae are anomalous communications between two or more body cavities or between a body cavity and the skin. The underlying etiology may be inflammatory, infectious, malignant, traumatic/iatrogenic, ischemic, congenital, or radiation associated.

Vesicovaginal fistulae

A special case of a fistula that occurs in women is *vesicovaginal fistulae (VVF)*. In developed countries, the most common etiology for a VVF is bladder injury during pelvic surgery, particularly abdominal hysterectomy, with the fistula occurring at the vaginal cuff. Other risk factors include prior pelvic radiation, cesarean section, and cervical conization [1]. In developing countries, the most common etiology is obstetric complication, particularly obstructed labor. A VVF due to obstructed labor tends to be larger and more distal in the vagina than VVF associated with other etiologies.

Evaluation

The most consistent symptom in patients with VVF is constant urine leakage per vagina. Patients with large fistulae may report absence of discrete voids, with urine drained entirely through the fistula.

Alternatively, there may be pooling of urine in the vagina upon standing. Other presenting complaints include recurrent urinary tract infections, skin breakdown, or pelvic pain.

The cornerstone of the VVF evaluation is a complete physical examination, including thorough speculum pelvic examination. The size, location, number of fistulae, vaginal dimensions, and presence of pelvic masses should be noted. Urine culture, and cytology as indicated, should be obtained. Cystoscopy is useful in determining the location of the VVF relative to the ureteral orifices. While VVF can be visualized cystoscopically, early on it may appear as a nonspecific bullous edema. Even mature fistula tracts may be challenging to identify due to adjacent pits; in such circumstances, a guidewire can be used to gently probe the different pits, and passage of the guidewire into the vagina confirms the exact location of the fistula tract [1]. If there is suspicion of malignancy or a prior history of malignancy, the fistula tract should be biopsied.

A dye test can confirm the diagnosis of VVF: after packing the vagina with clean sponges, instillation of methylene blue or indigo carmine into the bladder via a urethral Foley will often stain the vaginal packing blue. A "double dye test" may be also be used to evaluate for concomitant ureteral fistulae. In the double dye test, oral phenazopyridine is given and blue dye is instilled into the bladder. If the vaginal packing stains orange, this is suggestive of ureterovaginal fistula, but if it stains blue then it is suggestive of VVF.

A cystogram may also be performed. A lateral view should be obtained, as there is less superimposition of vagina on bladder, and thus a higher probability of demonstrating the fistula [1]. A voiding cystourethrogram may also be considered as the increased intravesical pressure on voiding may be necessary to force urine out of the fistula and into the vagina.

An upper tract study such as computed tomography (CT) urography is indicated in the evaluation of patients with VVF as a substantial proportion of these patients have an associated ureteral injury. If the distal ureter is not well visualized on CT urography, or there is high suspicion for a ureterovaginal fistula, retrograde pyelogram should be performed.

Management

A VVF may be managed conservatively with urethral catheter drainage for 3 weeks if it is new in onset and the tract is relatively small (<3 mm) and immature. For a small (<3 mm) but epithelialized VVF, consideration may be given to endoscopic fulguration of the tract, followed by bladder drainage for 3 weeks. It should be noted that fulguration of a fistula tract is associated with the risk of increasing the size of the tract and/or devitalizing adjacent tissue that could otherwise be used for a formal repair [1].

For patients who fail initial conservative management, timing of formal fistula repair depends on the etiology. It is generally accepted that repair of a VVF due to obstructed labor or radiation should be delayed for roughly 6 months to allow demarcation of ischemic tissue. For other uncomplicated VVF, immediate repair is appropriate.

VVF may be repaired transvaginally or transabdominally. The advantages of the transvaginal approach include decreased blood loss, shorter postoperative recovery, availability of adjacent local tissue flaps (peritoneal and martius flaps), and avoidance of adhesions in patients with prior multiple abdominal surgeries. The advantages of the transabdominal approach include better exposure of the surgical field in nulliparous patients with fistulae located high relative to the cuff, the ability to perform simultaneous transabdominal procedures as indicated, and the availability of rectus and peritoneal flaps. Regardless of the choice of surgical approach, the principles of fistula repair include nonoverlapping suture lines, multiple-layered tension-free closure, and postoperative bladder drainage.

Urethral diverticulum

Most urethral diverticula (UD) are acquired, and likely originate in the periurethral glands. Accordingly, most UD have an ostium located in the posterolateral part of the distal two-thirds of the urethra, which is where the ostium of most periurethral glands are also located. It is possible that infection of these periurethral glands, with obstruction and then rupture into the urethral lumen is the underlying mechanism for UD formation [1].

The classic presenting signs of UD have been described as the "3Ds": dysuria, dyspareunia, and dribbling. However, not all patients have these symptoms and some may be completely asymptomatic. Other presenting signs and symptoms include recurrent urinary tract infection, frequency, urgency, perineal pain, vaginal discharge, vaginal mass, and obstructive voiding symptoms. The differential diagnosis includes Skene's gland cyst, Gartner's duct abnormalities, urethral prolapse, urethral caruncle, vulvodynia, interstitial cystitis, and endometriosis.

Evaluation

In evaluating patients for UD, the physical examination should include: assessment of the size, location and number of any anterior vaginal masses; tenderness to palpation; and discharge from urethra upon "milking" the mass. A thorough pelvic examination should be performed including assessment for vaginal atrophy, stress incontinence, and POP. In cases where there is suspicion for associated malignancy, urine cytology should be performed. Urine analysis, urine culture, and cystoscopy are indicated to rule out underlying infection, as well as other lower urinary tract abnormalities. It may be possible to visualize the ostium of the UD on cystoscopy, and it is often located posterolaterally at the midurethra. Urodynamics may be performed in patients with associated significant voiding dysfunction or incontinence.

Imaging studies useful in confirming the diagnosis of UD are positive-pressure double-balloon urethrography, voiding cystourethrography (VCUG), and pelvic magnetic resonance imaging (MRI). In double-balloon positive-pressure urethrography, a catheter with two balloons and an infusing port located between the two balloons is placed in the urethra. One balloon is inflated at the bladder neck and the other is inflated just proximal to the urethral meatus. Contrast material is then injected through the infusing port to distend the urethra. Under this positive pressure, the UD fills with contrast and can be visualized radiographically. A VCUG is more widely available, but may be limited if the patient is unable to void and generate an adequate flow rate to fill the UD [1]. A pelvic MRI is an excellent technique for demonstrating UD; on T2 images, the UD is seen as a high-intensity signal while on T1 images, it has low signal intensity.

Management

Repair of UD is frequently accomplished through an inverted U incision on the anterior vaginal wall after placing a urethral catheter into the bladder. The incision is deepened to the space between the periurethral fascia and the anterior vaginal wall. A transverse incision is made on the periurethral fascia, exposing the diverticulum. The UD is then dissected free and completely excised at its ostium. The urethra and periurethral fascia are closed with absorbable suture with the suture lines for the two layers perpendicular to each other.

In patients in whom the periurethral fascia is not robust, or the risk of urethrovaginal fistula is deemed to be high, a martius flap may be laid over the periurethral fascia before closing the vaginal incision. A pericatheter VCUG is performed 2–3 weeks postoperatively and the catheter removed if no extravasation is demonstrated. Potential postoperative complications of urethral diverticulectomy are urethrovaginal fistula, stress incontinence, urethral stricture, and recurrence of UD. Malignancies may be detected on pathologic evaluation of urethral diverticulectomy specimens. Most commonly, adenocarcinoma is found, although transitional cell carcinoma and squamous cell carcinoma may also be found.

WHAT TO AVOID

- In repair of VVF, avoid overlapping suture lines; other principles of proper fistula repair include multiple-layered closure, tension-free closure, and postoperative bladder drainage.
- In evaluating patients with POP, avoid performing pelvic examination only in lithotomy as some defects may be demonstrated only when the patient is upright. Examine patients both in lithotomy and in standing position with one foot on a stool and legs apart.
- In evaluating patients with VVF, avoid missing an upper tract fistula; perform an upper tract study such as CT urography because a significant number of these patients have an associated ureteral injury.

KEY WEB LINK

American Urological Association (AUA)/Society Of Urodynamics, Female Pelvic Medicine & Urogenital Reconstruction (SUFU) Guideline (2012)
http://www.auanet.org/content/media/adult_urodynamics_guideline.pdf

Multiple choice questions

1 A 55-year-old woman complains of large volume continuous leakage of clear fluid from the vagina 6 days after abdominal hysterectomy. The next step is:

- a Reassurance that this is normal
- b CT of the abdomen and pelvis
- c Pelvic examination and double dye test
- d Immediate abdominal exploration

2 A 30-year-old female presents with a painful enlarging anterior vaginal mass which she first noted 2 months ago. The mass is associated with dyspareunia and post void dribbling. The least useful diagnostic tool of the following is:

- a Positive-pressure urethrography
- b Pelvic MRI
- c CT of the pelvis
- d Voiding cystourethrography

References

1 Campbell MF, Wein AJ, Kavoussi LR, ScienceDirect (Online service). *Campbell-Walsh Urology*. Philadelphia, PA; [Edinburgh]: Saunders Elsevier; 2007.

2 National Collaborating Centre for Women's and Children's Health (UK). London: RCOG Press;2006.

3 Machin SE, Mukhopadhyay S. Pelvic organ prolapse: review of the aetiology, presentation, diagnosis and management. *Menopause Int* 2011;17(4):132–136.

4 Maher CM, Feiner B, Baessler K, Glazener CM. Surgical management of pelvic organ prolapse in women: the updated summary version Cochrane review. *Int Urogynecol J* 2011;22(11):1445–1457.

5 Maher C, Baessler K, Glazener CM, Adams EJ, Hagen S. Surgical management of pelvic organ prolapse in women: a short version Cochrane review. *Neurourol Urodyn* 2008;27(1):3–12.

Answers to multiple choice questions

1 c The presentation is concerning for post hysterectomy urovaginal fistula. There is not enough information to determine if it is a VVF or ureterovaginal fistula. The diagnosis first needs to be made. Thus, the next most appropriate step is to perform the dye test. While a small amount of postoperative fluid leakage may occur initially after hysterectomy, persistent large volume leakage should prompt further investigation. Abdominal CT is unlikely to make the diagnosis without a cystogram/urogram component.

2 c The patient most likely has a urethral diverticulum. All the options listed except CT are useful in diagnosing urethral diverticulum.

15 Interstitial cystitis and chronic pelvic pain

Ifeanyichukwu Anusionwu

The James Buchanan Brady Urological Institute and Department of Urology, The Johns Hopkins School of Medicine, Baltimore, MD, USA

KEY POINTS

- The typical presentation of interstitial cystitis (IC) is a chronic pelvic pain perceived by the patient to originate in the bladder, exacerbated by bladder filling, and associated with urinary urgency and/or frequency.
- The classic findings of IC after cystoscopy and distention are glomerulations and/or Hunner's ulcers.
- Pathogenesis of IC is likely related to increased epithelial permeability, histamine release by mast cells, inhibition of bladder epithelial proliferation by antiproliferative factor (APF), and neurogenic inflammation.
- Oral therapies include pentosan polysulfate, amitriptyline, antihistamines, and analgesics. Intravesical therapies include hydrodistention, dimethyl sulfoxide (DMSO), and glycosaminoglycan instillations.
- Urinary diversion, with or without simple cystectomy, is a treatment of last resort which has fallen out of favor in recent years. Patients should be thoroughly counseled before undergoing an irreversible surgical procedure.

CASE STUDY

The patient is a 53-year-old female with a history of depression and dyspareunia who presented with complaint of significant urgency, frequency (four times per hour), nocturia (more than five times per night), and suprapubic pain (8/10). She could not identify exacerbating factors, but reported relief with wearing an analgesic patch. She denies incontinence related to the urge or otherwise. Bowel habits are normal with bowel movements daily or every other day.

The past medical history included congenital hip dysplasia, head injury after being hit by a car at age four, bilateral foot neuromas, insomnia, anxiety, depression, and chronic lower back pain. She was status post-neuroma surgeries, breast augmentation, liposuction, and excision of benign breast cyst. Medications included Valium, Lexapro, and Ambien. Physical and vaginal examinations were unremarkable. Urinalysis was within normal limits and urine culture which was sent returned negative. She was given a voiding diary and a brochure on dietary suggestions for IC.

During her return visit, she reported no improvement on the IC diet, which she found restrictive. The voiding diary did reflect her previously reported voiding complaints, with maximum voided volume of 8 ounces and interval between voids ranging from 15 minutes to 3 hours. She was referred to physical therapy where she was noted to have hypertonicity of the pelvic floor muscles and tenderness of levator ani. She underwent massage therapy, training in relaxation techniques, and biofeedback. She did have some improvement in her frequency and pain (down to 4/10 at baseline), but still had significant bother and unacceptable quality of life. She was started on pentosan polysulfate, but complained of significant diarrhea and vomiting so the medication was stopped. Gabapentin was started and she actually noted marked improvement of her pain. However, she felt that her quality of life was still not satisfactory. Gabapentin was continued and weekly intravesical instillation of pentosan polysulfate was started. With this regimen and continued physical therapy, the patient is functioning satisfactorily.

Handbook of Urology, First edition. J. Kellogg Parsons, John B. Eifler and Misop Han. © 2014 by John Wiley & Sons, Ltd.
Published 2014 by John Wiley & Sons, Ltd.

Clinical presentation

Interstitial cystitis (IC) presents with chronic pelvic pain, urgency, and frequency exacerbated by bladder filling [1]. IC is a diagnosis of exclusion, which means that these symptoms cannot be attributed definitively to urinary infection, radiation cystitis, urinary calculi, malignancy, or other diagnoses. Urgency in IC is different from urgency in overactive bladder because patients with overactive bladder often report the sudden desire to pass urine in order to avoid incontinence, while patients with IC report the desire to pass urine in order to relieve bladder pressure/discomfort.

The National Institute of Diabetes and Digestive and Kidney Disease (NIDDK) diagnostic criteria for IC [2] is restrictive and often used for research purpose but not for clinical diagnosis as many patients with IC do not meet the NIDDK criteria.

IC has a much higher prevalence in women, with a male to female ratio 1:5. Median age of onset is 40 years, but men tend to be diagnosed at an older age. Up to half of IC patients can experience temporary spontaneous remission [1]. Symptoms fluctuate over time but generally progress with older age. IC is associated with a number of other diagnoses including depression, allergies, fibromyalgia, chronic fatigue syndrome, vulvar vestibulitis, irritable bowel syndrome, inflammatory bowel disease, and Sjogren's syndrome.

Etiology

Several etiological models have been proposed, the most prominent and well documented of which is increased permeability at the bladder epithelial surface. This model posits that caustic urinary solutes (primarily potassium) diffuse through the leaky epithelium and into the bladder interstitium, in the process injuring tissue, stimulating sensory nerves, and generating symptoms. Mast cells also likely play a role in pathogenesis by producing histamine, which can cause pain, hyperemia, and fibrosis. It has also been suggested that IC may result from inhibition of bladder epithelial proliferation by antiproliferative factor (APF). APF suppresses production of growth factors, including heparin-binding epidermal growth factor-like growth factor. Activation of sensory pain fibers may lead to neuropathic inflammation; the resulting neuropathic pain can persist after the resolution of tissue damage [1]. Twin studies which showed greater concordance of IC in monozygotic twins than dizygotic twins suggest a contribution of genetics to susceptibility to IC [3].

Diagnosis

The differential diagnosis of IC includes tuberculous cystitis, carcinoma *in situ*, bladder cancer, and eosinophilic cystitis. Evaluation of patients with IC should include history, physical examination (including vaginal examination in females and digital rectal examination in males), urinalysis, urine culture, urine cytology (in high-risk patients or those with microhematuria), and voiding diary (including frequency and volume of voids).

A number of questionnaires and symptom indices have been developed to quantify symptoms in IC patients. The O'Leary-Sant Indices, composed of the IC symptom index and problem index measure pain and urinary symptoms and the degree of bother these symptoms cause to patients [4]. It has been shown to be useful in discriminating between IC patients and controls. Other instruments developed for use in IC include the University of Wisconsin symptom instrument and Pelvic Pain and Urgency/Frequency Patient Symptom Scale (PUF).

Cystoscopy with or without hydrodistention under anesthesia and bladder biopsy are performed at the discretion of the physician. Cystoscopic findings include Hunner's ulcers (erythematous patches of epithelium similar in appearance to carcinoma *in situ*) and diffuse glomerulations (prominent microvascular patterns in the bladder wall that become visible with bladder filling) [1]. Urodynamic studies are also optional, but when performed, may show decreased bladder capacity, pain on bladder filling, and normal compliance.

Pathological findings in bladder biopsy specimens of patients with IC are highly variable. They may be completely normal or demonstrate mastocytosis, submucosal inflammation, denuded epithelium, and/or epithelial ulceration.

Management

An initial course of antibiotic therapy is reasonable in patients who have not had such a trial, but repeated courses of antibiotics in the absence of documented infection should not be pursued.

Conservative strategies that may be useful include biofeedback, massage, and stress reduction exercises. Patients often note that certain foods, such as caffeine, alcohol, cranberry juice, citrus fruits, and spicy foods lead to exacerbation of their symptoms. Restricting the implicated foods from the diet may be worthwhile.

Different classes of medications have been used to manage IC. Pentosan polysulfate (trade name Elmiron), a heparin analogue which can work by repairing the defective glycosaminoglycan layer of the bladder, has demonstrated in clinical trials and meta-analysis of clinical trials to be highly efficacious in the treatment of IC. The usual dosage is 100 mg orally three times a day, but it can take up to 6 months of treatment before a therapeutic effect is seen.

Antihistamines including cimetidine and hydroxyzine, which can block neuronal activation of mast cells, is also efficacious [1]. The usual dose is 25 mg orally in the morning then 50 mg orally at bedtime.

Tricyclic antidepressants, particularly amitriptyline, are commonly used. The mechanism of action includes anticholinergic activity, antihistaminic activity, and serotonin and norepinephrine reuptake inhibition. The usual dose is 25–75 mg orally at bedtime, but the drug often needs to be titrated slowly to that dose over the course of several weeks.

Immunosuppresive drugs such as cyclosporine, azathioprine, and chloroquine derivatives have also been used for treatment of IC but are not routinely recommended as first-line oral therapy.

Acetaminophen, nonsteroidal anti-inflammatory agents, gabapentin, pregabalin, and opioid analgesics may be used cautiously, but are generally not as effective as pentosan polysulfate, antihistamines, or amitriptyline. Patients with refractory pain may warrant consultation with a chronic pain specialist.

Intravesically instilled glycosaminoglycans, which function by creating a permeability barrier in the bladder epithelium, have been used with some benefit in the treatment of IC, particularly when used in combination with lidocaine. Parsons and colleagues reported positive effect when heparin was used at a dose of 10,000 international units mixed in 10 mL sterile water and instilled intravesically three times a week [5]. The usual duration of instillation is 30–60 minutes. Pentosan polysulfate may also be administered intravesically at a dose of 300 mg in 50 mL of normal saline, twice a week. Hyaluronic acid at a dose of 40 mg in 40 mL of normal saline instilled intravesically once a week has been reported to be beneficial as well [6].

Intravesically instilled 50 cc of 50% dimethyl sulfoxide (DMSO) for 15 minutes has anti-inflammatory, analgesic, and muscle relaxant properties. It is also felt to modulate histamine release and desensitize nociceptive pathways [1]. The treatment has been shown to be beneficial, but often has to be repeated every couple of weeks.

Use of neuromodulation in treating IC has been reported, but this therapy appears to be most appropriate for patients with associated urgency, frequency, and pelvic floor dysfunction. Intradetrusor injection of botulinum toxin A is considered an investigational treatment for IC.

Hydrodistention, while a diagnostic tool, also provides symptomatic improvement to some patients. Under anesthesia, the bladder is distended to 80 cm H_2O for 8 minutes. Prolonged distention has no therapeutic benefit over distention for a few minutes and is not recommended. Transurethral fulguration of Hunner's ulcers may provide symptomatic relief to some patients with IC.

Major surgery—including urinary diversion with or without simple cystectomy and substitution cystoplasty—in carefully selected patients for whom all therapies have failed can potentially provide relief from urinary frequency, but may not alleviate the symptom of pain. It is important to thoroughly counsel the patient before undertaking an irreversible surgical procedure.

WHAT TO AVOID

1 Interstitial cystitis (IC) is a diagnosis of exclusion. In patients with the typical symptoms, avoid missing identifiable causes such as infection, malignancy, calculi, and other diagnoses.

2 For therapeutic hydrodistention, avoid distending the bladder for hours as this has no therapeutic benefit; distention to 80 cm H_2O for 8 minutes is sufficient.

3 Reserve major surgery (i.e., urinary diversion with or without simple cystectomy and substitution cystoplasty) only for those patients who have failed all other therapies.

KEY WEB LINK

AUA Clinical practice guideline for interstitial cystitis (IC)/bladder pain syndrome
http://www.auanet.org/content/clinical-practice-guidelines/clinical-guidelines.cfm

Multiple choice questions

1 A 45-year-old female presents with a 6-month history of suprapubic pain which she feels is from her bladder and is worse with a full bladder. She also complains of urinary urgency and has a past medical history of vulvar vestibulitis. Initial evaluation includes all of the following except:

a Voiding diary
b Urinalysis and urine culture
c Urodynamic testing
d Physical exam including vaginal speculum exam

2 A 50-year-old female with history of fibromyalgia presents with chronic pelvic pain, urgency, and frequency exacerbated by bladder filling. She has had one empiric course of antibiotics. Urinalysis shows 1 WBC/HPF, 8 RBC/HPF, and no bacteria. Urine culture is negative. The most appropriate next step is:

a Another course of antibiotics
b Amitriptyline
c Pentosan polysulfate
d Urine cytology

References

1 Campbell MF, Wein AJ, Kavoussi LR. *Campbell-Walsh Urology*. 9th ed. Philadelphia, PA: Saunders Elsevier; 2007.
2 Wein AJ, Hanno PM, Gillenwater JY. Interstitial cystitis: an introduction to the problem. In: Hanno PM, Staskin DR, Krane RJ, Wein AJ, editors. *Interstitial Cystitis: Current Concepts*. London: Springer-Verlag; 1990. pp. 13–15.
3 Warren JW, Keay SK, Meyers D, Xu J. Concordance of interstitial cystitis in monozygotic and dizygotic twin pairs. *Urology* 2001;57:22–25.
4 O'Leary MP, Sant GR, Fowler FJ, Jr., Whitmore KE, Spolarich-Kroll J. The interstitial cystitis symptom index and problem index. *Urology* 1997;49:58–63.
5 Parsons CL, Housley T, Schmidt JD, Lebow D. Treatment of interstitial cystitis with intravesical heparin. *Br J Urol* 1994;73:504–507.
6 Morales A, Emerson L, Nickel JC, Lundie M. Intravesical hyaluronic acid in the treatment of refractory interstitial cystitis. *J Urol* 1996;156:45–48.

Answers to multiple choice questions

1 **c** All the listed options are indicated in the initial evaluation of patients with interstitial cystitis except urodynamic testing. Urodynamics are optional and are reserved for complex cases.

2 **d** Interstitial cystitis is a diagnosis of exclusion. In patients suspected to have interstitial cystitis, the presence of hematuria or microhematuria should prompt further evaluation for an underlying malignancy. Carcinoma *in situ* can sometimes present similar to interstitial cystitis. While one empiric course of antibiotics may be tried in patients with interstitial cystitis, repeated antibiotic courses in the absence of documented infection is not recommended.

Section 6 Oncology

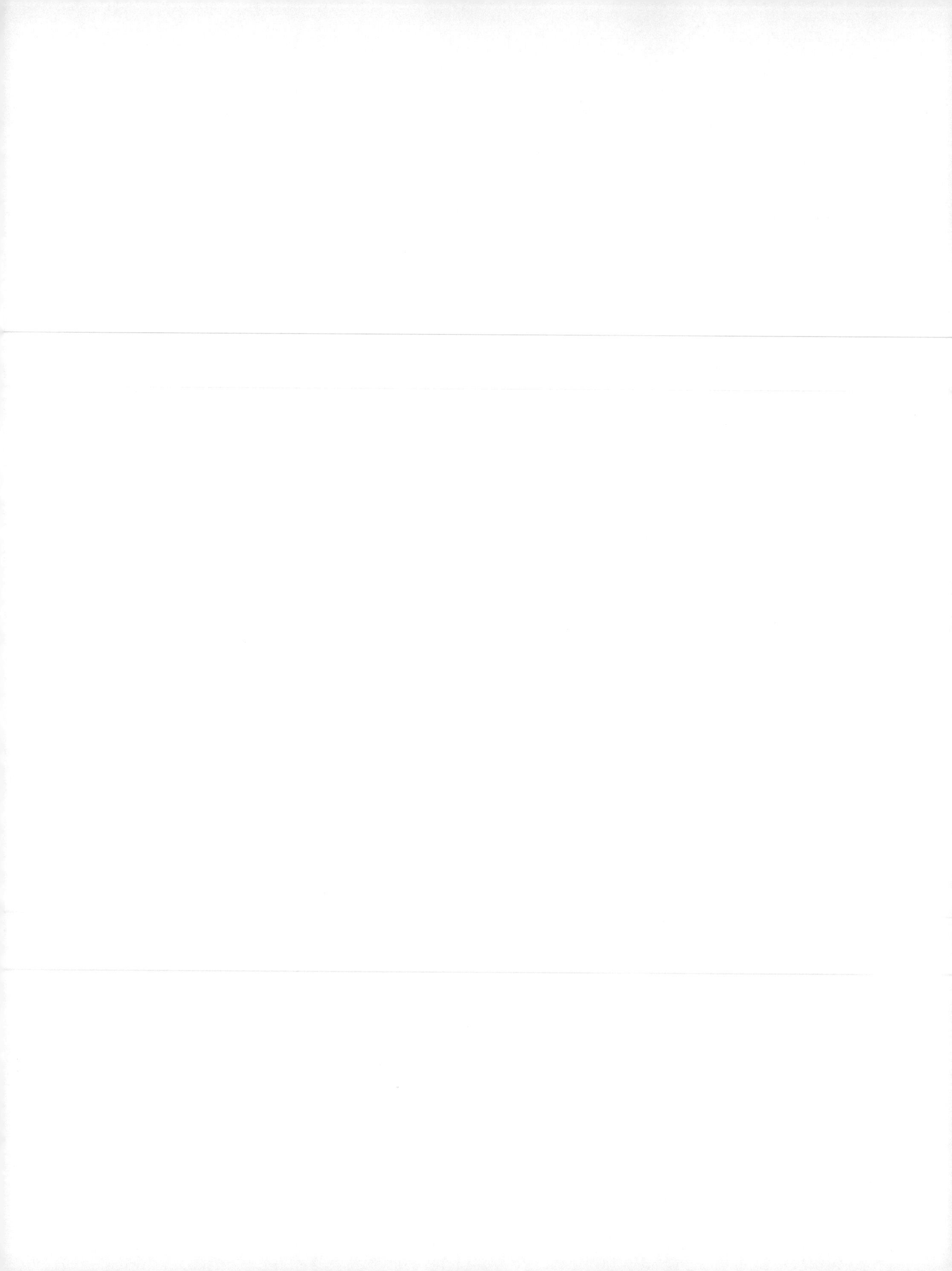

16 Prostate cancer screening and diagnosis

John B. Eifler

The James Buchanan Brady Urological Institute and Department of Urology, The Johns Hopkins School of Medicine, Baltimore, MD, USA

KEY POINTS

- Prostate cancer is the most common non-skin cancer malignancy in American men and the second leading cause of cancer death.
- Since the introduction of prostate-specific antigen (PSA) screening, the proportion of patients with local–regional disease has increased, while the proportion presenting with metastatic disease has decreased. Thus, PSA testing has allowed diagnosis of prostate cancer while the disease is more likely to be confined to the prostate.
- PSA screening remains controversial, and the risks and benefits of screening should be discussed with patients prior to initiating PSA screening.
- Transrectal ultrasound-guided prostate biopsy with 10–14 representative cores is the standard method for diagnosing prostate cancer.
- The grade of prostate cancer on biopsy (categorized by the Gleason score) carries the greatest prognostic information of any preoperative clinical variable currently available.
- Risk stratification using biopsy Gleason score, serum PSA, and clinical stage allows accurate pretreatment assessment of prognosis.
- The majority of patients do not require imaging prior to therapy for localized prostate cancer.

CASE STUDY 1

A 60-year-old man is found by his primary care provider to have a PSA of 6.5 with percentage free PSA of 9%. This is the patient's first PSA test. He is otherwise healthy with no comorbidities or previous surgeries, and he reports no lower urinary tract symptoms (LUTS) or erectile dysfunction. He denies ever having a urinary tract infection or urologic procedure. On digital rectal examination (DRE), his prostate is found to have a smooth contour with no palpable nodules or induration. A TRUS-guided prostate biopsy is performed which reveals atypical glands in three separate cores on the left side. Repeat biopsy is performed 6 weeks later and demonstrates Gleason 3 + 4 = 7 disease at the left apex in two of the two cores. The patient elects to undergo a radical prostatectomy.

CASE STUDY 2

A 55-year-old man is referred to the urology clinic for having an elevated PSA at 5.3. He has been healthy with the exception of a recent pneumonia treated with levofloxacin. He undergoes TRUS-guided prostate biopsy in the urology clinic. That night, the patient presents to the emergency department with fever of 103.1°C, rigors, and tachycardia of 120s. WBC count is 18.2, and urinalysis shows positive leukocyte esterase and positive nitrites. While awaiting culture results, he is placed on amikacin. Over the next 2 days, his fevers resolve and laboratory abnormalities normalize. He is discharged on IV amikacin to complete a 14-day course, and urine culture reveals ESBL-producing *E. coli* resistant to penicillin, cephalosporins, and fluoroquinolones.

Handbook of Urology, First edition. J. Kellogg Parsons, John B. Eifler and Misop Han. © 2014 by John Wiley & Sons, Ltd.
Published 2014 by John Wiley & Sons, Ltd.

Introduction

Prostate cancer is the most common non-skin cancer of American men, with over 240,000 cases expected in 2011. It is also the second leading cause of cancer death in American men behind lung cancer, with over 33,000 deaths projected in 2011 [1]. Approximately one in six men is diagnosed with prostate cancer in their lifetime. More than 90% of men are diagnosed with local or regional stage disease, which has a 5-year survival that approaches 100% [1].

Between 1990 and 2007, the mortality rate of prostate cancer has decreased by 39%, primarily due to improvements in diagnosis and treatment [1]. In addition to the potential benefits of prostate cancer screening, the decrease in mortality may be related to increased utility of aggressive prostate cancer treatment in the 1980s, including increases in the use of radical prostatectomy and external beam radiation therapy [2].

Age, race, and family history are the strongest risk factors for prostate cancer. The incidence of prostate cancer increases with age, with the median age of diagnosis of 67 years. Autopsy studies have suggested that 30% of men between the ages of 30 and 40 years as well as 90% of men between 70 and 90 years old may harbor the disease [3, 4]. Thus the majority of elderly men who harbor prostate cancer will not die of the disease. African-American men have the greatest risk of being diagnosed with prostate cancer (hazard ratio 1.6 compared to white American men) and dying (hazard ratio 2.4 compared to white men) from prostate cancer [1]. Other ethnic groups, including Asian Americans, American Indians, and Hispanics, do not have an increased probability of dying of prostate cancer [1]. Men with a first-degree relative diagnosed with prostate cancer are more than twice as likely to be diagnosed with the disease as men without an involved first-degree relative [5].

Since the adoption of prostate-specific antigen (PSA) screening, the stage of disease at the time of diagnosis has changed substantially [6, 7]. The proportion of patients with local–regional disease has increased, while the proportion presenting with metastatic disease has decreased accordingly [1]. Of men who undergo radical prostatectomy at Johns Hopkins, the proportion of men with organ-confined disease has also increased, from 54% in 1993 to 73% in 2007 [6].

Prostate-specific antigen

PSA is a serine protease of the kallikrein family produced by prostatic epithelium that is a component of seminal fluid. Elevation in serum levels of PSA is commonly associated with benign prostatic hyperplasia (BPH), prostate cancer, or prostatitis. However, serum PSA levels also increase with age, African-American ethnicity, and with increasing prostate volume [8]. PSA expression is also affected by androgen levels; 5α-reductase inhibitors (such as finasteride and dutasteride) and androgen-deprivation therapy may significantly decrease PSA and make it an unreliable marker for prostatic pathology. Other therapies that reduce prostate volume, such as radiation therapy or surgical therapy involving the prostate (including transurethral resection of the prostate, TURP) may reduce serum PSA as well [9]. In addition, the administration of antibiotics may decrease the serum PSA if the elevation is related to prostatitis [10]. These factors should always be considered when interpreting PSA levels. Furthermore, there is considerable variability in PSA level on repeat screening [11], and repeat PSA screening should be considered prior to prostate biopsy.

In men treated with 5α-reductase inhibitor, a baseline PSA measurement should be obtained prior to therapy. Of note, using low-dose finasteride treatment for male pattern baldness has the same effect [12]. Unfortunately, the change in PSA as a result of 5α-reductase inhibitor therapy is variable, and thus, the proper screening protocol for these patients remains controversial. In the Prostate Cancer Prevention Trial (PCPT), the PSA level was multiplied by 2.3 once the patient had taken the medication for >2 years [13], which is a good rule of thumb if the pretreatment PSA is unknown. Another proposed technique is to find the PSA nadir after initiating finasteride, then perform biopsy for *any* subsequent increase in PSA [14]. Complicating matters, the use of 5α-reductase inhibitors has been found in subset analyses to be associated with high-risk prostate cancers. These considerations should be discussed with patients prior to initiating 5α-reductase inhibitor therapy.

Total serum PSA is typically used in prostate cancer screening. The incidence of prostate cancer and the risk of future prostate cancer increase with increasing serum PSA, and a cut off of 4 ng/mL was initially used as a threshold for prostate biopsy. However, data from the PCPT demonstrate that there is no PSA cutoff below which men had an insignificant risk of cancer [15]. Thus, Thompson et al. recommend using PSA together with family history, race, and digital rectal examination (DRE) findings in deciding who should undergo prostate biopsy. Because of the lack of sensitivity and specificity using serum PSA alone, investigators have attempted to increase the accuracy by adjusting for prostate volume (PSA density), rate of change over time (PSA velocity), and percentage of PSA complexed with serine proteases in serum (percentage free PSA).

PSA density: because PSA is dependent on prostate volume and can be elevated in patients with BPH, PSA density (defined as serum PSA divided by prostate volume) has been proposed [16]. PSA density >0.15 has been associated with prostate cancer aggressiveness [17]. Like PSA, it lacks the accuracy to be used as a single screening test for prostate cancer, but it may serve as an additional tool to fully evaluate whether a patient requires a prostate biopsy.

PSA velocity: patients with prostate cancer also tend to have an increased rate of change in PSA over time than men with benign etiology of PSA elevation. Thus, PSA velocity (defined as change in PSA corrected for the elapsed time between measurements) is likely to be higher in men with prostate cancer. Men with a PSA between 4 and 10 with a PSA velocity >0.75 ng/mL/year have a high likelihood of harboring prostate cancer, and PSA velocity >0.35 ng/mL/year is associated with future risk of developing life-threatening prostate cancer [18]. However, some authors have found that PSA velocity offers little prognostic benefit over PSA alone [19].

Free PSA: PSA complexes with $\alpha 1$ antichymotrypsin in solution and the percentage of unbound PSA has been studied for its relationship with prostate cancer (percentage free PSA). Men with cancer tend to have a higher proportion of bound PSA, thus a lower percentage free PSA.

As a result of the association between increased serum PSA and prostate cancer, screening with serum PSA has become commonplace in the United States. Recently, two large randomized-controlled trials in the United States and Europe evaluating the effectiveness of PSA screening have presented interim results. The Prostate, Lung, Colorectal, and Ovarian Cancer (PLCO) trial randomized men to PSA screening arm or to a control arm without screening, finding no difference in prostate-cancer-specific mortality between the two arms with a median follow-up of 11 years. The trial suffered from a high contamination rate, that is, nearly half of the participants in the control arm had undergone PSA screening beforehand. Because men with a diagnosis of prostate cancer were excluded, this may have biased the study population toward men with low risk of prostate cancer. Furthermore, reanalysis of the data to compare mortality outcomes in men who actually underwent PSA screening and those who did not demonstrated a significant survival benefit for men who underwent PSA screening [20], though any secondary subset analysis should be closely scrutinized. In the European Randomized Prostate Cancer Screening trial (ERSPC), European men with no prior PSA screening were randomized to the screening arm (PSA) or the control arm in several trial locations throughout seven countries in the European Union. This trial demonstrated an ~20% decrease in relative risk of prostate-cancer-specific mortality with PSA screening after a median of 9 years of follow-up. However, it is estimated that 1055 need to be screened and 37 need to be treated to prevent one death with screening within this period [21]. The ERSPC study was not affected by the contamination seen in the control arm of the PLCO study, which may have allowed the statistical power to detect the relative risk reduction in prostate-cancer-specific mortality. Nonetheless, both studies highlight the risks of overdiagnosis and overtreatment associated with PSA screening. Given the long natural history of prostate cancer, longer follow-up of the ERSPC cohort may demonstrate a more impressive survival benefit in men who undergo screening.

Unfortunately, determining *which* men diagnosed with prostate cancer will benefit from treatment is not possible with contemporary technology. Thus, patients interested in being screened for prostate cancer should be informed of the risk of overdiagnosis and overtreatment as well as the potential side effects of prostate cancer treatments.

Currently, the AUA and American Cancer Society recommend annual screening beginning at age 50 years *in well-informed participants who understand the risk of overdiagnosis and overtreatment*, with earlier screening in men with a positive family history or black race [10, 22]. The United States Preventive Services Task Force recently posted a preliminary update to the recommendations on PSA screening, suggesting that most men should not undergo screening due to the risk of overdiagnosis and overtreatment [23]. As the differences in these recommendations make clear, the optimum schedule for PSA screening remains controversial. Before initiating PSA screening, patients should be counseled regarding the risks and benefits so that they can make an informed decision.

Other prostate cancer markers

PCA-3: PCA-3 is a noncoding mRNA expressed in all prostate cells but at higher levels in prostate cancer cells. The advantage over PSA is that PCA-3 is independent of prostate volume and age. Despite these advantages, some have suggested that PCA-3 level does not correlate with stage or grade of prostate cancer [24], and thus the clinical role of PCA-3 remains uncertain. Urine assays to detect PCA-3 are currently available, which are administered after patients undergo a prostate examination (prostatic massage).

TMPRSS2:ERG fusion protein: recent studies have demonstrated that gene rearrangements are common in patients with prostate cancer. An abnormal gene fusion involving the androgen regulated gene *TMPRSS2* and the *ETS* transcription factor gene has been found in ~50% of patients with prostate cancer [25]. A urine test can detect *TMPRSS2:ERG* fusion in the urine of men with prostate cancer with very high specificity. Unfortunately, some authors suggest that the fusion product is only found in 15% of prostate cancer patients, limiting its utility [26].

As the number of useful biomarkers increases, it is likely that future clinicians will have panels of biomarkers to assist in the decision to biopsy patients with suspected prostate cancer [27].

Transrectal ultrasound-guided prostate biopsy

Men who have an elevated PSA or abnormal DRE finding are recommended to undergo transrectal ultrasound-guided prostate biopsy to randomly sample prostate tissue from the peripheral zone of the prostatic base, mid, or apex from both sides. Prior to the procedure, patients should be counseled to stop antiplatelet agents 7–10 days prior to the biopsy, and those taking warfarin should be bridged with enoxaparin, stopping at least 24 hours prior to the procedure. Patients with significant coagulopathy, anorectal pathology, severe immunosuppression, as well as active acute prostatitis should be counseled not to undergo transrectal biopsy. The AUA recommends administering antibiotic therapy prior to the procedure, and a 1-day or 3-day course of fluoroquinolone has commonly been used [28]. Fluoroquinolone resistance has been increasing in several regions within the United States, and alternative agents used prior to prostate biopsy have been proposed, including first- or third-generation cephalosporins. Some authors recommend a tap water enema on the morning of the procedure to evacuate the rectum, which improves ultrasound acoustic performance and may decrease the risk of infectious complications.

The procedure is performed by placing patients in the left lateral decubitus position with knees tucked toward the chest. The ultrasound probe is introduced into the rectum, and the prostate volume is assessed using measurements in the transverse and sagittal planes. Lidocaine is typically administered at the base of the seminal vesicle under ultrasound guidance. The prostate is then surveyed for hypoechoic lesions, which would be suspicious for cancer and should be biopsied separately. A spring-driven needle core biopsy gun is used to sample the peripheral zone of the apex, mid, and base bilaterally under ultrasound guidance, which is where 85% of prostate tumors are found [27]. Contemporary extended core biopsy techniques typically utilize 10–14 cores.

It is estimated that this technique samples 1/1000 of the tissue of the prostate to assess for large cancers, and as a result may miss clinically significant prostate cancers. For men with elevated PSA between 4 and 10 ng/mL, ~22% will be found to harbor prostate cancer on sextant biopsy [29]. An additional 10% of patients with negative prostate biopsy who undergo repeat biopsy will be found to harbor prostate cancer. Furthermore, for men diagnosed with low-risk prostate cancer, ~30% will be upstaged or upgraded on repeat biopsy. **Patients with an elevated PSA and negative prostate biopsy represent a difficult management quandary. In these circumstances, a second biopsy is warranted, whereas third and fourth biopsies are unlikely to be positive and even then typically reveal low-grade and low-stage disease** [30].

The improved cancer detection rates with extended core techniques over sextant biopsy has led many to pursue "saturation" biopsy techniques, in which 20–50 cores may be taken from the prostate, which have been found to have increased cancer detection rates [31]. However, these typically carry an increased anesthetic requirement and the potential for greater morbidity.

Prostate biopsy complications

Though prostate biopsy carries a low risk of significant morbidity, systemic infections and hemorrhage may occur. Approximately 2% of patients will develop a febrile urinary tract infection despite prophylactic fluoroquinolone administration that requires hospitalization, and this rate may increase with time as the incidence of fluoroquinolone-resistant *Escherichia coli* (FREC) in the community increases [32]. Whether the use of alternative agents for prophylaxis such as third-generation cephalosporins in areas with high prevalence of FREC will decrease the risk remains uncertain. Rectal bleeding is typically minor and may be controlled with direct digital pressure. Occasionally, anoscopy is required to oversew a bleeding artery. Acute urinary retention may occur after biopsy in <1% of patients [33]. Hematospermia is common after the procedure and may cause significant anxiety for patients.

Results of biopsy—Gleason score, HGPIN, atypia

Each biopsy core is assessed by the pathologist, and if tumor is present, the grade of the tumor is categorized using the Gleason scoring system. The Gleason score is determined by pathologists by examining the histologic architecture of a tumor and assigning a score from 1 to 5, with 1 being least aggressive and 5 being most aggressive. The Gleason score reports the two most prevalent patterns in each biopsy core, with the most prevalent pattern reported first [34]. For instance, a biopsy core containing a large degree of pattern 3 and small amount of pattern 4 would be Gleason 3 + 4 = 7, whereas a patient with more pattern 4 would be Gleason 4 + 3 = 7. According to the most recent iteration of the Gleason scoring system, Gleason 3 + 3 = 6 represents the least aggressive histologic pattern [34]. **The grade of prostate cancer on biopsy carries the greatest prognostic information of any preoperative clinical variable currently available.**

Another entity frequently encountered in clinical practice is high-grade prostatic intraepithelial neoplasia (HGPIN), which is thought to be a precursor lesion of prostate cancer. Patients found to have this entity have a 26.4% risk of finding prostate cancer in subsequent biopsies [35], which is similar to men who have a benign finding on biopsy. Thus, only patients with extensive HGPIN are recommended to undergo repeat biopsy within a year [35]. Atypical small acinar proliferation (ASAP) is also associated with an increased risk of prostate adenocarcinoma on subsequent biopsy, and immediate repeat biopsy is recommended.

Clinical staging and prostate cancer risk stratification

After prostate biopsy, pretreatment parameters such as DRE findings (clinical stage), serum PSA, biopsy Gleason score, number and extent of positive biopsy cores may be used to predict the extent of disease (stage) as well as to stratify patients based on the risk of harboring aggressive disease.

Contemporary clinical staging of prostate cancer is based primarily on the DRE as specified by the American Joint Committee on Cancer (AJCC; see Table 16.1). Of note, if prostate cancer is the result of PSA screening and DRE is negative, the clinical stage is T1c. If the tumor is palpable (induration or palpable nodule on DRE), the clinical stage is T2 or greater.

Pretreatment parameters using data obtained from DRE, prostate biopsy, and serum PSA have been used to risk stratify patients with prostate cancer. A few approaches are frequently cited in the urologic literature and deserve special mention. The Partin tables use serum PSA, biopsy Gleason score, and clinical stage to predict the likelihood that cancer would be confined to the prostate (pT2), have extraprostatic extension (pT3), invade the seminal vesicles (pT3b), or spread to the pelvic lymph nodes (pN+) if the patient were to undergo radical prostatectomy [36, 37]. The Partin tables are useful for counseling patients about the predicted stage of their disease and in the decision to perform a pelvic lymphadenectomy. The Han and Kattan nomograms use serum PSA, biopsy Gleason, and clinical stage to predict the likelihood of biochemical recurrence (PSA elevation after radical prostatectomy), which is also helpful in counseling patients [38, 39]. Finally, a frequently used classification system for prostate cancer was created by D'Amico et al. which categorizes patients as low risk (PSA < 10, biopsy Gleason sum is ≤6, *and* clinical stage is T1c or T2a), intermediate risk (PSA ≥ 10

Table 16.1

AJCC TNM tumor classification system for prostate cancer		
	Tx	Cannot be assessed
	T0	No evidence of primary tumor
	T1a (TURP)	Incidental finding in ≤5% of tissue resected
T1: clinically inapparent (−DRE)	T1b (TURP)	Incidental finding in >5% of tissue resected
	T1c (PSA)	Tumor identified by needle biopsy
T2: palpable, confined to prostate	T2a (+DRE)	Tumor involves one-half of one lobe
	T2b (+DRE)	Tumor involves more than one-half of one lobe but not both lobes
	T2c (+DRE)	Tumor involves both lobes
T3: tumor beyond prostate	T3 (+DRE)	Tumor invades extraprostatic soft tissue (T3a) or SV (T3b)
T4: tumor invades adjacent structures	T4 (+DRE)	Tumor is fixed or invades adjacent structures (bladder, rectum, pelvic side wall)

but <20 *or* clinical stage T2b/T2c *or* biopsy Gleason sum of 7), or high risk (PSA ≥ 20 *or* clinical stage ≥T3a *or* biopsy Gleason sum ≥8) [40].

In addition to serum PSA, biopsy Gleason score, and clinical stage, other clinically available parameters may be used to predict the aggressiveness of prostate cancer, including the number (or percentage) of positive cores, the maximum percentage of any core involved with cancer, the presence of perineural invasion, and prostate volume. Imaging studies, particularly prostate MRI, may improve risk stratification further in carefully selected patients and is an area of active research.

Imaging for metastatic prostate cancer

Prostate cancer tends to metastasize first to the pelvic lymph nodes, then to bone and visceral organs. The NCCN recommends screening for bone metastases with radionuclide bone, which is currently the most sensitive modality for detecting skeletal metastasis, in all prostate cancer patients with PSA > 20, in those with palpable disease and PSA > 10, in any patient with Gleason score >7, in anyone with clinical T3 or T4 disease, and in patients who have bone pain [41]. Suspicious lesions found on bone scan should be imaged with MRI. CT scan should be performed to screen for metastatic disease to the lymph nodes or visceral organs in men with clinical T3/T4 disease or in those with nomogram risk of lymph node metastasis above 20% [41].

WHAT TO AVOID/KEY PITFALLS

- Most men diagnosed with prostate cancer should not undergo diagnostic bone scan unless they are symptomatic or have high-risk disease.
- Fever and the systemic inflammatory response syndrome in patients undergoing transrectal ultrasound-guided prostate biopsy with fluoroquinolone prophylaxis should raise suspicion for FREC, and amikacin or a third-generation cephalosporin should be administered while awaiting culture data.
- Men with a life expectancy of <10 years should not be offered PSA screening.
- Focal HGPIN on prostate biopsy is not associated with an increased risk of prostate cancer and does not merit repeat biopsy. If diffuse HGPIN is present, repeat biopsy should be performed within 1 year.

KEY WEB LINKS

National Comprehensive Cancer Network Guidelines in Oncology; Prostate Cancer
http://www.nccn.org/professionals/physician_gls/pdf/prostate.pdf

National Comprehensive Cancer Network Guidelines: Prostate Cancer Early Detection
http://www.nccn.org/professionals/physician_gls/pdf/prostate_detection.pdf

American Cancer Society: Early Detection, Diagnosis, and Staging
http://www.cancer.org/Cancer/ProstateCancer/DetailedGuide/prostate-cancer-detection

American Urologic Association Guidelines. Prostate-Specific Antigen Best Practice Statement: 2009 Update
http://www.auanet.org/content/media/psa09.pdf

Multiple choice questions

1 A 55-year-old man with a PSA of 5.5 ng/mL undergoes TRUS-guided prostate biopsy. Pathology reveals an atypical focus, suspicious for prostate cancer. The next step is:

- a Antibiotic therapy for 6 weeks
- b PSA surveillance
- c Repeat biopsy in 6–12 months
- d Repeat biopsy within 3 months
- e Initiate 5α-reductase inhibitor therapy

2 A 50-year-old man presents to the urology clinic with a PSA of 2.1 ng/mL. He has no past medical history and takes finasteride 1 mg daily for male pattern baldness. He reports normal libido and erectile function, no lower urinary tract symptoms (LUTS), and prostate examination is normal. He denies family history of prostate cancer. The next step is:

- a Immediate prostate biopsy
- b Repeat PSA in 1 year
- c Antibiotic therapy for 6 weeks, then recheck PSA
- d Measure serum testosterone level
- e Pelvic MRI with endorectal coil

References

1 Siegel R, Ward E, Brawley O, Jemal A. Cancer statistics, 2011: the impact of eliminating socioeconomic and racial disparities on premature cancer deaths. *CA Cancer J Clin* 2011;61(4):212–236.

2 Walsh PC. Cancer surveillance series: interpreting trends in prostate cancer–part I: evidence of the effects of screening in recent prostate cancer incidence, mortality, and survival rates. *J Urol* 2000;163:364–365.

3 Sakr WA, Haas GP, Cassin BF, Pontes JE, Crissman JD. The frequency of carcinoma and intraepithelial neoplasia of the prostate in young male patients. *J Urol* 1993;150:379–385.

4 Haas GP, Sakr WA. Epidemiology of prostate cancer. *CA Cancer J Clin* 1997;47:273–287.

5 Steinberg GD, Carter BS, Beaty TH, Childs B, Walsh PC. Family history and the risk of prostate cancer. *Prostate* 1990;17:337–347.

6 Makarov DV, Trock BJ, Humphreys EB, et al. Updated nomogram to predict pathologic stage of prostate cancer given prostate-specific antigen level, clinical stage, and biopsy Gleason score (Partin tables) based on cases from 2000 to 2005. *Urology* 2007;69(6):1095–1101.

7 Catalona WJ, Smith DS, Ratliff TL, Basler JW. Detection of organ-confined prostate cancer is increased through prostate-specific antigen-based screening. *JAMA* 1993;270:948–954.

8 Stamey TA, Yang N, Hay AR, McNeal JE, Freiha FS, Redwine E. Prostate-specific antigen as a serum marker for adenocarcinoma of the prostate. *N Engl J Med* 1987;317:909–916.

9 Loeb S, Carter HB. Early detection, diagnosis, and staging of prostate cancer. In: Wein AJ, Kavoussi LR, Novick AC, Partin AW, Peters CA, editors. *Campbell-Walsh Urology*. 10th ed. Philadelphia, PA: Elsevier Saunders; 2011.

10 Greene KL, Albertsen PC, Babaian RJ, et al. Prostate specific antigen best practice statement: 2009 update. *J Urol* 2009;182(5):2232–2241.

11 Greene KL, Albertsen PC, Babaian RJ, et al. Prostate specific antigen best practice statement: 2009 update. *J Urol* 2013;189:S2–S11.

12 D'Amico AV, Roehrborn CG. Effect of 1 mg/day finasteride on concentrations of serum prostate-specific antigen in men with androgenic alopecia: a randomised controlled trial. *Lancet Oncol* 2007;8:21–25.

13 Thompson IM, Chi C, Ankerst DP, et al. Effect of finasteride on the sensitivity of PSA for detecting prostate cancer. *J Natl Cancer Inst* 2006;98(16):1128–1133.

14 Morgentaler A. Re: The interpretation of serum prostate specific antigen in men receiving 5alpha-reductase inhibitors: a review and clinical recommendations. *J Urol* 2007;177:1954.

15 Thompson IM, Pauler DK, Goodman PJ, et al. Prevalence of prostate cancer among men with a prostate-specific antigen level < or = 4.0 ng per milliliter. *N Engl J Med* 2004;350(22):2239–2246.

16 Benson MC, Whang IS, Pantuck A, et al. Prostate specific antigen density: a means of distinguishing benign prostatic hypertrophy and prostate cancer. *J Urol* 1992;147:815–816.

17 Tosoian JJ, Trock BJ, Landis P, et al. Active surveillance program for prostate cancer: an update of the Johns Hopkins experience. *J Clin Oncol* 2011;29:2185–2190.

18 Carter HB, Ferrucci L, Kettermann A, et al. Detection of life-threatening prostate cancer with prostate-specific antigen velocity during a window of curability. *J Natl Cancer Inst* 2006;98(21):1521–1527.

19 Vickers AJ, Wolters T, Savage CJ, et al. Prostate-specific antigen velocity for early detection of prostate cancer:

result from a large, representative, population-based cohort. *Eur Urol* 2009;56(5):753–760.

20 Crawford ED, Grubb R, 3rd, Black A, et al. Comorbidity and mortality results from a randomized prostate cancer screening trial. *J Clin Oncol* 2011;29(4):355–361.

21 Schroder FH, Hugosson J, Roobol MJ, et al. Prostate-cancer mortality at 11 years of follow-up. *N Engl J Med* 2012;366(11):981–990.

22 Brooks DD, Wolf A, Smith RA, Dash C, Guessous I. Prostate cancer screening 2010: updated recommendations from the American Cancer Society. *J Natl Med Assoc* 2010;102(5):423–429.

23 Lin K, Croswell JM, Koenig H, Lam C, Maltz A. Prostate-Specific Antigen-Based Screening for Prostate Cancer: An Evidence Update for the U.S. Preventive Services Task Force. Evidence Synthesis No. 90. AHRQ Publication No. 12-05160-EF-1. Rockville, MD: Agency for Healthcare Research and Quality; October 2011.

24 Hessels D, Klein Gunnewiek JM, van Oort I, et al. DD3(PCA3)-based molecular urine analysis for the diagnosis of prostate cancer. *Eur Urol* 2003;44(1):8–15; discussion 15–16.

25 Perner S, Mosquera JM, Demichelis F, et al. TMPRSS2-ERG fusion prostate cancer: an early molecular event associated with invasion. *Am J Surg Pathol* 2007;31(6):882–888.

26 Demichelis F, Fall K, Perner S, et al. TMPRSS2:ERG gene fusion associated with lethal prostate cancer in a watchful waiting cohort. *Oncogene* 2007;26(31):4596–4599.

27 Wein AJ, Kavoussi LR, Campbell MF, ScienceDirect (Online service). In: Wein AJ, Kavoussi LR, Novick AC, Partin AW, Peters CA, editors. *Campbell-Walsh urology.* 10th ed. Philadelphia, PA: Elsevier Saunders; 2011.

28 Wolf JS, Jr., Bennett CJ, Dmochowski RR, Hollenbeck BK, Pearle MS, Schaeffer AJ. Best practice policy statement on urologic surgery antimicrobial prophylaxis. *J Urol* 2008;179:1379–1390.

29 Djavan B, Ravery V, Zlotta A, et al. Prospective evaluation of prostate cancer detected on biopsies 1, 2, 3 and 4: when should we stop? *J Urol* 2001;166(5):1679–1683.

30 Djavan B, Milani S, Remzi M. Prostate biopsy: who, how and when. An update. *Can J Urol* 2005; 12(Suppl 1):44–48; discussion 99–100.

31 Fleshner N, Klotz L. Role of "saturation biopsy" in the detection of prostate cancer among difficult diagnostic cases. *Urology* 2002;60:93–97.

32 Patel U, Kirby R. Infections after prostate biopsy and antibiotic resistance. *BJU Int* 2008;101:1201–1202.

33 Raaijmakers R, Kirkels WJ, Roobol MJ, Wildhagen MF, Schrder FH. Complication rates and risk factors of 5802 transrectal ultrasound-guided sextant biopsies of the prostate within a population-based screening program. *Urology* 2002;60:826–830.

34 Epstein JI, Allsbrook WC, Jr., Amin MB, Egevad LL. The 2005 International Society of Urological Pathology (ISUP) Consensus Conference on Gleason Grading of Prostatic Carcinoma. *Am J Surg Pathol* 2005;29: 1228–1242.

35 Epstein JI, Herawi M. Prostate needle biopsies containing prostatic intraepithelial neoplasia or atypical foci suspicious for carcinoma: implications for patient care. *J Urol* 2006;175:820–834.

36 Partin AW, Yoo J, Carter HB, et al. The use of prostate specific antigen, clinical stage and Gleason score to predict pathological stage in men with localized prostate cancer. *J Urol* 1993;150:110–114.

37 Eifler J, Feng Z, Lin B, et al. An updated prostate cancer staging nomogram (Partin tables) based on cases from 2006 to 2011. *BJU Int* 2013;111(1):22–29.

38 Kattan MW, Eastham JA, Stapleton AM, Wheeler TM, Scardino PT. A preoperative nomogram for disease recurrence following radical prostatectomy for prostate cancer. *J Natl Cancer Inst* 1998;90:766–771.

39 Han M, Partin AW, Zahurak M, Piantadosi S, Epstein JI, Walsh PC. Biochemical (prostate specific antigen) recurrence probability following radical prostatectomy for clinically localized prostate cancer. *J Urol* 2003;169: 517–523.

40 D'Amico AV, Whittington R, Malkowicz SB, et al. Pretreatment nomogram for prostate-specific antigen recurrence after radical prostatectomy or external-beam radiation therapy for clinically localized prostate cancer. *J Clin Oncol* 1999;17:168–172.

41 Mohler J, Bahnson RR, Boston B, et al. NCCN clinical practice guidelines in oncology: prostate cancer. *J Natl Compr Canc Netw* 2010;8:162–200.

Answers to multiple choice questions

1 d Repeat biopsy within 3 months. An atypical focus diagnosed by prostate biopsy is associated with an increased risk of prostate cancer on subsequent biopsy. Repeat biopsy should be performed in these patients. On the contrary, HGPIN does not increase the risk of prostate cancer on repeat biopsy, and only men with extensive HGPIN should undergo repeat biopsy within 6–12 months. Men with symptoms of chronic prostatitis and an elevated PSA may benefit from prolonged antibiotic therapy. 5α-reductase inhibitor therapy is not indicated in patients with an atypical focus.

2 a Immediate prostate biopsy. 5α-reductase inhibitors decrease serum PSA approximately twofold, and low-dose finasteride used to treat male pattern baldness is also noted to have this effect. Thus, his adjusted PSA would be 4.2 ng/mL and prostate biopsy is indicated. Repeating PSA in 1 year risks a delay in diagnosis, but this would be appropriate in a patient with extensive HGPIN. Antibiotic therapy for 6 weeks may be considered in a patient presenting with symptoms of prostatitis. Serum testosterone level is not necessary in this patient with normal libido and erectile function. Pelvic MRI with endorectal coil is in clinical testing, but is currently not indicated in the diagnosis of prostate cancer.

17 Prostate cancer: localized

Stacy Loeb

Department of Urology, New York University School of Medicine and Manhattan Veterans Affairs Medical Center, New York, NY, USA

KEY POINTS

- Prostate cancer is a leading cause of cancer mortality.
- Localized prostate cancer is typically asymptomatic, and the presence of symptoms usually suggests advanced disease.
- Screening of asymptomatic men for prostate cancer can be done using the prostate-specific antigen (PSA) blood test and digital rectal examination (DRE).
- Screening has been shown to reduce metastasis and death from prostate cancer, but also leads to overdiagnosis and overtreatment.
- Prostate biopsy is necessary to make a histological diagnosis of prostate cancer.
- Staging of prostate cancer may include the PSA and DRE results prior to diagnosis, in conjunction with the histological findings on biopsy and results of imaging.
- Numerous nomograms and risk classification schemes are available to help guide treatment decisions.
- For men with clinically localized prostate cancer, treatment options include active surveillance, radical prostatectomy, radiation therapy, and cryotherapy.
- The selection of treatment depends upon risk classification, life expectancy, and patient preferences.

CASE STUDY

A 55-year-old African American man with no significant past medical history undergoes his first prostate-specific antigen (PSA) test as a part of a routine physical examination, which comes back at 8.5 ng/mL. Repeat measurement by his primary care physician is 8.6 ng/mL. On digital rectal examination (DRE), there is a small nodule on the left. He has no family history of prostate cancer, minimal lower urinary tract symptoms (International Prostate Symptom Score [IPSS] 5), and normal erectile function (Sexual Health Inventory for Men [SHIM] 25).

He undergoes an uneventful 12-core transrectal ultrasound-guided prostate biopsy, which reveals a prostate volume of 30 cc and no suspicious findings. The pathology comes back as Gleason 4 + 4 = 8 in one core from the left base (20%) and two additional cores of Gleason 3 + 3 = 6 (10% right base, 20% right mid). CT scan and bone scan reveal no evidence of metastatic disease.

The patient is counseled about management options for localized prostate cancer, and he expresses that maintaining sexual function is a priority. Active surveillance is discussed but is not recommended due to his young age, absence of comorbidities, and the presence of high-risk features. Other management options are also discussed, including radical prostatectomy, radiation therapy with concomitant hormonal therapy, and whole-gland cryotherapy. The patient is concerned about his sexual function with hormonal therapy or cryotherapy, so elects to undergo open nerve-sparing radical prostatectomy.

His perioperative course is uneventful and he is discharged home on postoperative day 1. The final pathology reveals Gleason 4 + 3 = 7 organ-confined disease with negative surgical margins. The patient does not receive any adjuvant therapy. Nine months later, he is continent, has an undetectable PSA, and his erectile function has almost returned to baseline (SHIM 23).

Handbook of Urology, First edition. J. Kellogg Parsons, John B. Eifler and Misop Han. © 2014 by John Wiley & Sons, Ltd. Published 2014 by John Wiley & Sons, Ltd.

Statistics and epidemiology

According to data from the World Health Organization, there were 272,223 deaths from prostate cancer worldwide in 2008 [1]. In 2013, there are an estimated 238,590 new prostate cancer cases and 29,720 disease-specific deaths in the United States.

Incidence and mortality rates of prostate cancer vary widely across the globe [1]. For example, the United States and Scandinavia have high incidence rates; whereas the incidence and mortality rates are lower in Asia. Within the United States, rates of prostate cancer also differ by ethnic heritage. Specifically, African Americans have an increased risk of prostate cancer diagnosis and advanced disease [3]. Conversely, Asian Americans have lower incidence and mortality from prostate cancer.

Autopsy studies have shown that the prevalence of histological prostate cancer shows a direct increase with age [4]. Similar trends are seen in clinical practice, such that age is used as one of the key variables to guide prostate cancer screening and management decisions [5].

There are several other well-established risk factors for prostate cancer, including a positive family history. A meta-analysis showed that men with a first-degree family history of prostate cancer have a 2.5-fold increased risk, and a greater risk with younger age at the relative's diagnosis [6]. However, it should be noted that family history encompasses both shared genetic and environmental factors. Moreover, men with a family history of prostate cancer may be more likely to undergo prostate-specific antigen (PSA) testing, thereby increasing the risk of screen-detected disease [7].

Overall, studies of concordance rates for prostate cancer between twins have estimated that heritable factors account for 42% of prostate cancer susceptibility [8]. In recent years, innovations in genetics research have led to the identification of numerous single-nucleotide polymorphisms which are associated with prostate cancer risk [9, 10].

Several environmental factors have also been studied for a relationship to prostate cancer risk. For example, studies have shown an association between increased sunlight exposure with decreased prostate cancer risk. Although some dietary and environmental factors have been studied for a possible association with increased prostate cancer risk (e.g., charred meat, calcium intake, and pesticides), these associations remain speculative and causality has not been proven [11–13].

Prostate cancer screening

Early prostate cancer does not typically cause symptoms. Current screening protocols incorporate PSA and digital rectal examination (DRE). PSA is a serine protease which liquefies the seminal coagulum and was first utilized in forensics to identify human semen. It was later discovered to also serve as a useful marker for prostatic disease [14]. Indeed, the risk of overall and aggressive prostate cancer increases directly with increasing PSA levels. In men from a clinical trial undergoing empiric biopsies with PSA <4 ng/mL, prostate cancer was detected in 6.6%, 10.1%, 17.0%, 23.9%, and 26.9% with PSA levels ≤0.5, 0.6–1.0, 1.1–2.0, 2.1–3.0, and 3.1–4.0 ng/mL, respectively [15]. Thus, even at low levels, PSA represents a valid marker for the presence of prostate cancer.

The problem is that serum PSA levels may also be elevated with manipulation (such as cystoscopic procedures, catheterization, and prostate biopsy) and in nonmalignant conditions such as benign enlargement and prostatitis; as such, it is not cancer specific [16]. Other factors may also affect PSA levels, including medications (e.g., 5-α-reductase inhibitors and statins), genetic factors, as well as the type of assay platform used in the measurement [17–22].

Despite these issues, PSA remains the foundation of prostate cancer screening. A randomized trial from Europe reported that PSA screening reduced the rate of disease-specific mortality by 21% at 11 years [23]. A smaller randomized trial in the United States showed no difference in prostate cancer mortality between men randomized to the screening and control arms [24]. However, several issues with this study, such as widespread PSA testing among "controls," may be responsible for the negative findings. Additional follow-up from these studies will provide more long-term data on mortality in the future.

In addition to the benefits of early detection and reduced mortality, PSA-based screening also has potential harms including the cost, anxiety, and possible side effects of unnecessary biopsies [25]. Due to concerns about the relative benefits and harms of prostate cancer screening, there are a wide range of professional organization guidelines. These range from initiating a conversation about screening at age 40 to discouraging population-based screening [26–30].

Other tools for screening

PSA exists in two forms in the circulation—a free form ("free PSA") or bound to proteins such as α-1-antichymotrypsin [31]. Studies in the 1990s showed that prostate cancer was significantly more likely with a lower percent-free PSA (%fPSA) [32]. Additionally, several isoforms exist which may be differentially expressed in benign and malignant tissues. Specifically, the "B-PSA" isoform has been associated with BPH, whereas proPSA is associated with a higher risk of total and aggressive prostate cancer [33]. The [-2] proPSA isoform and prostate health index (combining it with total and free PSA) are now approved as an adjunct in screening. [34, 35].

Aside from free PSA and isoforms, other variations on the PSA test may help increase specificity for prostatic malignancy. These include PSA density (dividing PSA by prostate volume) and PSA density of the transition zone (PSA divided by transition zone volume) [36, 37]. Another way to use the PSA test is to study changes over time, such as PSA velocity and PSA doubling time [38, 39]. In the future, genetic factors may also be used to adjust PSA levels or help determine the need for prostate biopsy, although their incremental utility has not been definitively shown and requires further evaluation [40]. Alternate markers have also been investigated for prostate cancer screening, including PCA3 [41]. Numerous studies have shown an association between PCA3 with prostate cancer detection on initial and repeat biopsy although many studies do not show an association with aggressiveness [42, 43].

Overall, screening increasingly involves the simultaneous consideration of multiple risk factors to make clinical decisions. This may be facilitated by multivariable nomograms or risk calculators [44, 45]. These are prediction tools which formally combine PSA with other risk factors such as age, family history, and DRE findings to provide more precise estimates of prostate cancer risk.

Prostate biopsy

Prostate biopsy remains the gold standard for histological diagnosis of prostate cancer. A declining number of cases are diagnosed in other ways such as transurethral resection of the prostate.

Prostate biopsy is typically performed transrectally using ultrasound guidance; however, a perineal approach is also possible in the United States. More recently, MRI-guided biopsies are being evaluated for patients particularly those with prior negative biopsy and persistent PSA elevations [46].

The 2012 National Comprehensive Cancer Network (NCCN) Guidelines recommend considering prostate biopsy for suspicious DRE, a PSA >2.5 ng/mL, or a PSA velocity ≥0.35 ng/mL/year [29]. Free PSA may also be used to aid in the decision for patients where the risks of biopsy and/or diagnosis are outweighed by comorbid conditions.

Although routine antimicrobial prophylaxis is recommended for men undergoing prostate biopsy, an increasing risk of hospitalization has been observed during the past decade in the United States and other countries [25, 47]. This may be related to increasing antimicrobial resistance. Noninfectious complications are also possible after biopsy. In a European screening trial, persistent hematuria, hematospermia, urinary retention, and pain were reported in 22.6%, 50.4%, 0.4%, and 7.5% of biopsies, respectively, although the vast majority were mild and self-limited [48]. In the future, improved biomarkers or imaging technology may help reduce or even avoid the need for invasive biopsy procedures in some men. In particular, there is active investigation into a role for MRI in this setting.

Once prostate biopsy is done, each core should be reviewed individually for the presence and extent of prostate cancer. Other possible diagnoses on prostate biopsy include prostatitis, high-grade prostatic intraepithelial neoplasia (a putative premalignant lesion), and atypical glands suspicious for carcinoma (for which prompt repeat biopsy is recommended) [49].

The majority of prostate cancers are adenocarcinoma, although other tumor types (e.g., small cell, sarcoma) are rarely identified on prostate biopsy [49]. Since management differs for these unusual histologies, this chapter specifically deals with adenocarcinoma. Grading for adenocarcinoma is based upon the Gleason grading system, which involves assigning a score from 1 to 5 to two most common histologic patterns which are then summed together. In instances where a higher grade tertiary pattern is present, a 2005 consensus conference recommended assigning the biopsy Gleason score based on the most common and highest grade patterns for clinical decision making [49].

Prostate cancer staging

Once a diagnosis of prostate cancer is made on biopsy, staging is necessary to determine the extent of disease and decide upon treatment. In this regard, a plethora of nomograms and tables are available to help assess prognosis. In 1993, the Partin tables were created using PSA, Gleason score, and clinical stage to predict pathologic features [50]. Other tables and nomograms are available using clinical and/or pathologic variables to predict biochemical recurrence and prostate cancer-specific mortality after treatment [51–54].

Alternatively, patients may be categorized into risk groups, which is useful to predict prognosis and guide therapy. These include the D'Amico risk groups: low (PSA ≤10 ng/mL, Gleason score ≤6, and clinical stage T1/T2a), intermediate (PSA 10–20 ng/mL, Gleason score 7, or clinical stage T2b), and high (PSA >20 ng/mL, Gleason score 8–10, or clinical stage ≥T2c) [55]. The 2013 NCCN guidelines use a similar classification scheme with an additional subcategory for "very low-risk" disease (clinical stage T1c, Gleason score ≤6, PSA <10 ng/mL, fewer than three positive biopsy cores with ≤50% cancerous involvement, and PSA density <0.15 ng/mL/g) [29].

Since regional and distant metastases are rare in low-risk patients, imaging is not required before proceeding to active surveillance or definitive therapy. However, for patients with higher risk features, imaging studies should be performed. For example, the NCCN recommends bone scan for clinical stage T1 disease with a PSA >20 ng/mL, clinical stage T2 disease with a PSA >10 ng/mL or Gleason score ≥8, clinical stage ≥T3, or symptoms [56]. Additionally, a CT or an MRI is recommended for patients with clinical stage ≥T3, or clinical stage T1/T2 disease with >10% predicted probability of lymph node metastases. Despite the availability of such guidelines on patient selection for pretreatment imaging studies, inappropriate imaging for low-risk disease is common.

Treatment for localized disease

For localized disease, there are many different management options [57]. Two of the most important considerations for treatment selection are risk classification and life expectancy [56]. Other essential factors in treatment selection are patient-specific characteristics and preferences. These variables are critical due to substantial differences in side-effect profiles, time commitment, and follow-up protocols between the various management options.

At one end of the spectrum is active surveillance. In the 2013 NCCN guidelines, this is the treatment of choice for men with low- or very low-risk disease and a life expectancy <10 years [56]. It is also an alternative to radiation therapy for intermediate-risk patients with a life expectancy <10 years, as well as low-risk patients with a life expectancy >10 years who wish to defer definitive therapy.

Although active surveillance has enrolled more patients over time, still the majority of men diagnosed with low-risk disease in the United States undergo initial definitive therapy [58]. Selection criteria for active surveillance vary between protocols, but are typically based on some combination of PSA, clinical stage, and Gleason score. The Johns Hopkins Active Surveillance Program was initiated in 1995 and includes men with clinical stage T1c prostate cancer, a PSA density <0.15, Gleason score ≤6, and a maximum of two positive cores on biopsy with ≤50% cancerous involvement. In a recent update, the 10-year freedom from intervention was 41% and there were no deaths from prostate cancer [59].

Another large active surveillance program from Canada includes men with clinical stage T1 or T2 disease and a PSA <15 ng/mL. During the early phase of the study, men older than 70 years with Gleason 7 disease were also included. However, due to a higher risk of progression in this population, the current protocol only includes men with a Gleason score ≤6 [60].

Advantages of active surveillance are the avoidance or delay of definitive treatment with its associated side effects. Although close follow-up is necessary, there is debate over the best triggers for intervention during active surveillance. At Johns Hopkins, annual surveillance biopsies are performed [61], whereas other programs also use PSA kinetics to evaluate for progressive disease [62]. Also, limitations in current diagnostic modalities result in understaging or undergrading in some cases. For example, in a population of men who would meet criteria for active surveillance but chose radical prostatectomy, 28% had adverse pathology features [63].

Another option for management of localized disease is radical prostatectomy, which may be offered to men with low-, intermediate-, and high-risk disease with at least a 10-year life expectancy [29]. There are many different approaches to this procedure [64]. The initial description in 1904 by Hugh Hampton Young employed a perineal approach. The retropubic approach was first used in 1947, but it was not frequently performed until the pioneering discoveries of Dr. Patrick Walsh in the early 1980s led the anatomic retropubic prostatectomy to become the gold standard for surgical management of prostate cancer [65].

Laparoscopic approaches to radical prostatectomy were subsequently developed but widespread utilization did not occur due to the technical difficulty [66, 67]. However, the development of a robotic platform to assist in laparoscopic radical prostatectomy helped to overcome these challenges and has rapidly accelerated in popularity in advance of long-term oncologic data [68]. Early comparisons suggest decreased intraoperative blood loss with robotic-assisted laparoscopic radical prostatectomy [69]; whereas many other metrics of surgical outcome are similar when the procedures are performed by experienced surgeons.

A Swedish randomized trial showed that radical prostatectomy, as compared to watchful waiting, was associated with a 38% relative reduction in prostate cancer mortality ($p = 0.01$) [70]. However, potential side effects of radical prostatectomy include incontinence and erectile dysfunction, regardless of approach. Rates of urinary and sexual dysfunction after radical prostatectomy vary based on surgical factors (e.g., nerve sparing) and importantly, patient-specific factors (e.g., preoperative functional status, age, and comorbidities) [71]. Bladder neck contracture is another possible urologic complication of radical prostatectomy. Thromboembolic complications are uncommon and perioperative mortality is rare [72].

Another management option for localized prostate cancer is radiation therapy, which is an option for patients with low- to high-risk disease [56]. Radiation therapy is available in two main forms. The first type is external beam radiation therapy, which uses linear accelerators to deliver photons to the prostate while minimizing dosage to surrounding tissues. Alternate forms of external beam radiation therapy are currently available using heavy particles (e.g., proton beam) instead of photons; however, these techniques are expensive and incremental value has not been proven.

The second main form of radiation therapy is brachytherapy, in which radioactive seeds (palladium 103 or iodine 125) are implanted into the prostate. Historically, this was performed freehand, but the technique has since been revolutionized with the use of image guidance (most commonly with transrectal ultrasound). Indeed, precise seed placement is critical for the oncologic efficacy of this technique.

With regard to side effects, radiation may potentially lead to progressive erectile dysfunction. Although radiation therapy has a lower risk of incontinence than radical prostatectomy [73], it may be associated with different genitourinary sequelae (e.g., radiation cystitis), as well as bowel dysfunction due to the proximity of the rectum to the radiation field.

For higher risk patients, concomitant androgen deprivation therapy is recommended in conjunction with radiation therapy [56]. Indeed, long-term outcomes from the randomized European Organisation for Research and Treatment of Cancer (EORTC) trial were recently reported, demonstrating a significant improvement in 10-year clinical disease-free survival and cancer-specific survival with combined therapy compared to radiation therapy alone in this patient population [74]. Nevertheless, hormonal therapy itself has numerous possible side effects including gynecomastia, hot flashes, and sexual dysfunction [57].

As with radical prostatectomy, there is substantial long-term data demonstrating the oncologic efficacy of radiation therapy for clinically localized prostate cancer. Contemporary randomized trials have not directly compared radical prostatectomy versus radiation therapy for clinically localized disease. Though there are numerous observational studies comparing surgery and radiation [75, 76], interpretation is hindered by differences in patient selection as well as the definition of biochemical recurrence [77].

Unlike radical prostatectomy where the main source of PSA has been removed, monitoring for PSA recurrence after radiation therapy is more complex. This is particularly true since transient "PSA bounces" may occur (especially after brachytherapy), which subsequently decline spontaneously. In 1996, American Society for Radiation Oncology (ASTRO) defined biochemical recurrence after radiation therapy as three consecutive PSA rises, and the time of failure was backdated to midway between the nadir and first PSA rise. Due to a lack of specificity for clinical outcomes, a subsequent consensus conference in 2005 adopted the Phoenix criteria (PSA rise by ≥2 ng/mL above the nadir value without backdating) as the new standard for defining biochemical recurrence after radiation therapy [78].

Another treatment modality for prostate cancer is cryotherapy, which uses cold temperatures to induce coagulative necrosis. According to an AUA Best Practice Statement (2008), cryotherapy is an option for men with clinically localized disease of any grade with a negative metastatic evaluation, and also for the treatment of locally recurrent disease after radiation therapy [79].

As with radical prostatectomy and radiation therapy, technological advances have significantly increased the safety and feasibility of cryotherapy over time. These include switching from liquid nitrogen to inert gas, the development of smaller cryoprobes, real-time imaging and temperature monitoring, and the use of urethral warming devices [79].

Currently, the technique is performed as a same-day surgery. Using transrectal ultrasound guidance, cryoneedles are placed into the prostate using a perineal template. Freeze–thaw cycles are performed with a urethral warmer in place, and the patient is discharged with a urinary catheter.

Although the cryotherapy procedure itself is generally well tolerated, the most significant functional side effect is erectile dysfunction [80, 81]. For example, in the Cryo On-Line Database (COLD) registry, only 32.3% of men who were potent prior to treatment had successful intercourse afterward. Accordingly, this procedure is best reserved for patients with preexisting impotence or who are not interested in preservation of sexual function [79]. The risk of side effects is greater when cryotherapy is used in the salvage setting for radio-recurrent disease.

With respect to oncologic outcomes, there is controversy over the appropriate definition for biochemical failure after cryotherapy. In some series, post-cryotherapy biopsies are also used as a way to identify treatment failure. In 4099 patients from the observational COLD registry, the 2-year recurrence-free survival rate was 75.5% [80]. This group also showed that the likelihood of a positive posttreatment biopsy varied based upon the presence of a rising PSA. In another study from the COLD registry including men aged >75 years, the 5-year progression-free survival was 79% using the ASTRO and 62.6% using the Phoenix definition, which differed based on D'Amico risk category [82].

Finally, there are several investigational treatment options for prostate cancer. One of these options is high-intensity focused ultrasound (HIFU), which causes coagulative necrosis of tissue using focused ultrasound waves. Similar to cryotherapy, it has been used both in the primary setting, as well as in the management of recurrent disease after radiation therapy. One of the largest series of HIFU in clinically localized disease reported a 5-year recurrence-free survival rate of 72% using the Phoenix criteria [83]. This treatment may be associated with urinary obstruction, leading some centers to perform a bladder outlet procedure in conjunction with HIFU [84]. Overall, a synthesis of the evidence by the United States Preventive Services Task Force concluded that there was insufficient evidence to fully compare the benefits and harms of HIFU [57]. It has been primarily used in Europe and Japan, and is not currently approved for use as a prostate cancer treatment in the United States [85].

Another investigational option is focal therapy, which involves treatment of a portion of the prostate instead of the whole gland (conceptually similar to a "lumpectomy" for breast cancer). Although organ-sparing procedures have become a standard of care for other forms of malignancy such as renal cell cancer, in this instance, it is complicated by the well-documented multifocality of prostate cancer. For example, among patients with unilateral low-risk disease on biopsy who underwent radical prostatectomy, 65% had prostate cancer on the contralateral side in the final pathologic specimen, with aggressive features present in 20% [86].

Despite the absence of high-quality data demonstrating its utility, there has been a significant increase in utilization of focal cryotherapy over time [80]. Compared to whole-gland cryotherapy, focal treatment is associated with a lower risk of erectile dysfunction [80], although long-term oncologic efficacy is uncertain. Other modalities are also being explored for focal therapy (HIFU, photodynamic therapy, radio frequency ablation and laser therapy [87]) and remain investigational. Overall, clinical trials are necessary to assess the safety and cost-effectiveness of focal therapy compared to other management strategies.

In conclusion, the treatment options for clinically localized prostate cancer have greatly expanded and improved over time. Since numerous management options are available with different relative advantages and disadvantages, the use of risk assessment tools and informed patient–physician discussions can aid in the optimal selection.

COMMON PITFALLS/WHAT TO AVOID

- PSA screening should not be performed in men with <10-year life expectancy who will not benefit from early detection.
- Imaging studies are not necessary for staging of low-risk prostate cancer patients.
- Treatment should be tailored to patient-specific characteristics.

KEY WEB LINKS

www.nccn.org
www.auanet.org
http://seer.cancer.gov

Multiple choice questions

1 Which of the following populations has the lowest prostate cancer incidence?
  a US Caucasian
  b African American
  c Asian
  d Scandinavian

2 All of the following are risk factors for prostate cancer except
  a Positive family history
  b Increased sunlight exposure
  c Increasing age
  d African American

3 Which of the following screening results is *not* associated with an increased risk of overall prostate cancer and aggressive disease?
  a High PSA density
  b High percent free PSA
  c High PSA
  d High PSA velocity

References

1 World Health Organization Global Health Observatory Repository Data. Available at http://apps.who.int/ghodata/?vid=10011 (Last accessed 17 November 2011).
2 American Cancer Society. Cancer Facts & Figures 2013. Available at http://www.cancer.org/acs/groups/content/@epidemiologysurveilance/documents/document/acspc-036845.pdf (Last accessed 1 June 2013).
3 Cancer of the Prostate- SEER Stat Fact Sheet. Available at http://seer.cancer.gov/statfacts/html/prost.html#incidence-mortality (Last accessed 28 November 2011).
4 Sakr WA, Grignon DJ, Crissman JD, et al. High grade prostatic intraepithelial neoplasia (HGPIN) and prostatic adenocarcinoma between the ages of 20–69: an autopsy study of 249 cases. *In Vivo* 1994;8(3):439–443.
5 Oesterling JE, Jacobsen SJ, Chute CG, et al. Serum prostate-specific antigen in a community-based population of healthy men. Establishment of age-specific reference ranges. *JAMA* 1993;270(7):860–864.
6 Johns LE, Houlston RS. A systematic review and meta-analysis of familial prostate cancer risk. *BJU Int* 2003;91(9):789–794.
7 Bratt O, Garmo H, Adolfsson J, et al. Effects of prostate-specific antigen testing on familial prostate cancer risk estimates. *J Natl Cancer Inst* 2010;102(17):1336–1343.
8 Lichtenstein P, Holm NV, Verkasalo PK, et al. Environmental and heritable factors in the causation of cancer—analyses of cohorts of twins from Sweden, Denmark, and Finland. *N Engl J Med* 2000;343(2):78–85.
9 Eeles RA, Kote-Jarai Z, Giles GG, et al. Multiple newly identified loci associated with prostate cancer susceptibility. *Nat Genet* 2008;40(3):316–321.
10 Zheng SL, Sun J, Wiklund F, et al. Cumulative association of five genetic variants with prostate cancer. *N Engl J Med* 2008;358(9):910–919.

11 Chan JM, Gann PH, Giovannucci EL. Role of diet in prostate cancer development and progression. *J Clin Oncol* 2005;23(32):8152–8160.
12 Punnen S, Hardin J, Cheng I, Klein EA, Witte JS. Impact of meat consumption, preparation, and mutagens on aggressive prostate cancer. *PLoS One* 2011;6(11):e27711.
13 John EM, Dreon DM, Koo J, Schwartz GG Residential sunlight exposure is associated with a decreased risk of prostate cancer. *J Steroid Biochem Mol Biol* 2004;89–90(1–5):549–552.
14 Stamey TA, Yang N, Hay AR, et al. Prostate-specific antigen as a serum marker for adenocarcinoma of the prostate. *N Engl J Med* 1987;317(15):909–916.
15 Thompson IM, Pauler DK, Goodman PJ, et al. Prevalence of prostate cancer among men with a prostate-specific antigen level < or =4.0 ng per milliliter. *N Engl J Med* 2004;350(22):2239–2246.
16 Tchetgen MB, Oesterling JE. The effect of prostatitis, urinary retention, ejaculation, and ambulation on the serum prostate-specific antigen concentration. *Urol Clin North Am* 1997;24(2):283–291.
17 Chang SL, Harshman LC, Presti JC, Jr. Impact of common medications on serum total prostate-specific antigen levels: analysis of the National Health and Nutrition Examination Survey. *J Clin Oncol* 2010;28(25): 3951–3957.
18 D'Amico AV, Roehrborn CG. Effect of 1 mg/day finasteride on concentrations of serum prostate-specific antigen in men with androgenic alopecia: a randomised controlled trial. *Lancet Oncol* 2007;8(1):21–25.
19 Etzioni RD, Howlader N, Shaw PA, et al. Long-term effects of finasteride on prostate specific antigen levels: results from the prostate cancer prevention trial. *J Urol* 2005;174(3):877–881.
20 Loeb S, Carter HB, Walsh PC, et al. Single nucleotide polymorphisms and the likelihood of prostate cancer at a given prostate specific antigen level. *J Urol* 2009;182(1):101–104; discussion 105.
21 Gudmundsson J, Besenbacher S, Sulem P, et al. Genetic correction of PSA values using sequence variants associated with PSA levels. *Sci Transl Med* 2010;2(62):1–9.
22 Loeb S, Chan DW, Sokoll L, et al. Prostate specific antigen assay standardization bias could affect clinical decision making. *J Urol* 2008;180(5):1959–1962; discussion 1962–3.
23 Schroder FH, Hugosson J, Roobol MJ, et al. Prostate-Cancer Mortality at 11 Years of Followup. *N Engl J Med* 2012;366(11):981–990.
24 Andriole GL, Crawford ED, Grubb RL, et al. Prostate cancer screening in the randomized Prostate, Lung, Colorectal, and Ovarian Cancer Screening Trial: mortality results after 13 years of follow-up. *J Natl Cancer Inst* 2012;104(2):125–132.
25 Loeb S, Carter HB, Berndt SI, Ricker W, Schaeffer EM. Complications after prostate biopsy: data from SEER-Medicare. *J Urol* 2011;186(5):1830–1834.
26 Heidenreich A, Aus G, Bolla M, et al. EAU guidelines on prostate cancer. *Eur Urol* 2008;53(1):68–80.
27 Schroder FH. Stratifying risk—the U.S. Preventive Services Task Force and prostate-cancer screening. *N Engl J Med* 2011;365(21):1953–1955.
28 U.S. Preventive Services Task Force. Screening for Prostate Cancer: Draft Recommendation Statement. Available at http://www.uspreventiveservicestaskforce.org/draftrec3.htm (Last accessed 29 October 2011).
29 National Comprehensive Cancer Network Clinical Practice Guidelines in Oncology. Available at http://www.nccn.org/professionals/physician_gls/pdf/prostate_detection.pdf (Last accessed 1 June 2013).
30 Carter HB, Albertsen PC, Barry MJ, et al. Early Detection of Prostate Cancer: AUA Guideline. Available at http://www.auanet.org/education/guidelines/prostate-cancer-detection.cfm. (Last accessed 1 June 2013).
31 Lilja H, Christensson A, Dahlen U, et al. Prostate-specific antigen in serum occurs predominantly in complex with alpha 1-antichymotrypsin. *Clin Chem* 1991;37(9): 1618–1625.
32 Catalona WJ, Partin AW, Slawin KM, et al. Use of the percentage of free prostate-specific antigen to enhance differentiation of prostate cancer from benign prostatic disease: a prospective multicenter clinical trial. *JAMA* 1998;279(19):1542–1547.
33 Canto, E.I., H. Singh, S.F. Shariat, et al. Serum BPSA outperforms both total PSA and free PSA as a predictor of prostatic enlargement in men without prostate cancer. *Urology* 2004;63(5):905–910; discussion 910-911.
34 Catalona WJ, Partin AW, Sanda MG, et al. A multicenter study of [-2] pro-prostate specific antigen combined with prostate specific antigen and free prostate specific antigen for prostate cancer detection in the 2.0 to 10.0 ng/ml prostate specific antigen range. *J Urol* 2011;185: 1650–1655.
35 Sokoll LJ, Wang Y, Feng Z, et al. [-2]proenzyme prostate specific antigen for prostate cancer detection: a national cancer institute early detection research network validation study. *J Urol* 2008;180(2):539–543; discussion 543.
36 Benson MC, Whang IS, Pantuck A, et al. Prostate specific antigen density: a means of distinguishing benign prostatic hypertrophy and prostate cancer. *J Urol* 1992;147(3 Pt 2):815–816.
37 Djavan, B., A. Zlotta, C. Kratzik, et al. PSA, PSA density, PSA density of transition zone, free/total PSA ratio, and PSA velocity for early detection of prostate cancer in men with serum PSA 2.5 to 4.0 ng/mL. *Urology* 1999;54(3):517–522.
38 Carter HB, Pearson JD, Metter EJ, et al. Longitudinal evaluation of prostate-specific antigen levels

in men with and without prostate disease. *JAMA* 1992;267(16):2215–2220.

39 Loeb S, Kettermann A, Ferrucci L, et al. PSA doubling time versus PSA velocity to predict high-risk prostate cancer: data from the Baltimore Longitudinal Study of Aging. *Eur Urol* 2008;54(5):1073–1080.

40 Nam RK, Zhang WW, Trachtenberg J, et al. Utility of incorporating genetic variants for the early detection of prostate cancer. *Clin Cancer Res* 2009;15(5): 1787–1793.

41 de Kok JB, Verhaegh GW, Roelofs RW, et al. DD3(PCA3), a very sensitive and specific marker to detect prostate tumors. *Cancer Res* 2002;62(9):2695–2698.

42 de la Taille A, Irani J, Graefen M, et al. Clinical evaluation of the PCA3 assay in guiding initial biopsy decisions. *J Urol* 2011;185(6):2119–2125.

43 Marks LS, Fradet Y, Deras IL, et al. PCA3 molecular urine assay for prostate cancer in men undergoing repeat biopsy. *Urology* 2007;69(3):532–535.

44 Roobol MJ, Steyerberg EW, Kranse R, et al. A risk-based strategy improves prostate-specific antigen-driven detection of prostate cancer. *Eur Urol* 2010;57(1):79–85.

45 Thompson IM, Ankerst DP, Chi C, et al. Assessing prostate cancer risk: results from the Prostate Cancer Prevention Trial. *J Natl Cancer Inst* 2006;98(8):529–534.

46 Lee SH, Chung MS, Chung BH. Magnetic resonance imaging targeted biopsy in men with previously negative prostate biopsies. *J Endourol* 2011;26(7):787–791.

47 Nam RK, Saskin R, Lee Y, et al. Increasing hospital admission rates for urological complications after transrectal ultrasound guided prostate biopsy. *J Urol* 2010;183(3):963–968.

48 Raaijmakers R, Kirkels WJ, Roobol MJ, Wildhagen MF, Schrder FH. Complication rates and risk factors of 5802 transrectal ultrasound-guided sextant biopsies of the prostate within a population-based screening program. *Urology* 2002;60(5):826–830.

49 Epstein JI, Allsbrook WC, Jr., Amin MB, Egevad LL. Update on the Gleason grading system for prostate cancer: results of an international consensus conference of urologic pathologists. *Adv Anat Pathol* 2006;13(1):57–59.

50 Partin AW, Yoo J, Carter HB, et al. The use of prostate specific antigen, clinical stage and Gleason score to predict pathological stage in men with localized prostate cancer. *J Urol* 1993;150(1):110–114.

51 Kattan MW, Eastham JA, Stapleton AM, Wheeler TM, Scardino PT. A preoperative nomogram for disease recurrence following radical prostatectomy for prostate cancer. *J Natl Cancer Inst* 1998;90(10):766–771.

52 Han M, Partin AW, Zahurak M, et al. Biochemical (prostate specific antigen) recurrence probability following radical prostatectomy for clinically localized prostate cancer. *J Urol* 2003;169(2):517–523.

53 Stephenson AJ, Kattan MW, Eastham JA, et al. Prostate cancer-specific mortality after radical prostatectomy for patients treated in the prostate-specific antigen era. *J Clin Oncol* 2009;27(26):4300–4305.

54 Eggener SE, Scardino PT, Walsh PC, et al. Predicting 15-year prostate cancer specific mortality after radical prostatectomy. *J Urol* 2011;185(3):869–875.

55 D'Amico AV, Whittington R, Malkowicz SB, et al. Biochemical outcome after radical prostatectomy, external beam radiation therapy, or interstitial radiation therapy for clinically localized prostate cancer. *JAMA* 1998;280(11):969–974.

56 National Comprehensive Cancer Network Clinical Practice Guidelines in Oncology version 2013. Available at http://www.nccn.org/professionals/physician_gls/pdf/prostate.pdf (Last accessed 1 June 2013).

57 Wilt TJ, MacDonald R, Rutks I, et al. Systematic review: comparative effectiveness and harms of treatments for clinically localized prostate cancer. *Ann Inter Med* 2008;148(6):435–448.

58 Miller DC, Gruber SB, Hollenbeck BK, Montie JE, Wei JT. Incidence of initial local therapy among men with lower-risk prostate cancer in the United States. *J Natl Cancer Inst* 2006;98(16):1134–1141.

59 Tosoian JJ, Trock BJ, Landis P, et al. Active surveillance program for prostate cancer: an update of the Johns Hopkins experience. *J Clin Oncol* 2011;29(16): 2185–2190.

60 Klotz L, Zhang L, Lam A, et al. Clinical results of long-term follow-up of a large, active surveillance cohort with localized prostate cancer. *J Clin Oncol* 2009;28(1):126–131.

61 Ross AE, Loeb S, Landis P, et al. Prostate-specific antigen kinetics during follow-up are an unreliable trigger for intervention in a prostate cancer surveillance program. *J Clin Oncol* 2010;28(17):2810–2816.

62 Klotz LH, Choo R, Morton G, Danjoux C Expectant management with selective delayed intervention for favorable-risk prostate cancer. *Can J Urol* 2002; 9(Suppl 1):2–7.

63 Suardi N, Briganti A, Gallina A, et al. Testing the most stringent criteria for selection of candidates for active surveillance in patients with low-risk prostate cancer. *BJU Int* 2010;105(11):1548–1552.

64 Schaeffer EM, Loeb S, Walsh PC. The case for open radical prostatectomy. *Urol Clin North Am.* 37(1):49–55, Table of Contents.

65 Walsh PC, Lepor H, Eggleston JC. Radical prostatectomy with preservation of sexual function: anatomical and pathological considerations. *Prostate* 1983;4(5):473–485.

66 Schuessler WW, Schulam PG, Clayman RV, Kavoussi LR. Laparoscopic radical prostatectomy: initial short-term experience. *Urology* 1997;50(6):854–857.

67 Guillonneau B, Vallancien G. Laparoscopic radical prostatectomy: initial experience and preliminary assessment after 65 operations. *Prostate* 1999;39(1):71–75.

68 Kang DC, Hardee MJ, Fesperman SF, Stoffs TL, Dahm P. Low quality of evidence for robot-assisted laparoscopic prostatectomy: results of a systematic review of the published literature. *Eur Urol* 2010;57(6):930–937.
69 Farnham SB, Webster TM, Herrell SD, Smith JA, Jr. Intraoperative blood loss and transfusion requirements for robotic-assisted radical prostatectomy versus radical retropubic prostatectomy. *Urology* 2006;67(2):360–363.
70 Bill-Axelson A, Holmberg L, Ruutu M, et al. Radical prostatectomy versus watchful waiting in early prostate cancer. *N Engl J Med* 2011;364(18):1708–1717.
71 Alemozaffar M, Regan MM, Cooperberg MR, et al. Prediction of erectile function following treatment for prostate cancer. *JAMA* 2011;306(11):1205–1214.
72 Secin FP, Jiborn T, Bjartell AS, et al. Multi-institutional study of symptomatic deep venous thrombosis and pulmonary embolism in prostate cancer patients undergoing laparoscopic or robot-assisted laparoscopic radical prostatectomy. *Eur Urol* 2008;53(1):134–145.
73 Hoffman RM, Hunt WC, Gilliland FD, Stephenson RA, Potosky AL. Patient satisfaction with treatment decisions for clinically localized prostate carcinoma. Results from the Prostate Cancer Outcomes Study. *Cancer* 2003;97(7):1653–1662.
74 Bolla M, Van Tienhoven G, Warde P, et al. External irradiation with or without long-term androgen suppression for prostate cancer with high metastatic risk: 10-year results of an EORTC randomised study. *Lancet Oncol* 2010;11(11):1066–1073.
75 Cooperberg MR, Vickers AJ, Broering JM, Carroll PR. Comparative risk-adjusted mortality outcomes after primary surgery, radiotherapy, or androgen-deprivation therapy for localized prostate cancer. *Cancer* 116(22):5226–5234.
76 Zelefsky MJ, Eastham JA, Cronin AM, et al. Metastasis after radical prostatectomy or external beam radiotherapy for patients with clinically localized prostate cancer: a comparison of clinical cohorts adjusted for case mix. *J Clin Oncol* 2010;28(9):1508–1513.
77 Nielsen ME, Makarov DV, Humphreys E, et al. Is it possible to compare PSA recurrence-free survival after surgery and radiotherapy using revised ASTRO criterion—"nadir +2"? *Urology* 2008;72(2):389–393; discussion 394–395.
78 Roach M, 3rd, Hanks G, Thames H, Jr., et al. Defining biochemical failure following radiotherapy with or without hormonal therapy in men with clinically localized prostate cancer: recommendations of the RTOG-ASTRO Phoenix Consensus Conference. *Int J Radiat Oncol Biol Phys* 2006;65(4):965–974.
79 Babaian RJ, Donnelly B, Bahn D, et al. Best practice statement on cryosurgery for the treatment of localized prostate cancer. *J Urol* 2008;180(5):1993–2004.
80 Ward JF, Jones JS. Focal cryotherapy for localized prostate cancer: a report from the national Cryo On-Line Database (COLD) Registry. *BJU Int* 2011;109(11): 1648–1654.
81 Caso JR, Tsivian M, Mouraviev V, Kimura M, Polascik TJ. Complications and postoperative events after cryosurgery for prostate cancer. *BJU Int* 2011;109(6): 840–845.
82 Dhar N, Ward JF, Cher ML, Jones JS. Primary full-gland prostate cryoablation in older men (> age of 75 years): results from 860 patients tracked with the COLD Registry. *BJU Int* 2011;108(4):508-12.
83 Uchida T, Shoji S, Nakano M, et al. Transrectal high-intensity focused ultrasound for the treatment of localized prostate cancer: eight-year experience. *Int J Urol* 2009;16(11):881-6.
84 Vallancien G, Prapotnich D, Cathelineau X, Baumert H, Rozet F Transrectal focused ultrasound combined with transurethral resection of the prostate for the treatment of localized prostate cancer: feasibility study. *J Urol* 2004;171(6 Pt 1):2265–2267.
85 Uchida T, Nakano M, Hongo S, et al. High-intensity focused ultrasound therapy for prostate cancer. *Int J Urol* 2011;19(3):187–201.
86 Yoon GS, Wang W, Osunkoya AO, et al. Residual tumor potentially left behind after local ablation therapy in prostate adenocarcinoma. *J Urol* 2008;179(6): 2203–2206; discussion 2206.
87 Eggener SE, Scardino PT, Carroll PR, et al. Focal therapy for localized prostate cancer: a critical appraisal of rationale and modalities. *J Urol* 2007;178(6): 2260–2267.

Answers to multiple choice questions

1 c
2 b
3 b

18 Prostate cancer: treatment of metastatic disease

John B. Eifler

The James Buchanan Brady Urological Institute and Department of Urology, The Johns Hopkins School of Medicine, Baltimore, MD, USA

KEY POINTS

- Prostate cancer cells are exquisitely sensitive to androgen.
- Castration leads to clinical improvement in the majority of men with metastatic prostate cancer.
- Chronic activation of the luteinizing hormone-releasing hormone (LHRH) receptor leads to downregulation of the receptor, resulting in low serum LH and testosterone levels.
- Antiandrogens inhibit the androgen receptor directly and can be steroidal or nonsteroidal agents.
- The majority of patients do not require imaging prior to therapy for localized prostate cancer.
- Androgen deprivation has long-term adverse effects, including osteoporosis, erectile dysfunction, decreased libido, decreased muscle mass, gynecomastia, increased risk of metabolic syndrome, and cardiovascular events.
- For men who fail androgen deprivation, taxane-based chemotherapy has been shown to improve disease-specific survival.
- Abiraterone inhibits androgen synthesis and has been shown to improve survival in men who fail docetaxel-based regimens.
- Sipuleucel-T is an immunotherapy recently approved by the FDA for men with asymptomatic or minimally symptomatic metastatic prostate cancer.
- Bisphosphonate therapy has been shown to decrease osteoporosis and skeletal-related events in men on androgen deprivation therapy.
- Spinal cord compression should be treated with immediate high-dose dexamethasone.

CASE STUDY 1

A 60-year-old man is diagnosed with Gleason 4 + 4 = 8 prostate cancer with PSA 108 ng/mL. Bone scan and CT scan are negative for metastatic disease. He is started on an LHRH agonist (leuprolide) and his PSA decreases to the undetectable range. Serum testosterone is 49 ng/dL. After 8 months of therapy, his serum PSA rises to 9 ng/mL. Bicalutamide is added to his regimen and again his PSA returns to undetectable levels, though the patient reports fatigue, lethargy, decreased muscle mass, gynecomastia, and erectile dysfunction. After 18 months, his PSA is seen to rise to 30 ng/mL. Repeat bone scans and CT scans are negative. Bicalutamide is discontinued, and his serum PSA decreases to 15 ng/mL. On re-check 3 months later, his PSA has risen to 50 ng/mL, and abiraterone is initiated with prednisone, resulting in undetectable PSA. His PSA begins rising after 6 months of abiraterone therapy, and by 12 months, it reaches 250 ng/mL. Bone scan reveals several metastases throughout the lumbar vertebrae as well as the right ischium. Abiraterone is discontinued, and he begins docetaxel chemotherapy as well as alendronate to decrease pathologic fractures. His PSA decreases to 100 ng/mL and his vertebral metastases decrease in size. On repeat imaging after 3 months, several new osteoblastic lesions are seen throughout the bony skeleton, and CT reveals multiple enlarged pelvic and retroperitoneal lymph nodes. The patient's creatinine has risen to 3.5, precluding further chemotherapy. He elects to enter home hospice, and 3 weeks later he expires.

CASE STUDY 2

A 55-year-old man with widely metastatic prostate cancer presents to the emergency department with severe back pain and leg weakness. PSA is 588 ng/mL in the ED, and MRI of the thoracic and lumbar spine reveals epidural metastasis with spinal cord compression. High-dose IV dexamethasone is administered. Over the subsequent 2 weeks, the dexamethasone is tapered, and the patient undergoes palliative radiation therapy 1 week after presentation.

Introduction

Suppression of gonadal testosterone is the mainstay of treatment of metastatic prostate cancer and is effective in decreasing tumor burden and serum prostate-specific antigen (PSA). However, almost all patients will develop progression of disease, even if testosterone is kept at castrate levels (<50 ng/dL). Unfortunately, combination chemotherapy has been largely unsuccessful for metastatic prostate cancer to date. With effective therapy, the progression-free survival for patients with metastatic prostate cancer ranges from 12 to 20 months, while the overall survival ranges from 24 to 36 months.

How does prostate cancer survival escape androgen deprivation therapy (ADT)? Evidence suggests that surviving cells possess somatic alterations in the androgen receptor which may allow activation in the absence of androgens [1].

Detection of metastatic disease

The most common site of metastasis is bone, and almost all patients with metastatic disease will have bone metastases. Visceral metastases are rare with prostate cancer, even late in the disease course. They are found in <10% of patients in most chemotherapy studies, while lymph node metastases are present in roughly 20% of affected patients. When visceral metastases are present, lung and liver are the most prevalent sites [2, 3].

The National Comprehensive Cancer Network recommends bone scan in men with high-risk prostate cancer by D'Amico criteria as well as in men with serum PSA > 10 and palpable disease. Furthermore, men should undergo pelvic CT or MRI to evaluate for lymph node metastasis if a prostate cancer nomogram (e.g., Partin tables) predicts a probability of lymph node metastasis >20% [4].

In men with rising PSA after definitive therapy for localized disease, the timing of initiation of ADT remains controversial (early vs. delayed). At our institution, delayed therapy is favored to prevent the side effects of ADT without compromising survival (for detailed analysis, see later). In our experience, the serum PSA at which patients will demonstrate bone scan-detectable metastases is variable, with a median PSA level at detection of metastasis of 31.9 ng/mL. However, 25.9% of men were found to have bone metastases when PSA was below 10 ng/mL, precluding a cut-off at which men should be screened for metastasis [5]. Thus, men with biochemical recurrence should be screened with regular bone scans so that ADT may be initiated in a timely fashion.

Hormone-naïve disease

Benign and malignant prostatic epithelia atrophy in the absence of androgens. Charles Huggins demonstrated clinical improvement in 21 patients with advanced or metastatic prostate cancer after castration in 1941, providing the precedent for the contemporary management of patients with advanced or metastatic disease, ADT [6]. Huggins received the Nobel Prize for this discovery in 1966. In patients receiving ADT, androgens originating from the adrenal gland (17-ketosteroids) are elevated in serum, and the wide majority of patients treated with ADT eventually fail. The following discussion highlights major classes of pharmaceuticals used for androgen deprivation, as well as the side-effect profile.

Initial ADT commonly involved disruption of the hypothalamic–pituitary axis by decreasing the release of luteinizing hormone (LH). The initial pharmaceuticals used for ADT were estrogen derivatives, taking advantage of the potent inhibition of LH secretion caused by estrogen. Diethylstilbestrol was widely used for this purpose, though cardiac toxicity is significant and limits the utility of these agents [7].

Bilateral orchiectomy

Traditionally, ADT was effected with bilateral surgical orchiectomy, which rapidly reduces serum testosterone and alleviates symptoms of metastatic disease. However, randomized clinical trials demonstrated that diethylstilbestrol had similar efficacy to surgical castration [8, 9].

Luteinizing hormone-releasing hormone agonists and antagonists

Luteinizing hormone-releasing hormone (LHRH) agonists were discovered in the early 1970s, and though the initial effect is a surge in LH secretion, long-term administration leads to castrate levels of testosterone. Chronic activation of the LHRH receptors leads to downregulation, resulting in selective medical hypophysectomy [10]. LHRH agonists remain the mainstay of ADT and are often the first agents employed [11]. Examples include leuprolide and goserelin. Long-term results of these therapies have been found to be similar to surgical castration [12].

Initiation of LHRH agonist therapy should be avoided in men with impending spinal cord compression or bone pain due to the testosterone flare effect, which lasts 10–20 days. Coadministration of an antiandrogen will ameliorate the flare phenomenon though not eliminate it [13]. Alternatively, one could choose an LHRH antagonist (e.g., abarelix), which prevents the release of LH and has no flare phenomenon. Rarely, severe side effects have been associated with abarelix use, and it was only approved for use in patients who cannot take other hormonal agents and refuse surgical castration. However, recently another LHRH antagonist, degarelix, was shown to be equivalent to leuprolide monotherapy and was approved in the United States [14].

Antiandrogens

A second effective strategy involves competitively inhibiting the binding of testosterone to the androgen receptor using a class of molecules termed antiandrogens. Antiandrogens are further classified as steroidal or nonsteroidal, with nonsteroidal agents having an improved side-effect profile (less loss of libido or erectile dysfunction).

Steroidal agents inhibit central receptors in the hypothalamus as well as peripheral androgen receptors (AR) and are associated with low testosterone levels. The most prominent of these agents is cyproterone acetate. Side effects include erectile dysfunction, loss of libido, and up to 10% of patients can have severe cardiac complications, limiting the utility of these agents.

Nonsteroidal agents block the binding of AR not only in target organs but also in the hypothalamus and pituitary, inhibiting the negative feedback loop and resulting in increased LH and testosterone, which is converted to estrogens in the periphery. One benefit of the increased testosterone is maintenance of erectile function; however, the increased estrogen level may cause painful gynecomastia. Other side effects may include diarrhea and liver toxicity. Examples include flutamide, bicalutamide, and nilutamide. A couple of notes on antiandrogen studies warrant mention here. Antiandrogen monotherapy has been shown to be inferior to medical or chemical castration [15, 16], though high-dose bicalutamide (15 mg/day) has been shown to have equivalent efficacy to castration [17]. However, in men with low-risk, localized prostate cancer, overall survival is worse with bicalutamide than with watchful waiting (see later).

A novel androgen receptor antagonist, MDV3100, binds to the androgen receptor and blocks translocation of the AR to the nucleus. Unlike other antiandrogens (see later the discussion of antiandrogen withdrawal syndrome), MDV3100 does not have agonist properties for the androgen receptor. Phase III studies evaluating the efficacy of this agent are ongoing [18].

Inhibition of androgen synthesis

Ketoconazole, the widely used antifungal agent, interferes with the cytochrome P450 pathway and potently inhibits androgen synthesis, blocking the conversion of C21 to C19 steroids [19]. Castrate levels of testosterone are reached within 4 hours of administration, faster than either antiandrogens or LHRH agonists [20]. Ketoconazole is commonly used in two settings. First, men who fail first-line ADT will often respond to ketoconazole. Secondly, men with metastatic disease with impending catastrophe (e.g., spinal cord compression or severe bone pain) will often receive ketoconazole due to the rapid decrease seen in serum testosterone. Side effects include gynecomastia, weakness, hepatic dysfunction, and visual changes [21]. It should be administered with hydrocortisone to prevent adrenal insufficiency.

A potent inhibitor of androgen synthesis, **abiraterone**, is a pregnenolone derivative that inhibits cytochrome P17, causing an increase in aldosterone and a simultaneous decrease in cortisol and androgens. Testosterone levels fall to <1 ng/mL, less than that seen with any other pharmaceutical or surgical castration. Side effects have included hypertension, hypokalemia, and peripheral edema [22].

Side effects of androgen ablation

Androgen deprivation causes profound systemic changes, including osteoporosis, hot flashes, erectile dysfunction, decreased libido, decreased muscle mass, gynecomastia, anemia, increased risk of metabolic syndrome (>50%) [23], and cardiovascular events. A large, population-based cohort study suggested that men receiving ADT for at least 1 year had a 20% increased risk of cardiovascular morbidity to matched prostate cancer patients not on ADT [24]. **ADT causes significant morbidity and mortality and must be used discriminately.**

Natural history of response to androgen deprivation

Though the majority of men with metastatic prostate cancer will have a clinical response to ADT, most will eventually fail ADT. Factors that predict the durability of response include the magnitude of drop in PSA as well as the speed with which the PSA decreases. For instance, patients are far more likely to show no sign of PSA progression if they reach an undetectable PSA with ADT [25], and rate of PSA declines after ADT predicts cancer-specific mortality [26]. It remains unclear whether early use of ADT (before men are symptomatic or have bone scan-demonstrated metastasis) improves survival over delaying therapy until onset of symptoms [27].

When should androgen deprivation treatment be initiated?

While ADT clearly lowers PSA and can lead to clinical responses, adverse effects of ADT can be onerous and affect quality of life. Some authors have recommended delaying initiation of ADT until patients have demonstrated metastatic disease to delay onset of the side effects [28].

It remains unclear whether early use of ADT (before men are symptomatic or have bone scan-demonstrated metastasis) improves survival over delayed therapy only with symptomatic disease [27]. Perhaps, this was best demonstrated in the Veterans Administration study of early ADT (VACURG I and II). Men treated prior to developing symptoms had no difference in cancer-specific survival when compared to men who initiated therapy late [9]. In men who fail after radical prostatectomy, the median time to metastasis was 8 years and median time to prostate cancer-specific mortality was 14 years [29, 30]. Thus, delaying ADT may prevent the side effects of treatment for many years. Furthermore, men without metastatic disease may be harmed by treatment. Iversen et al. randomized men with localized disease to bicalutamide or placebo, finding an overall survival benefit to placebo [17].

Nonmetastatic castration-resistant disease

Ultimately, the majority of men with metastatic prostate cancer will fail ADT. The term "castration-resistant prostate cancer" (CRPC) refers to disease that continues to progress despite castrate levels of testosterone. CRPC is typically characterized by a rising PSA despite therapy with antiandrogen and LHRH agonist. In these patients, information that should be ascertained includes number and sites of metastasis, serum PSA level, and prior therapy.

When patients become castration resistant, they can remain without metastasis as well, and it may take many years before evidence of metastasis develops [31]. In one particular study, only 33% of patients had bone scan-positive lesions after 2 years [31].

Treatment for patients with castration-resistant disease is controversial, and few randomized trials are presently available to guide treatment. Fortunately, several new agents designed to treat CRPC have recently been approved by the FDA and are entering clinical practice (see later).

Once a patient on LHRH agonists and/or antiandrogens has a rising PSA (and the finding is reproduced with repeat PSA testing), a frequently utilized technique is to continue LHRH agonists while discontinuing antiandrogens.

Cessation of antiandrogen therapy may be associated with a clinically significant decrease in PSA and occasionally decreased tumor burden for patients with bone or visceral metastases [32]. Thus, in patients on combined LHRH agonists and antiandrogens with a rising PSA, the antiandrogen should be discontinued before attempting other therapies. The median duration of this effect is 3.5–5 months [33]. After PSA begins to rise, either second-line ADT (ketoconazole or abiraterone) or cytotoxic chemotherapy has traditionally been considered. For patients with low metastatic burden, second-line androgen deprivation is often preferred.

Recently, sipuleucel-T has been approved by the FDA for treatment of patients with asymptomatic or minimally symptomatic metastatic CRPC. This agent is an immunotherapy, produced by harvesting a patient's circulating mononuclear cells and incubating with GM-CSF and a purified prostate cancer antigen (PA2024, based on prostatic acid phosphatase) [34]. The agent is hypothesized to stimulate the immune system to slow the progress of prostate cancer. In a phase 3 randomized, placebo-controlled trial (IMPACT), sipuleucel-T improved median overall survival from 21.7 to 25.8 months (HR 0.78, p = 0.03) [35]. Some authors have questioned the study design and hypothesized that the results may have a previously unrecognized bias [36], that dead cells may have been given to controls and lead to an artifactual benefit for patients receiving sipuleucel-T. Side effects of sipuleucel-T included fever and chills, headaches, myalgia, flu-like symptoms, hyperhidrosis, and groin pain [35].

Chemotherapy for metastatic or hormone-refractory prostate cancer

Chemotherapy with docetaxel and prednisone has been shown to improve survival in patients with metastatic prostate cancer. Docetaxel is thought to inhibit microtubule elongation and promote apoptosis preferentially in tumor cells. In a large randomized-controlled trial (RCT) (TAX 327) comparing docetaxel to the previous mainstay of chemotherapy, mitoxantrone, docetaxel improved median survival from 16.4 to 17.8 months (HR 0.83, p = 0.03) for weekly dosing to 19.2 months when the agent was given every 3 weeks [3].

In patients who have progressed after using docetaxel, mitoxantrone and prednisone have traditionally been the mainstay of treatment. Recently, a novel taxane chemotherapeutic agent, cabazitaxel, was approved by the FDA for metastatic CRPC in patients who previously failed docetaxel. In a phase 3 RCT (TROPIC), patients taking cabazitaxel had a median overall survival of 15.1 months, compared to 12.7 months for those taking mitoxantrone (HR 0.70, $p < 0.0001$) [37]. Side effects of cabazitaxel included neutropenia (82%), febrile neutropenia (8%), and diarrhea (6%).

A CYP17A inhibitor, abiraterone, has also been approved by the FDA for men with CRPC who fail docetaxel. In the COU 301 trial, men with CRPC who failed docetaxel were randomized to abiraterone + prednisone versus prednisone alone. Abiraterone improved overall survival from 10.9 to 14.8 months (HR 0.54, $p < 0.001$) [38]. Side effects of abiraterone included fluid retention, hypokalemia, severe hypertension, cardiac abnormalities, and elevated liver function enzymes.

Use of agents to decrease skeletal-related events

Bone metastasis requires disruption of the normal bone homeostasis. ADT is associated with bone mineral loss. Metastatic prostate cancer cells may lead to bone matrix resorption, and cytokines induced by systemic malignancy may increase osteoclast and osteoblast activities. Pharmacologic approaches to decrease bone metastases and morbidity from skeletal-related events (SRE), such as pain and pathologic fractures, are an important consideration in patients with advanced disease.

Bisphosphonate therapy, using compounds such as zoledronate, has been shown to improve bone mineral density in men on long-term androgen deprivation [39] and to decrease the incidence of SRE in men with CRPC metastatic to bone [40]. Saad et al. evaluated the incidence of SRE for 122 patients with CRPC metastatic to bone randomized to zoledronate or placebo, finding after 2 years a decreased incidence of SRE in men who received zoledronate (38% vs. 49%, p = 0.028) [40]. In general, bisphosphonate therapy is only indicated in patients demonstrated to have bony metastases. Side effects of bisphosphonates include myalgias and fatigue, though rarely osteonecrosis of the mandibular bone may occur with these medications, particularly in those who undergo dental work or have poor dentition.

In recent years, inhibitors of the receptor activator of NFκB ligand (RANKL) have gained prominence in an effort to decrease SRE. These agents decrease osteoclast activity *in vitro* and *in vivo*. In a phase 3 RCT, a monoclonal antibody against RANKL (denosumab) was compared to zoledronate in bisphosphonate-naïve patients with metastatic CRPC. Men using denosumab had increased time to their first SRE compared to men using zoledronate (20.7 vs. 17.1 months, p = 0.008) [41]. Side effects of denosumab include fatigue, hypocalcemia, hypophosphatemia, nausea, and osteonecrosis of the jaw (2%). Patients taking denosumab should concurrently take calcium and Vitamin D.

Palliative measures

Bone pain

Men with CRPC and skeletal metastases may face focal bone pain, which is typically controlled by external beam radiation therapy. Of note, lesions on bone scan should be assessed with X-ray or MRI to assess for pathologic fractures [42].

Treatment of cord compression

Signs of cord compression include problems with ambulation (leg weakness), fecal and/or urinary incontinence, and back pain. Prompt treatment is critical to prevent irreparable damage. Typically, these lesions arise from the vertebrae and are seen on bone scan, but lesions arising from the soft tissue surrounding the spinal cord are missed with bone scan. Thus, patients with signs and symptoms of cord compression and negative bone scan should undergo spinal MRI [42].

When cord compression is confirmed, high-dose dexamethasone is used for initial management. Ultimately, radiation therapy is used for definitive management. For men whose lesions are refractory to radiation or for recurrent disease, surgery may be indicated depending on prognosis [43].

WHAT TO AVOID/KEY PITFALLS

- LHRH agonists initially cause testosterone levels to increase. Thus, LHRH agonist monotherapy should be avoided in patients with bone pain or other symptoms of metastatic disease.
- Nonsteroidal antiandrogens such as bicalutamide and flutamide cause an increase in serum testosterone levels. Men taking these agents will maintain erectile function, though they may face loss of libido.
- For men on an antiandrogen who experience a rise in PSA, the next step in management should be discontinuation of the antiandrogen.
- Men on ADT and bisphosphonates who present with jaw pain should be worked up for osteonecrosis of the jaw and should stop bisphosphonate therapy immediately.
- Men presenting with severe bone pain or impending spinal cord compression should be given high-dose dexamethasone.

KEY WEB LINKS

National Comprehensive Cancer Network Guidelines in Oncology; Prostate Cancer
http://www.nccn.org/professionals/physician_gls/pdf/prostate.pdf

American Cancer Society: Hormone (Androgen Deprivation) Therapy for Prostate Cancer
http://www.cancer.org/Cancer/ProstateCancer/DetailedGuide/prostate-cancer-treating-hormone-therapy

American Cancer Society: Chemotherapy for Prostate Cancer
http://www.cancer.org/Cancer/ProstateCancer/DetailedGuide/prostate-cancer-treating-chemotherapy

Multiple choice questions

1 A 55-year-old man was started on bicalutamide for metastatic prostate cancer. Three months after initiation of therapy, his serum LH, testosterone, and estradiol levels should be

a LH increased, testosterone increased, estradiol increased
b LH increased, testosterone increased, estradiol decreased
c LH decreased, testosterone decreased, estradiol decreased
d LH decreased, testosterone increased, estradiol increased
e LH increased, testosterone decreased, estradiol decreased

2 A 50-year-old man with metastatic prostate cancer is treated with leuprolide and bicalutamide. Three years after starting therapy, his PSA increases from undetectable to 5.5. Bone scan remains negative. The next step is

a Continue current therapy, start docetaxel and prednisone
b Stop current therapy, start docetaxel and prednisone
c Stop current therapy, start ketoconazole and prednisone
d Continue leuprolide, stop bicalutamide
e Sipuleucel-T, acetaminophen, and diphenhydramine

References

1 Nelson WG, De Marzo AM, Isaacs WB. Prostate cancer. *N Engl J Med* 2003;349:366–381.

2 Hudes GR, Greenberg R, Krigel RL, et al. Phase II study of estramustine and vinblastine, two microtubule inhibitors, in hormone-refractory prostate cancer. *J Clin Oncol* 1992;10:1754–1761.

3 Tannock IF, de Wit R, Berry WR, et al. Docetaxel plus prednisone or mitoxantrone plus prednisone for advanced prostate cancer. *N Engl J Med* 2004;351: 1502–1512.

4 Mohler J, Bahnson RR, Boston B, et al. NCCN clinical practice guidelines in oncology: prostate cancer. *J Natl Compr Canc Netw* 2010;8:162–200.

5 Loeb S, Makarov DV, Schaeffer EM, Humphreys EB, Walsh PC. Prostate specific antigen at the initial diagnosis of metastasis to bone in patients after radical prostatectomy. *J Urol* 184:157–161.

6 Huggins C, Hodges CV. Studies on prostatic cancer: I. The effect of castration, of estrogen and of androgen injection on serum phosphatases in metastatic carcinoma of the prostate. *Cancer Res* 1941;1:293–297.

7 Nelson JB. Hormone therapy for prostate cancer. In: Wein AJ, Kavoussi LR, Novick AC, Partin AW, Peters CA. *Campbell-Walsh Urology.* 10th ed. Philadelphia, PA: Elsevier; 2011; pp. 2934–2953.

8 Robinson MR, Smith PH, Richards B, Newling DW, de Pauw M, Sylvester R. The final analysis of the EORTC Genito-Urinary Tract Cancer Co-Operative Group phase III clinical trial (protocol 30805) comparing orchidectomy, orchidectomy plus cyproterone acetate and low dose stilboestrol in the management of metastatic carcinoma of the prostate. *Eur Urol* 1995;28:273–283.

9 Byar DP. Proceedings: The Veterans Administration Cooperative Urological Research Group's studies of cancer of the prostate. *Cancer* 1973;32:1126–1130.

10 Moul JW, Evans CP, Gomella LG, Roach M, 3rd, Dreicer R. Traditional approaches to androgen deprivation therapy. *Urology* 2011;78:S485–S493.

11 Loblaw DA, Virgo KS, Nam R, et al. Initial hormonal management of androgen-sensitive metastatic, recurrent, or progressive prostate cancer: 2006 update of an American Society of Clinical Oncology practice guideline. *J Clin Oncol* 2007;25:1596–1605.

12 Seidenfeld J, Samson DJ, Hasselblad V, et al. Single-therapy androgen suppression in men with advanced prostate cancer: a systematic review and meta-analysis. *Ann Intern Med* 2000;132:566–577.

13 Brawer MK, Crawford ED, Labrie F, Mendoza-Valdes A, Miller PD, Petrylak DP. Androgen deprivation and other treatments for advanced prostate cancer. *Rev Urol* 2001;3(Suppl 2):S59–S68.

14 Klotz L, Boccon-Gibod L, Shore ND, et al. The efficacy and safety of degarelix: a 12-month, comparative, randomized, open-label, parallel-group phase III study in patients with prostate cancer. *BJU Int* 2008;102:1531–1538.

15 Chang A, Yeap B, Davis T, et al. Double-blind, randomized study of primary hormonal treatment of stage D2 prostate carcinoma: flutamide versus diethylstilbestrol. *J Clin Oncol* 1996;14:2250–2257.

16 Kolvenbag GJ, Nash A. Bicalutamide dosages used in the treatment of prostate cancer. *Prostate* 1999;39:47–53.

17 Iversen P, Johansson JE, Lodding P, et al. Bicalutamide (150 mg) versus placebo as immediate therapy alone or as adjuvant to therapy with curative intent for early nonmetastatic prostate cancer: 5.3-year median follow-up from the Scandinavian Prostate Cancer Group Study Number 6. *J Urol* 2004;172:1871–1876.

18 Higano CS, Crawford ED. New and emerging agents for the treatment of castration-resistant prostate cancer. *Urol Oncol* 2011;29:S1–S8.

19 Pont A, Williams PL, Azhar S, et al. Ketoconazole blocks testosterone synthesis. *Arch Intern Med* 1982;142: 2137–2140.

20 Trachtenberg J, Halpern N, Pont A. Ketoconazole: a novel and rapid treatment for advanced prostatic cancer. *J Urol* 1983;130:152–153.

21 Scholz M, Jennrich R, Strum S, Brosman S, Johnson H, Lam R. Long-term outcome for men with androgen independent prostate cancer treated with ketoconazole and hydrocortisone. *J Urol* 2005;173:1947–1952.

22 Attard G, Reid AH, Yap TA, et al. Phase I clinical trial of a selective inhibitor of CYP17, abiraterone acetate, confirms that castration-resistant prostate cancer commonly remains hormone driven. *J Clin Oncol* 2008;26:4563–4571.

23 Braga-Basaria M, Dobs AS, Muller DC, et al. Metabolic syndrome in men with prostate cancer undergoing long-term androgen-deprivation therapy. *J Clin Oncol* 2006;24:3979–3983.

24 Saigal CS, Gore JL, Krupski TL, et al. Androgen deprivation therapy increases cardiovascular morbidity in men with prostate cancer. *Cancer* 2007;110:1493–1500.
25 Benaim EA, Pace CM, Lam PM, Roehrborn CG. Nadir prostate-specific antigen as a predictor of progression to androgen-independent prostate cancer. *Urology* 2002;59:73–78.
26 D'Amico AV, McLeod DG, Carroll PR, Cullen J, Chen MH. Time to an undetectable prostate-specific antigen (PSA) after androgen suppression therapy for postoperative or postradiation PSA recurrence and prostate cancer-specific mortality. *Cancer* 2007;109:1290–1295.
27 Ryan CJ, Small EJ. Early versus delayed androgen deprivation for prostate cancer: new fuel for an old debate. *J Clin Oncol* 2005;23:8225–8231.
28 Walsh PC, DeWeese TL, Eisenberger MA. A structured debate: immediate versus deferred androgen suppression in prostate cancer-evidence for deferred treatment. *J Urol* 2001;166:508–515.
29 Pound CR, Partin AW, Eisenberger MA, Chan DW, Pearson JD, Walsh PC. Natural history of progression after PSA elevation following radical prostatectomy. *JAMA* 1999;281:1591–1597.
30 Makarov DV, Humphreys EB, Mangold LA, et al. The natural history of men treated with deferred androgen deprivation therapy in whom metastatic prostate cancer developed following radical prostatectomy. *J Urol* 2008;179:156–161.
31 Smith MR, Kabbinavar F, Saad F, et al. Natural history of rising serum prostate-specific antigen in men with castrate nonmetastatic prostate cancer. *J Clin Oncol* 2005;23:2918–2925.
32 Kelly WK, Scher HI. Prostate specific antigen decline after antiandrogen withdrawal: the flutamide withdrawal syndrome. *J Urol* 1993;149:607–609.
33 Scher HI, Kelly WK. Flutamide withdrawal syndrome: its impact on clinical trials in hormone-refractory prostate cancer. *J Clin Oncol* 1993;11:1566–1572.
34 Small EJ, Fratesi P, Reese DM, et al. Immunotherapy of hormone-refractory prostate cancer with antigen-loaded dendritic cells. *J Clin Oncol* 2000;18:3894–3903.
35 Kantoff PW, Higano CS, Shore ND, et al. Sipuleucel-T immunotherapy for castration-resistant prostate cancer. *N Engl J Med* 2010;363:411–422.
36 Huber ML, Haynes L, Parker C, Iversen P. Interdisciplinary critique of sipuleucel-T as immunotherapy in castration-resistant prostate cancer. *J Natl Cancer Inst* 2012;104:273–279.
37 de Bono JS, Oudard S, Ozguroglu M, et al. Prednisone plus cabazitaxel or mitoxantrone for metastatic castration-resistant prostate cancer progressing after docetaxel treatment: a randomised open-label trial. *Lancet* 2010;376:1147–1154.
38 de Bono JS, Logothetis CJ, Molina A, et al. Abiraterone and increased survival in metastatic prostate cancer. *N Engl J Med* 2011;364:1995–2005.
39 Smith MR, Eastham J, Gleason DM, Shasha D, Tchekmedyian S, Zinner N. Randomized controlled trial of zoledronic acid to prevent bone loss in men receiving androgen deprivation therapy for nonmetastatic prostate cancer. *J Urol* 2003;169:2008–2012.
40 Saad F, Gleason DM, Murray R, et al. Long-term efficacy of zoledronic acid for the prevention of skeletal complications in patients with metastatic hormone-refractory prostate cancer. *J Natl Cancer Inst* 2004;96:879–882.
41 Fizazi K, Carducci M, Smith M, et al. Denosumab versus zoledronic acid for treatment of bone metastases in men with castration-resistant prostate cancer: a randomised, double-blind study. *Lancet* 2011;377:813–822.
42 Antonarakis ES, Carducci MA, Eisenberger MA. Treatment of castration-resistant prostate cancer. In: Wein AJ, Kavoussi LR, Novick AC, Partin AW, Peters AC. *Campbell-Walsh Urology*. Philadelphia, PA: Elsevier; 2011.
43 Patchell RA, Tibbs PA, Regine WF, et al. Direct decompressive surgical resection in the treatment of spinal cord compression caused by metastatic cancer: a randomised trial. *Lancet* 2005;366:643–648.

Answers to multiple choice questions

1 a LH increased, testosterone increased, estradiol increased. Bicalutamide is a nonsteroidal antiandrogen, which competitively inhibits the AR. Men taking these agents (bicalutamide, flutamide, nilutamide) should expect an increase in LH and testosterone due to inhibition of the feedback loop in the hypothalamus and pituitary. As a result, men taking bicalutamide will typically have maintained erectile function, though libido will be decreased significantly. Increased estradiol levels lead to gynecomastia.

2 d Continue leuprolide, stop bicalutamide. Leuprolide is an LHRH agonist, while bicalutamide is a (nonsteroidal) antiandrogen. Antiandrogens have slight agonist effects on the AR, and discontinuation of antiandrogens in this setting often result in a decrease in PSA level that may last 3–5 months (the antiandrogen withdrawal phenomenon). After discontinuing bicalutamide, if PSA levels begin to rise again, ketoconazole or abiraterone should be initiated.

19 Benign prostatic hyperplasia

John B. Eifler

The James Buchanan Brady Urological Institute and Department of Urology, The Johns Hopkins School of Medicine, Baltimore, MD, USA

KEY POINTS

- Benign prostatic hyperplasia (BPH) is a histologic diagnosis characterized by an increased number of prostatic stromal cells within the transition zone of the prostate.
- Testosterone is converted to dihydrotestosterone (DHT) in prostate cells by the enzyme 5α-reductase. Inhibition of this enzyme reduces the size of the prostate.
- Initial evaluation of BPH should include history and physical examination including digital rectal examination, as well as urinalysis.
- Treatment options include watchful waiting, medical therapy, and surgical therapy.
- Combination therapy with an α-blocker and a 5α-reductase inhibitor is superior to therapy with either agent alone.
- Prostate surgery should be considered in men with moderate-to-severe lower urinary tract symptoms (LUTS) with a high degree of urinary bother who have either failed or declined medical management. Indications for surgery also include recalcitrant urinary retention, recurrent urinary infections, bladder stones, persistent gross hematuria secondary to BPH, and renal insufficiency secondary to BPH.
- Surgical options include transurethral procedures or simple prostatectomy.

CASE STUDY 1

A 65-year-old man presents to the urology clinic with incomplete emptying, weak stream, urinary frequency, urgency, and frequency. The symptoms have been increasing in severity over the past 9 months. He denies fevers, chills, gross hematuria, and has no history of previous urinary tract infection. Past medical history is significant for diabetes mellitus with peripheral neuropathy. Physical examination reveals no abdominal distention while digital rectal examination (DRE) demonstrates a 50 cc prostate which is smooth in contour with no palpable masses. A urinalysis is negative for blood, leukocyte esterase, and nitrites. An International Prostate Symptom Score (I-PSS) questionnaire is given to the patient, demonstrating a score of 19. After discussing treatment options, he is started on tamsulosin.

After 5 hours, the patient comes to the emergency department for inability to urinate. A Foley catheter is inserted with difficulty and 950 cc of clear yellow urine is drained from the bladder. The patient reports taking dextromethorphan for cold symptoms earlier in the evening. He is discharged home with the Foley catheter in place.

Ten days after his ED visit, he presents in the urology clinic. His bladder is filled with 200 cc sterile normal saline and the catheter is removed. After 3 hours, he remains unable to void. Pressure flow studies demonstrate a peak flow rate of 5 mL/s with detrusor pressure and maximum flow of 60 cm water. The patient is scheduled for photovaporization of the prostate.

Handbook of Urology, First edition. J. Kellogg Parsons, John B. Eifler and Misop Han. © 2014 by John Wiley & Sons, Ltd. Published 2014 by John Wiley & Sons, Ltd.

CASE STUDY 2

A 78-year-old man presents to the ED with urinary retention. Bladder scan demonstrates 600 cc in the bladder. A catheter is inserted and copious dark red urine drains along with clots. The catheter is irrigated, evacuating a large clot burden. He is placed on continuous bladder irrigation (CBI) and after discussing risks and benefits of a variety of treatments, he is started on finasteride. After 3 days, his urine is yellow and his CBI has been stopped. His catheter is removed and he voids without difficulty. He is continued on finasteride and scheduled for follow-up in the urology clinic.

Introduction

Benign prostatic hyperplasia (BPH) is a pathologic entity common in older men. The prostate tissue is composed of two basic elements: a glandular element composed of secretory ducts and acini and a stromal element composed primarily of collagen and smooth muscle. In BPH, unregulated cellular proliferation leads to increased prostate volume and increased stromal smooth muscle tone; this, in turn, causes physical compression of the urethra and mechanical obstruction of the bladder outlet. Obstruction of the bladder outlet induces two pathological changes in the structure of the bladder, which produce lower urinary tract symptoms (LUTSs). First, decreased bladder compliance causes urinary frequency and urgency. Second, decreased bladder muscle contractility—resulting from chronic tonicity as the bladder labors to overcome increased urethral pressure—causes urinary hesitancy, deterioration in the urinary stream, and increased residual urine.

Etiology

Histologically, an increased number of stromal and epithelial cells are seen in the transition zone of the prostate. Thus, hyperplasia is the appropriate term rather than hypertrophy. The causes for hyperplasia are multifactorial. Androgens promote cell proliferation and inhibit cell death in the prostate epithelium [1]. Furthermore, men who are castrated before puberty will not develop BPH, emphasizing the role on androgens during this time period [2, 3].

An analogue of testosterone, dihydrotestosterone (DHT), is the principal androgen within prostatic cells. Testosterone entering prostate cells is converted to DHT by an enzyme imbedded within the nuclear membrane called 5α-reductase (5-AR) [4]. Men lacking 5-AR have atrophic prostate glands and female external genitalia [5]. Type 2 5-AR is the predominant enzyme in the prostate tissue, whereas type 1 5-AR is present in skin and liver. Inhibition of type 2 5-AR (e.g., by finasteride) is effective in reducing the size of the prostate for men with BPH, and additional inhibition of the type 1 receptor (by the nonselective inhibitor dutasteride) shows no additional reduction in prostate volume. Surprisingly, immunohistochemistry (IHC) studies have demonstrated that the type 2 5-AR is expressed primarily in prostatic stromal cells, not in prostatic epithelial cells [6]. Thus, stromal cells affect prostatic epithelial cells through a paracrine mechanism, and some hypothesize that interruptions of this relationship may result in BPH.

Both testosterone and DHT bind to the androgen receptor, though DHT binds with higher affinity. The complex then enters the nucleus and alters the DNA expression profile of the cell [7]. Surprisingly, DHT levels are not higher in patients with BPH. Walsh et al. demonstrated that DHT levels were nearly identical in normal prostate tissue and in BPH tissue obtained from men who underwent open surgical procedures.

Clearly there is a genetic component to BPH as well. Partin et al. studied the rate of BPH in monozygotic and dizygotic twins, finding the relative risk of BPH for monozygotic twins was 3.3 over dizygotic twins [8]. Young men with BPH are more likely than older men to have an inherited form of the disease [9]. Sanda et al. categorized men with three or more affected family members as having familial BPH, finding these men more likely to have large prostate size (mean 82 vs. 55 cc for men with sporadic disease) [9]. Other factors hypothesized to play a role in the development of BPH include dysregulation of growth factors (such as FGF and IGF) and prostate inflammation.

Pathophysiology

Prostatic growth impinges upon the prostatic urethra and increases the pressure the bladder must overcome during micturition. Many symptoms from BPH are related to the chronic changes in the architecture of the bladder caused by this obstruction of the urethra.

BPH leads to nodule formation in the transition zone of the prostate, the region between the periurethral glands and the peripheral zone. The so-called "median lobe" enlargement that is often seen in BPH results from nodular formation in the periurethral glands at the bladder neck. As the prostate grows in size, it is compressed by the prostatic capsule, transmitting pressure to the urethra. Still, the relationship between the prostate size and symptoms is complex—not all men with an enlarged prostate will experience LUTS, and not all men with LUTS will have an enlarged prostate. Shapiro et al. demonstrated that this observation may be partly explained by differences in stromal–epithelial ratios between prostate nodules [10]. Histologic analysis of prostate nodules also demonstrates a significant amount of smooth muscle tissue [11], which likely also contributes to increased urethral resistance. Thus, BPH stroma is composed of both muscle elements and extracellular matrix and increased urethral resistance is both an active and passive process.

Urethral resistance is also modulated by adrenergic stimulation in the prostate. In human prostate samples from prostatectomy specimens, exposure to α_1-adrenergic agonists led to smooth muscle contraction in the specimen [12]. Other studies demonstrated the predominance of the α_{1A}-adrenergic receptor in mediating this response [13].

Obstruction leads to chronic changes in the bladder and progression of LUTS. Ultimately, if untreated, bladder decompensation may occur. Initially, the bladder responds with detrusor hypertrophy and is able to maintain the ability to empty. Over time, collagen deposition within the detrusor musculature occurs; these depositions appear as thick cords, called "trabeculations," jutting from the bladder wall that are visible on cystoscopy. Collagen deposition leads to decreased bladder contractility and compliance [14]. Often, frequency and urgency symptoms occur in a decompensated bladder with decreased compliance. Relief of obstruction will reverse this process early in the disease course, but at some point, irreversible changes occur. In animal models of partial obstruction, the time until this decompensation occurs is variable [14].

Complications of long-standing bladder obstruction *include bladder calculi, recurrent urinary tract infections (UTI), acute urinary retention, and irreversible kidney injury* [15]. If left untreated, LUTS tend to worsen with time. In the placebo arm of the Medical Therapy of Prostatic Symptoms (MTOPS) study of men with intermediate or severe symptoms as measured by the International Prostate Symptom Score (I-PSS), 14% of men in the placebo arm experienced >4 point increases in the I-PSS after 4 years, <1% had UTIs, and none experienced renal failure related to BPH [16]. Bladder calculi are rare, with only 1 of 276 people followed for 3 years with watchful waiting in one study [17]. *Urinary incontinence* is not uncommon in men with BPH, though it also occurs relatively commonly as a result of normal aging. *Gross hematuria* is a known complication of severe BPH and responds well to finasteride. In the MTOPS study, 2% developed *acute urinary retention.* Risk factors include age, higher I-PSS, low max flow rate, high serum PSA, and enlarged prostate size. In patients who are followed for BPH, these complications are rare.

Epidemiology

Strictly speaking, BPH is a histologic diagnosis, defined by stromoglandular hyperplasia [18]. Data from autopsy specimens suggest that men younger than 30 years rarely develop BPH, whereas roughly 90% of men older than 80 years will have evidence of the disease [19]. The autopsy prevalence of BPH is similar in all countries and cultures that have been studied, though I-PSS scores vary substantially between cultures [18].

BPH manifests clinically as LUTS. In recent decades, validated questionnaires have quantified LUTS and allowed comparison between individuals. The most widely used questionnaire is the I-PSS (previously known as the American Urological Association Symptom Index). The prevalence of LUTS, as measured by the I-PSS, increases with age and prostate size. Men in the Olmsted County Study cohort were found to have a 50% prevalence of moderate-to-severe

LUTS by their 70s [20]. Prostate size tends to increase throughout life, from approximately 25 cc for a man in his 30s to 45 cc for a man in his 70s. Though prostate size correlates significantly with the I-PSS score, the correlation is weak [21].

Several studies have evaluated the association between sedentary lifestyle and BPH. In the Health Professionals Follow-up Study, obesity was associated with simple prostatectomy (OR 2.38), whereas walking more than 2 hours per week was associated with a decreased prevalence (OR 0.73) [22]. Men with obesity, diabetes, or elevated fasting plasma glucose were also found to be more likely to have an enlarged prostate in the Baltimore Longitudinal Study of Aging [23].

Diagnosis

For a patient with LUTS, evaluation begins with a detailed **history and physical examination** as well as a **urinalysis** according to the AUA Guidelines [24]. History and physical examination is usually sufficient to establish the diagnosis. In the history, one should assess the history of LUTS, hematuria, UTI, urinary retention, exacerbation of symptoms by cold medications or anticholinergics. A digital rectal examination (DRE) should be performed to estimate the prostate size and assess for advanced prostate cancer. Also, neurologic status should be assessed by the anal sphincter tone, ambulatory status, and lower extremity motor function. Urinalysis should be performed to screen for UTI or hematuria, either of which suggests a non-BPH etiology.

Serum PSA testing should be offered to men with a greater than 10-year life expectancy for whom the result will inform the clinical plan of care. In addition to prostate cancer risk stratification, serum PSA also correlates with the risk of BPH progression and the need for surgery. The benefits and risks of PSA testing should be discussed.

Men with storage symptoms (frequency, urgency, and nocturia) as the predominant component of their LUTS should have a **urine cytology** to screen for urothelial cell carcinoma. Serum creatinine and pressure flow studies are not recommended for routine initial evaluation in patients with LUTS [24].

The **I-PSS** quantifies the extent of symptoms and establishes a baseline prior to surgical or pharmacologic therapy. By definition, men with I-PSS scores of 0–7 have mild, 8–19 moderate, and >19 severe LUTS, respectively. Patient bother, measured with a single question on the I-PSS, is very important for selecting a management strategy. Bother scores of >3 suggest that treatment may be indicated. BPH may also be associated with frequent UTI, urinary retention requiring catheterization, acute renal failure, bladder calculi, or gross hematuria.

Urinary flow studies are often useful in patients presenting with LUTS. Peak flow rates (Qmax) <10 cc/s are abnormal and consistent with obstruction if the patient voids at least 150 mL.

A **postvoid residual (PVR)** is a measure of how much urine remains in the bladder after the patient voids. It is not mandatory in all patients but should be considered in patients complaining of incomplete emptying. Of note, a large PVR may be associated with a higher failure rate with watchful waiting, though what PVR cutoff portends a poorer outcome remains unclear.

A **pressure flow study**, or urodynamics, is an invasive test that may provide additional information about obstruction but is not indicated for routine evaluation of BPH. If the differential diagnosis includes detrusor hyporeflexia (e.g., in elderly men with diabetes), pressure flow study can assist in determining whether the patient has adequate detrusor function. Urodynamics may also demonstrate uninhibited detrusor contractions, which are associated with rapid BPH progression. Also, long-standing BPH may irreversibly injure the detrusor musculature, and men with persistent retention should have urodynamics to assess for detrusor contractility.

Cystoscopy is not routinely performed for BPH but should be performed in men with hematuria, history of stricture disease or prior urinary tract surgery (to rule out stricture).

Transrectal ultrasound (TRUS) may also be used to delineate volume and anatomy for surgical planning, particularly in men with very large prostates who may be candidates for simple prostatectomy.

Treatment

The treatment for BPH should aim to reduce LUTS and prevent adverse consequences of the disease such as acute urinary retention, UTI, bladder stones, and renal insufficiency. Noninvasive or surgical therapies may be appropriate depending on the individual circumstances.

Watchful waiting

Men with elevated LUTS without substantial bother (usually bother score <4 on the I-PSS) may appropriately select watchful waiting. Behavioral modifications with limiting fluid intake (particularly in the evening), eliminating caffeine intake, and double voiding prior to bedtime will reduce symptoms in many men. Some authors have found that intensive behavioral modifications with weekly group sessions improved symptoms for men with BPH.

Medical therapy

α-Blockers

Smooth muscle is a large component of prostatic stroma and responds to norepinephrine (α-adrenergic agonist). The α_1-adrenergic receptor is the predominant subtype in the prostate, and α-adrenergic inhibitors are a major class of medications used to treat BPH. It should be noted that α_1-adrenergic receptors also line the trigone and bladder neck, so the efficacy of α-adrenergic inhibitors may not be entirely related to prostatic smooth muscle relaxation.

Pharmacologic inhibitors of adrenergic innervations of prostatic smooth muscle are classified according to specificity, including nonspecific α-adrenergic inhibitors (e.g., phenoxybenzamine) and selective α_1-adrenergic inhibitors (e.g., prazosin, terazosin, and tamsulosin). These agents have similar efficacy in reducing LUTS, though α_1-specific inhibitors have fewer side effects. Further studies demonstrated three subtypes of the α_1-adrenergic receptor, with the α_{1A}-subtype most common in prostate smooth muscle [25]. Silodosin, an α_{1A}-subtype specific inhibitor, has been shown to have similar efficacy to tamsulosin in reducing I-PSS scores [26].

Side effects of the α-blockers include orthostatic hypotension, dizziness, fatigue, rhinitis, retrograde ejaculation, and floppy iris syndrome. Intraoperative floppy iris syndrome occurs in approximately 2% of patients undergoing cataract surgery, causes billowing of the iris, and is associated with increased surgical complication rate [27]. Of note, floppy iris syndrome may occur several years after the α-blocker is discontinued. Patients should be counseled that they must notify the ophthalmologist of their α-blocker use prior to any eye surgery.

5α-Reductase inhibitors

The second major class of pharmaceutical agents used to treat BPH is 5α-reductase inhibitors (5αRi), which inhibit the conversion of testosterone to DHT, the primary androgen in the prostate. 5αRi reduce prostate volume slowly, reaching maximal effect 6 months after initiating therapy [28]. Thus, men with LUTS and *relatively large prostates* may benefit most from 5αRi therapy. The two common drugs used in this setting are finasteride, a selective type 2 5αRi, and dutasteride, a type 1 and type 2 inhibitor. Finasteride has been shown to significantly improve peak flow rate, I-PSS, and decrease prostate volume in randomized controlled trials [28], and also to *reduce incidence of acute urinary retention and need for surgery* [29]. Finasteride is also effective in *treating gross hematuria caused by BPH* [30].

Finasteride and dutasteride are well tolerated with *few side effects*. There is a slight increase in *sexual dysfunction* with use of finasteride—primarily loss of libido and ejaculatory dysfunction. There is also a 1–2% prevalence of gynecomastia. Use of 5αRi reduces serum PSA by roughly 50%, and any increase in PSA after initiating therapy should trigger prostate biopsy to evaluate for prostate cancer. These agents reduce the risk of incident, biopsy-detectable prostate cancer by 25% [31, 32]. While some data have suggested that finasteride and dutasteride also increase the risk of higher-grade prostate cancer, this issue is controversial and remains unresolved [33].

The mainstay of medical management for BPH is a combination of a 5αRi and an α-blocker. In the MTOPS trial, 3047 patients were randomized to finasteride, doxazosin, a combination of both, or placebo. Men taking combination therapy were less likely to experience disease progression (defined as acute retention, increased I-PSS by 4 points, 50% increase in creatinine, multiple UT, or new incontinence) when compared to men taking finasteride or doxazosin alone [16]. In particular, I-PSS and peak flow rate improved considerably in the combination arm when compared to monotherapy. Also, the men who achieved the greatest benefit from medical therapy had large prostate size.

Treatment of storage symptoms

Either as a result of bladder changes from BPH or *de novo* pathologic process, many men with LUTS have a predominance of storage symptoms: frequency, urgency, and nocturia. The mainstay of treatment for storage symptoms is an anticholinergic medication. Combination therapy with an α-blocker and a bladder-selective anticholinergic is effective in reducing symptoms in men with LUTS and prominent storage symptoms consistent with overactive bladder [34]. The use of anticholinergic medications in men with BPH is unlikely to cause retention [34, 35].

Phosphodiesterase inhibitors

Recently, evidence from randomized controlled trials has demonstrated that phosphodiesterase inhibitors (PDEi) are effective in reducing I-PSS scores in men with BPH [36]. Interestingly, patients using PDEi have no improvement in peak flow rate. The combination of PDEi and α-blockers may cause hypotension, so patients stable on α-blockers should be given low doses of PDEi and titrated up, with careful monitoring for hypotension.

Phytotherapy

Several supplements are used to treat LUTS, though the most common is saw palmetto (*Serenoa repens*). Two recent high-quality, placebo-controlled trials demonstrated no benefit to saw palmetto over placebo for treatment of LUTS [37, 38]. Other supplements have been studied but none have demonstrated improvement over placebo.

Surgical therapy

Men with moderate-to-severe LUTS with a high degree of urinary bother who have either failed or declined medical management should consider surgery. Indications for surgery also include recalcitrant urinary retention, recurrent urinary infections, bladder stones, persistent gross hematuria secondary to BPH, and renal insufficiency secondary to BPH. Men with *peak flow rates* >15 cc/s have been found to have worse outcomes with surgical procedures [39]. However, men in retention may not be able to void an adequate volume and should be assessed by urodynamics. Appearance on cystoscopy should not be used to determine need for surgery.

Some of the more common types of surgery are as follows:

Transurethral resection of the prostate (TURP). This procedure is performed endoscopically via a 26- or 28F cystoscope and an Iglesias resectoscope. A monopolar cutting loop is the element used for tissue dissection and requires the use of nonionic irrigation solution, such as sterile water or 1.5% glycine. In many instances, a continuous flow system is used to improve bladder drainage and to prevent overfilling the bladder during the procedure. The patient is placed in a lithotomy position and given appropriate antibiotics. Once adequate visualization is achieved, prostate tissue is excised by dragging the loop through the tissue in a stepwise manner. Care must be taken to avoid the ureteral orifices and to remain proximal to the verumontanum, which is the anatomic structure at which the ejaculatory ducts connect to the urethra. Resection distal to the verumontanum risks injury to the external urinary sphincter and thus urinary incontinence [40]. A Foley catheter is left in place for 1–3 days and may be placed on traction in the event of excessive hematuria. Continuous bladder irrigation may be considered.

Complications of the procedure include urinary extravasation, clot retention, and transurethral resection (TUR) syndrome. TUR syndrome refers to a constellation of symptoms—mental confusion, nausea, vomiting, hypertension, bradycardia, and visual disturbances—that may occur due to hyponatremia as a result of a prolonged operation with hypotonic irrigation solution. When patients are under general anesthesia, the first signs may be hypertension and bradycardia. Resection time should be limited to less than 90 minutes to avoid this complication. The success rate of TURP is excellent, reducing the rate of secondary complications of BPH (e.g., bladder calculi, urinary retention, renal failure, etc.) by 50% over watchful waiting with few side effects [17].

Photovaporization of the prostate (PVP) utilizes a similar approach to TURP, but rather than resecting tissue with a monopolar loop, the tissue is vaporized by a laser (most commonly the Greenlight, or KTP laser). As cautery is not used, the irrigation solution may be an electrolyte solution such as normal saline, alleviating the risk of TUR syndrome. The benefit of PVP is decreased bleeding intraoperatively and postoperatively, with fewer patients requiring continuous irrigation or postoperative transfusion [41]. Long-term outcomes of PVP have not been reported, though functional intermediate term outcomes (up to 5 years) are similar to TURP in carefully selected patients.

In *simple prostatectomy*, the surgeon removes the prostatic adenoma through abdominal incisions. The procedure may be performed either robotically or open through a suprapubic (incising the bladder) or a retropubic (incising the prostate capsule) approach. Though more invasive than TURP or PVP, rates of retreatment are lower for simple prostatectomy [42]. It remains an excellent option, particularly for patients with a severely enlarged prostate (>75 cc) for whom TURP and PVP may require multiple operations to remove entirely, for men with large bladder diverticula (which could be removed concurrently), large bladder calculi, or joint problems which may preclude prolonged lithotomy position [43]. Complication rates are low but include urinary extravasation, urinary incontinence, and erectile dysfunction.

Holmium laser enucleation of the prostate (HoLEP) utilizes laser technology to enucleate the prostate rather than vaporize it. The prostate tissue is released into the bladder after enucleation and morcellated with a separate device. The holmium laser is a contact laser (as opposed to noncontact lasers such as the Greenlight laser), so the target must be in contact with the fiber for energy transfer to occur. HoLEP is favored over PVP or TURP for very large prostates (>100 cc), which traditionally have been treated with open prostatectomy [44]. Compared to open prostatectomy, HoLEP is associated with decreased length of hospitalization and less catheterization time.

Thermotherapy includes transurethral needle ablation (TUNA) of the prostate, which involves delivering radiofrequency energy to the prostatic adenoma via needles inserted endoscopically with the intention of inducing prostatic necrosis, and transurethral microwave therapy, which involves inserting a specialized catheter device to deliver microwave energy to prostatic tissue. Neither is as effective as TURP and thus both are considered second-line therapy at the current time.

WHAT TO AVOID/KEY PITFALLS

- LUTS do not correlate well with prostate volume: not all patients with LUTS have enlarged prostates, and not all patients with enlarged prostates have LUTS.
- Only patients with *bothersome* LUTS (as measured by validated questionnaire) should consider medical or surgical therapy.
- Pressure flow studies for BPH should be reserved for patients in whom the etiology of LUTS is unclear, such as patients with neurological disorders or very elderly men.
- α-Blocker therapy is associated with floppy iris syndrome, which may complicate ophthalmologic procedures.
- Saw palmetto has been shown to have no benefit in the treatment of BPH when compared to placebo and is not recommended for treatment.

KEY WEB LINKS

WebMD Guide to BPH
http://www.webmd.com/prostate-cancer/enlarged-prostate

NIH Guide to BPH
http://www.ncbi.nlm.nih.gov/pubmedhealth/PMH0001419/

I-PSS
http://www.usrf.org/questionnaires/AUA_SymptomScore.html

Multiple choice questions

1 A 64-year-old man with a history of DVT on warfarin therapy has acute urinary retention refractory to tamsulosin. What is the best management option?
a Finasteride
b TURP
c Photovaporization of the prostate
d SP tube placement and finasteride therapy
e UroLume stent

2 A 70-year-old man with long-standing BPH treated with tamsulosin has an increasing I-PSS score and starts finasteride. Which of the following is true regarding combination therapy with α-blockers and 5αRi?
a It is associated with significant less PVR when compared to monotherapy

b It is associated with decreased likelihood of acute urinary retention when compared to monotherapy
c It is the treatment of choice in patients with chronic renal insufficiency secondary to BPH
d It is associated with significant improved peak flow rate compared with monotherapy
e It is contraindicated in the elderly individuals due to the risk of clinically significant hypotension.

References

1 Isaacs JT. Antagonistic effect of androgen on prostatic cell death. *Prostate* 1984;5:545–557.
2 Peters CA, Walsh PC. The effect of nafarelin acetate, a luteinizing-hormone-releasing hormone agonist, on benign prostatic hyperplasia. *N Engl J Med* 1987;317:599–604.
3 Isaacs JT. Prostate stem cells and benign prostatic hyperplasia. *Prostate* 2008;68:1025–1034.
4 McConnell JD. Benign prostatic hyperplasia. Hormonal treatment. *Urol Clin North Am* 1995;22:387–400.
5 Walsh PC, Madden JD, Harrod MJ, Goldstein JL, MacDonald PC, Wilson JD. Familial incomplete male pseudohermaphroditism, type 2. Decreased dihydrotestosterone formation in pseudovaginal perineoscrotal hypospadias. *N Engl J Med* 1974;291:944–949.
6 Silver RI, Wiley EL, Davis DL, Thigpen AE, Russell DW, McConnell JD. Expression and regulation of steroid 5 alpha-reductase 2 in prostate disease. *J Urol* 1994;152:433–437.
7 Chatterjee B. The role of the androgen receptor in the development of prostatic hyperplasia and prostate cancer. *Mol Cell Biochem* 2003;253:89–101.
8 Partin AW, Page WF, Lee BR, Sanda MG, Miller RN, Walsh PC. Concordance rates for benign prostatic disease among twins suggest hereditary influence. *Urology* 1994;44:646–650.
9 Sanda MG, Beaty TH, Stutzman RE, Childs B, Walsh PC. Genetic susceptibility of benign prostatic hyperplasia. *J Urol* 1994;152:115–119.
10 Shapiro E, Becich MJ, Hartanto V, Lepor H. The relative proportion of stromal and epithelial hyperplasia is related to the development of symptomatic benign prostate hyperplasia. *J Urol* 1992;147:1293–1297.
11 Shapiro E, Hartanto V, Lepor H. Quantifying the smooth muscle content of the prostate using double-immunoenzymatic staining and color assisted image analysis. *J Urol* 1992;147:1167–1170.
12 Lepor H, Tang R, Shapiro E. The alpha-adrenoceptor subtype mediating the tension of human prostatic smooth muscle. *Prostate* 1993;22:301–307.
13 Lepor H, Tang R, Meretyk S, Shapiro E. Alpha 1 adrenoceptor subtypes in the human prostate. *J Urol* 1993;149:640–642.
14 Levin RM, Haugaard N, O'Connor L, et al. Obstructive response of human bladder to BPH vs. rabbit bladder response to partial outlet obstruction: a direct comparison. *Neurourol Urodyn* 2000;19:609–629.
15 Flanigan RC, Reda DJ, Wasson JH, Anderson RJ, Abdellatif M, Bruskewitz RC. 5-year outcome of surgical resection and watchful waiting for men with moderately symptomatic benign prostatic hyperplasia: a Department of Veterans Affairs cooperative study. *J Urol* 1998;160:12–16; discussion 6–7.
16 McConnell JD, Roehrborn CG, Bautista OM, et al. The long-term effect of doxazosin, finasteride, and combination therapy on the clinical progression of benign prostatic hyperplasia. *N Engl J Med* 2003;349:2387–2398.
17 Wasson JH, Reda DJ, Bruskewitz RC, Elinson J, Keller AM, Henderson WG. A comparison of transurethral surgery with watchful waiting for moderate symptoms of benign prostatic hyperplasia. The Veterans Affairs Cooperative Study Group on Transurethral Resection of the Prostate. *N Engl J Med* 1995;332:75–79.
18 Roehrborn CG. Chapter 91: Benign prostatic hyperplasia: etiology, pathophysiology, epidemiology, and natural history. In: Wein AJ, Kavoussi LR, Novick AC, Partin AW, Peters CA, editors. *Campbell-Walsh Urology.* Vol. 11. Philadelphia, PA: Elsevier; 2011. pp. 2570–2610.
19 Berry SJ, Coffey DS, Walsh PC, Ewing LL. The development of human benign prostatic hyperplasia with age. *J Urol* 1984;132:474–479.
20 Wei JT, Calhoun E, Jacobsen SJ. Urologic diseases in America project: benign prostatic hyperplasia. *J Urol* 2005;173:1256–1261.
21 Bosch JL, Hop WC, Bangma CH, Kirkels WJ, Schroder FH. Prostate specific antigen in a community-based sample of men without prostate cancer: correlations with prostate volume, age, body mass index, and symptoms of prostatism. *Prostate* 1995;27:241–249.
22 Giovannucci E, Rimm EB, Chute CG, et al. Obesity and benign prostatic hyperplasia. *Am J Epidemiol* 1994;140:989–1002.
23 Parsons JK, Carter HB, Partin AW, et al. Metabolic factors associated with benign prostatic hyperplasia. *J Clin Endocrinol Metab* 2006;91:2562–2568.
24 McVary KT, Roehrborn CG, Avins AL, et al. Update on AUA guideline on the management of benign prostatic hyperplasia. *J Urol* 2011;185:1793–1803.
25 Forray C, Bard JA, Wetzel JM, et al. The alpha 1-adrenergic receptor that mediates smooth muscle contraction in human prostate has the pharmacological properties of the cloned human alpha 1c subtype. *Mol Pharmacol* 1994;45:703–708.

26 Chapple CR, Montorsi F, Tammela TL, Wirth M, Koldewijn E, Fernandez Fernandez E. Silodosin therapy for lower urinary tract symptoms in men with suspected benign prostatic hyperplasia: results of an international, randomized, double-blind, placebo- and active-controlled clinical trial performed in Europe. *Eur Urol* 2011;59:342–352.

27 Chang DF, Campbell JR. Intraoperative floppy iris syndrome associated with tamsulosin. *J Cataract Refract Surg* 2005;31:664–673.

28 Gormley GJ, Stoner E, Bruskewitz RC, et al. The effect of finasteride in men with benign prostatic hyperplasia. The Finasteride Study Group. *N Engl J Med* 1992;327: 1185–1191.

29 McConnell JD, Bruskewitz R, Walsh P, et al. The effect of finasteride on the risk of acute urinary retention and the need for surgical treatment among men with benign prostatic hyperplasia. Finasteride Long-Term Efficacy and Safety Study Group. *N Engl J Med* 1998;338:557–563.

30 Foley SJ, Soloman LZ, Wedderburn AW, et al. A prospective study of the natural history of hematuria associated with benign prostatic hyperplasia and the effect of finasteride. *J Urol* 2000;163:496–498.

31 Thompson IM, Goodman PJ, Tangen CM, et al. The influence of finasteride on the development of prostate cancer. *N Engl J Med* 2003;349:215–224.

32 Andriole GL, Crawford ED, Grubb RL 3rd, et al. Mortality results from a randomized prostate-cancer screening trial. *N Engl J Med* 2009;360:1310–1319.

33 Walsh PC. Chemoprevention of prostate cancer. *N Engl J Med* 2010;362:1237–1238.

34 Kaplan SA, Roehrborn CG, Rovner ES, Carlsson M, Bavendam T, Guan Z. Tolterodine and tamsulosin for treatment of men with lower urinary tract symptoms and overactive bladder: a randomized controlled trial. *JAMA* 2006;296:2319–2328.

35 Abrams P, Kaplan S, De Koning Gans HJ, Millard R. Safety and tolerability of tolterodine for the treatment of overactive bladder in men with bladder outlet obstruction. *J Urol* 2006;175:999–1004; discussion 1004.

36 McVary KT, Monnig W, Camps JL, Jr., Young JM, Tseng LJ, van den Ende G. Sildenafil citrate improves erectile function and urinary symptoms in men with erectile dysfunction and lower urinary tract symptoms associated with benign prostatic hyperplasia: a randomized, double-blind trial. *J Urol* 2007;177:1071–1077.

37 Barry MJ, Meleth S, Lee JY, et al. Effect of increasing doses of saw palmetto extract on lower urinary tract symptoms: a randomized trial. *JAMA*;306:1344–1351.

38 Bent S, Kane C, Shinohara K, et al. Saw palmetto for benign prostatic hyperplasia. *N Engl J Med* 2006;354: 557–566.

39 McConnell JD, Barry MJ, Bruskewitz RC. Benign prostatic hyperplasia: diagnosis and treatment. Agency for Health Care Policy and Research. *Clin Pract Guidel Quick Ref Guide Clin* 1994;1–17.

40 Fitzpatrick JM. Chapter 93: Minimally invasive and endoscopic management of benign prostatic hyperplasia. In: Wein AJ, Kavoussi LR, Novick AC, Partin AW, Peters CA, editors. *Campbell-Walsh Urology*. Vol. 3. Philadelphia, PA: Elsevier; 2011. pp. 2655–2694.

41 Gravas S, Bachmann A, Reich O, Roehrborn CG, Gilling PJ, De La Rosette J. Critical review of lasers in benign prostatic hyperplasia (BPH). *BJU Int* 2011;107: 1030–1043.

42 Mebust WK, Holtgrewe HL, Cockett AT, Peters PC. Transurethral prostatectomy: immediate and postoperative complications. A cooperative study of 13 participating institutions evaluating 3,885 patients. *J Urol* 1989;141:243–247.

43 Han M, Partin, AW. Chapter 94: Retropubic and suprapubic open prostatectomy. In: Wein AJ, Kavoussi LR, Novick AC, Partin AW, Peters CA, editors. *Campbell-Walsh Urology*. Vol. 3. Philadelphia, PA: Elsevier; 2011. pp. 2695–2703.

44 Matlaga BR, Kim SC, Kuo RL, Watkins SL, Lingeman JE. Holmium laser enucleation of the prostate for prostates of >125 mL. *BJU Int* 2006;97:81–84.

Answers to multiple choice questions

1 c Acute urinary retention refractory to α-blocker therapy is an indication for surgical intervention. When compared to TURP, photovaporization of the prostate (PVP) has decreased risk of bleeding complications and transfusion requirements. It may also be performed safely in patients on anticoagulation. Finasteride would be unlikely to relieve his retention in the short term. A UroLume stent is typically reserved for patients with extensive comorbidities that preclude prostatic surgery.

2 d Combination therapy with α-blockers and 5αRi has been shown to be superior to either therapy alone. In particular, I-PSS score and peak flow rates are significantly lower in men on combination therapy. There was no significant benefit seen in PVR or the likelihood of developing acute urinary retention. Chronic renal insufficiency secondary to BPH should undergo surgical intervention. Combination therapy has no increased risk of orthostatic hypotension when compared to α-blockers alone.

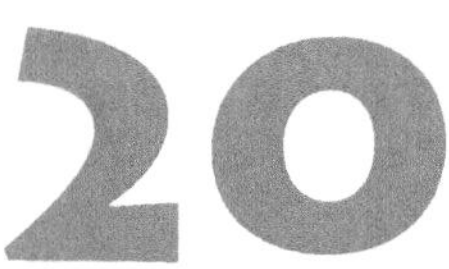

Bladder cancer: superficial

Ashley E. Ross and Trinity J. Bivalacqua

The James Buchanan Brady Urological Institute and Department of Urology, The Johns Hopkins School of Medicine, Baltimore, MD, USA

KEY POINTS

- Bladder cancer is the second most common genitourinary malignancy.
- Approximately 70% are nonmuscle invasive.
- Most present with gross or microscopic painless hematuria.
- Work up should include physical examination, urine culture and analysis, urine cytology, upper tract imaging and cystoscopy.
- Use of tumor markers and fluorescence cystoscopy may aid in diagnosis, treatment, and surveillance.
- First-line therapy for a bladder lesion is transurethral resection with the aggressiveness of superficial lesions being determined primarily by its grade.
- Recurrence of low-grade lesions can be prevented with adjuvant intravesical chemotherapy.
- Recurrence and progression of high-grade lesions may be prevented by intravesical immunotherapy.
- Refractory high-grade disease and high-grade nonmuscle invasive bladder cancer with aggressive features may require extirpative treatment.

CASE STUDY

A 72-year-old gentleman with a history of previous tobacco use and coronary artery disease presented with intermittent, painless, gross hematuria. Urine culture was negative as was a renal protocol multi-phase CT scan. Cystoscopy revealed a moderately enlarged prostate with trilobar hypertrophy and areas of the bladder that appeared somewhat injected and friable but not overtly cancerous. Efflux from bilateral ureteral orifices was clear. Cytology was sent at that time. Cytology was consistent with high-grade carcinoma and he was taken to the operating room for bilateral ureteral/renal pelvis washings, bilateral retrograde pyelograms and random biopsies of the bladder mucosa, and biopsy of the prostatic urethra. Biopsies of all suspicious friable areas were also acquired. He tolerated the procedure well and pathology revealed negative upper tract cytology and bladder biopsies consistent with CIS. He began intravesical BCG therapy 3 weeks following the procedure and tolerated a 6-week course fairly well with the exception of a few episodes of low-grade fevers. At 3 months, cystoscopy and cytology remained negative and he was started on maintenance BCG for a 3-week course. Unfortunately, in week 2 of this course he developed persistent high-grade fevers and required hospital admission for IV antibiotics. While he did not develop frank sepsis, he did have an arrhythmia causing cardiac strain (but not a frank myocardial infarction) during that admission which was managed with medications and resolved. During his admission for BCGosis, isoniazid was also initiated and continued for a 3-month course. At that time he continued his surveillance with cystoscopy and cytology every 3 months; however, maintenance BCG was discontinued given his previous adverse reaction and overall frail state. At 9 months following his initial transurethral biopsies he remained presumably tumor free, with negative cytology and biopsies.

Handbook of Urology, First edition. J. Kellogg Parsons, John B. Eifler and Misop Han.
Published 2014 by John Wiley & Sons, Ltd.

Introduction

Bladder cancer is the second most common genitourinary malignancy and its development is contributed to greatly by environmental exposure and advancing age. As such, the incidence of bladder cancer has been rising over the last 70 years, driven mostly by increases in industrializing nations where carcinogenic exposure is common [1]. In the United States, bladder cancer accounts for 7% of all diagnosed cancers. Among these cancers the overwhelming majority are of urothelial origin with ~70% of tumors being nonmuscle invasive, superficial disease [2]. With regards to superficial bladder cancer, grade is the critical distinguishing feature with low-grade cancers rarely showing invasion or progression and high-grade lesions having a high chance of progression, sometimes even having metastatic disease present despite the absence of local muscle invasion [3, 4]. As such, low-grade cancers are most often managed by resection and surveillance while high-grade lesions necessitate intravesical therapy, close surveillance, and sometimes cystectomy.

Grade, stage, and tumor biology

The bladder consists of three histological layers which from superficial to deep include the urothelium, the lamina propria (sub-urothelium connective tissue also containing muscularis mucosae), and the muscularis propria or detrusor muscle. Superficial bladder cancer refers to bladder cancer which does not involve the muscularis propria and is also called nonmuscle invasive bladder cancer. Among superficial bladder cancer, stages include Ta (papillary tumor confined to the urothelium), T1 (tumor invading the lamina propria), and Tis or carcinoma *in situ* (CIS) which is a flat, high-grade lesion confined to the urothelium.

Tumor grade is the most important predictor of disease progression [4]. Previous classification systems used designations of grades 1–3 to classify malignant tumors; however, more recent recommendations have been to simplify classifications into low grade or high grade. Low-grade tumors have cells that appear relatively normal but with some cellular structure irregularity. In contrast, high-grade lesions demonstrate severe irregularity and nuclear pleomorphism (Plate 20.1, see page 300). Papillary tumors with orderly cellular arrangement and minimal architectural or cellular abnormalities are now designated papillary urothelial neoplasm of low malignant potential (PUNLMP). PUNLMP tumors are considered by many to be benign. However, as these patients can recur, sometimes with cancerous lesions, most recommend routine patient follow-up [5].

Low-grade Ta lesions often recur but rarely progress (about 5% of cases). In contrast, high-grade T1 lesions recur in more than 80% of cases and progress over half of the time [6]. In addition, when cystectomy is performed for high-grade superficial lesions, 8–20% will have lymph node metastasis [3]. Molecularly, high- and low-grade cancers differ as well, with low-grade papillary tumors having relatively few chromosomal abnormalities (primarily loss of all or part of chromosome 9) and high-grade tumors having a high degree of aneuploidy (at chromosomes 7, 9,17, etc.) [7, 8].

Diagnosis

Gross (macroscopic), painless hematuria is the most common presenting symptom of bladder cancer (reported rates of 13–34%) with microscopic hematuria associated with a 0.5–10.5% rate of diagnosis [9]. In addition to hematuria, CIS may present with irritative symptoms, sometimes in the absence of any hematuria [10]. As a result, patients with hematuria or unexplained irritative voiding symptoms should be investigated by cystoscopy and upper tract imaging as well as urine culture and urine cytology.

Urine cytology is a highly specific test (positive test indicates the presence of malignancy regardless of radiologic and visual findings) [11]. The overall sensitivity of urine cytology is poor however, (~16%) but it does increase with tumor grade being as high as 60% in high-grade tumors in some studies [12, 13]. Therefore, in an attempt to complement cytology, investigators have developed other urine-based markers. Among these are the BTA stat and BTA TRAK tests which test for human complement H-related protein, immunocyst which uses labeled antibodies targeted against two bladder mutants and a bladder variant of carcinoembryonic antigen, NMP22 Bladder Check Test, and multiprobe fluorescence *in situ* hybridization (FISH, UroVysion) which identifies cellular aneuploidy of chromosomes 3, 7, and 17 as well as alterations at 9p21 [14]. Widespread use of these tests has been limited due to a lack of prospective trials demonstrating clinical value; that said, UroVysion has perhaps the most promising data with superior sensitivity over cytology [15].

In addition to attempts to improve diagnosis of bladder cancer via tumor markers, efforts have been made to augment white light cystoscopy. Most notable among these has been the intravesical use of photoactive porphyrins such as 5-aminolevulinic acid (5-ALA) or hexaminolevulinate (HAL) which accumulates preferentially in neoplastic tissue and fluoresces red under blue light [16].

Surgical management

Visible lesions in the bladder are initially treated by transurethral resection. This can be carried out under regional or general anesthesia. An examination under anesthesia should be carried out prior to the procedure as well as after the procedure for a large and/or invasive tumor. Doing so allows both for staging of the patient (fixation of a mass after resection suggests locally advanced disease) as well as detection of possible bladder perforation (indicated by increased abdominal girth).

Positioning for resection is in lithotomy. This puts the patient at risk for sciatic nerve injury (results in the inability to flex the knee), femoral nerve injury (inability to flex the hip or extend the knee), and common peroneal nerve injury (foot drop). These can be prevented by avoiding excessive external hip rotation and avoiding compression of the lateral knee at the fibular head.

Visualization can be aided by a 70 degree lens which allows for maintenance of anatomical relationships and improved surveillance of the bladder neck. Resection, however, is carried out with a 30 degree lens with which the resection loop can better be seen. Traditionally, resection is carried out in a nonconducting solution (such as sterile water or glycine; note that there is no evidence that glycine is superior to sterile water) [17]. Over the last decade, introduction of bipolar electroresection has allowed for resection in saline as well [18].

Resection of all visual tumors should be performed. Pure cutting current allows for minimal scaring and can be performed near the ureteral orifice with even resection of the orifice as needed. After resecting visible tumor, an additional resection or biopsy of the tumor base should be sent to pathology separately to determine muscle invasion. Complications include uncontrolled hematuria and clinically evident perforation that occur in <5% of cases. The incidence of perforation can be reduced by avoiding bladder over distention and using paralysis to limit the obturator reflex response when resecting laterally. Finally, staged resection can be considered for large, bulky tumors.

Following resection, an adjuvant intravesical chemotherapy can be given perioperatively to prevent tumor implantation and reduce the risk of recurrence in patients suspected to have low-risk disease. Mitomycin C appears to be the most effective agent; however, epirubicin is used commonly in Europe. With either agent, a single dose is administered postoperatively, preferably within 6 hours and can lessen recurrence of low-grade lesions up to 40% [19]. Importantly, perioperative adjuvant therapy should not be given in patients with extensive resection or suspected perforation as this can have serious sequelae and in rare instances has lead to death (similarly, BCG therapy should never be given within 2 weeks of resection).

Even when complete resection is thought to have occurred, re-resection in 1–6 weeks is recommended for T1 and high-grade Ta tumors [20]. This is because many of these tumors on repeat resection will demonstrate worse prognostic findings; particularly, if muscle was not present in the original specimen (almost two-thirds of patients where muscle was not present were upstaged on repeat resection while around one-third of those with muscle identified at the original surgery were upstaged) [21].

Immunotherapy

Intravesical immunotherapy has three roles: the treatment of CIS, the treatment of residual tumor, and for prophylaxis against the recurrence of high-grade lesions. Immunotherapy is primarily carried out using intravesical Bacillus Chalmette–Guerin (BCG) which has proven more effective than other immunologic-based therapies such as interferon. BCG is an attenuated mycobacterium that was developed as a vaccine for tuberculosis and works by the direct binding to fibronectin within the bladder, which then riggers a T-helper type-1 immune response [22, 23].

Treatment is typically begun several weeks following resection to allow for healing of the bladder mucosa which will limit the potential for intravasation of bacteria and systemic infection. Additionally, BCG therapy should be delayed in the presence of infection or if there is a traumatic catheterization. BCG is instilled and allowed to dwell in the bladder for 2 hours and then voided out [24]. A typical induction course involves one instillation of BCG per week for 6 weeks. After the induction course, BCG maintenance is carried out by three weekly instillations at 3 and 6 months and then every 6 months thereafter for 3 years. This provides the best recurrence free survival but is tolerated by only about 15% of patients.

BCG should be considered the first-line treatment for CIS with initial tumor free responses as high as 84% and ~50% being tumor free at 4 years [25]. BCG also is effective in decreasing the recurrence rates of T1 tumors as well as their rate of progression; however, superior results for progression were primarily seen with maintenance therapy [26]. Finally, BCG has been shown to treat residual papillary lesions but it should not be used as a substitute for surgery.

BCG-related toxicity includes low-grade symptoms, fevers (sometimes referred to as BCGosis) and BCG sepsis. In cases of low-grade fevers, treatment can be instituted with NSAIDs, phenazopyridine, or anticholinergics. If symptoms last longer than 24 hours, the provider can consider delaying therapy until symptoms improve and then reducing the BCG dose and giving isoniazid the day before, of, and after instillation [27]. If fevers (above 38.5°C) persist for 24 hours without signs of sepsis, BCG instillations should be stopped and urine cultures for bacteria and acid-fast bacilli obtained. Broad-spectrum antibiotics should be started and isoniazid 300 mg by mouth every day should be given for a 3-month course, resuming BCG when the patient is asymptomatic. Note that, when treating urinary tract infections, avoidance of quinolones should be attempted as they can affect the viability of BCG [28]. BCG sepsis can occur in a minority of patients. It should be aggressively treated with broad-spectrum antibiotics, anti-tuberculosis drugs (isoniazid, rifampin, and ethambutol; continued for 6 months with consideration of giving cycloserine, a faster acting agent, in particularly severe cases) and prednisone.

A number of novel agents for bladder cancer immunotherapy are being developed; however, they have not yet reached clinical practice. The goal of these agents is to reproduce the efficacy of BCG without the use of live bacteria, thus limiting its toxicity. Examples include nonspecific immune stimulants such as keyhole limpet hemocyanin (KLH) and mycobacterial cell wall extract mixed with immunostimulatory DNA [29, 30].

Intravesical chemotherapy

As mentioned above, intravesical chemotherapy instilled within 6 hours of resection has a dramatic impact on recurrence of low-grade lesions. The role for chemotherapy in treating high-grade lesions however is less clear with practice patterns in the United States favoring the use of BCG due to its higher efficacy, and those in Europe favoring chemotherapy as infectious complications are minimized. Intravesical chemotherapies include mitomycin C (MMC), thiotepa, and doxorubicin. MMC is a cross-linking agent that inhibits DNA synthesis and can allow for reasonable reductions in disease recurrence (though not to the level of BCG) [31]. Though systemic absorption can cause myelosuppression, this is rare due to its high molecular weight. Thiotepa is also an alkylating agent (and is the only chemotherapeutic approved by the FDA specifically for the intravesical treatment of papillary bladder cancer). Its use does reduce disease recurrence but, due to its lower molecular weight, is associated with a higher risk of systemic side effects [32]. Doxorubicin, an anthracycline antibiotic which inhibits topoisomerase II and protein synthesis has also shown improvements in preventing tumor recurrence (but not progression) following endoscopic resection [33]. A semisynthetic analog of doxorubicin, valrubicin, has recently become available and FDA approved in the United States for BCG refractory CIS in patients who cannot tolerate cystectomy, having a 21% complete response in this group [34].

Cystectomy for aggressive superficial and refractory high-grade disease

Up to 20% of patients with CIS will die of urothelial cancer within 10 years. In addition, an early recurrence following BCG or a T1 recurrence is associated with muscle invasive disease in over 80% of cases and carries with it an increased risk of metastasis for each occurrence [35]. Additionally, some studies suggest that patients treated after progression to muscle invasive disease have a poorer prognosis than those presenting initially with invasive disease [36]. Despite this risk, because of the morbidity of cystectomy, intravesical therapy for high-grade superficial lesions is reasonable. In addition to factors that would sway urologists toward early radical cystectomy (noninvasive disease with deep invasion to the lamina propria, presence of lymphovascular invasion or micropapillary features, association with diffuse CIS, presence of T1 disease in a diverticula, young patient age), molecular markers are also being explored. Perhaps the most studied is P53 status. Though its overexpression has been correlated to increased risk of progression, its use remains investigational [37].

As opposed to these cases that might prompt "early cystectomy," radical cystectomy should be considered first-line therapy for refractory high-grade disease (CIS or persistent high-grade papillary tumors refractory to two courses of BCG). In these individuals, 80% will fail if treated again with intravesical therapy and many experience rapid progression. In patients unfit for cystectomy with superficial recurrence, valrubicin or BCG combined with interferon may be considered [38].

Surveillance

Most relapses occur within 2 years of the original transurethral resection. Therefore close surveillance is warranted, particularly in the early period (recurrence within the first 3 months is a particularly poor prognostic sign). There is little evidence to support commonly practiced surveillance algorithms; however, general recommendations do exist and are based on the features of the initial tumor. For low-grade Ta lesions, cystoscopy should be performed at 3-month intervals and then annually starting at 9 months if there is no recurrence with cessation strongly considered at 5 years. For multifocal low-grade Ta lesions, very large low-grade lesions, or low-grade lesions that recur at 3 months, cystoscopy should be conducted every 3 months for 2 years and then semiannually or annually after that with a return to more frequent cystoscopy if a recurrence is found. Upper tract imaging can also be considered if a recurrence is found or if there is any hematuria. For high-grade lesions, cystoscopy should be performed every 3 months for 2 years and then semiannually for 2 years, and annually for life with cytology sent at each cystoscopy and upper track imaging annually for 2 years and then at less frequent intervals. All patients on surveillance should be encouraged not to smoke, increase their fluid intake, and reduce the fat in their diet.

WHAT TO AVOID

- Intravesical chemotherapy should not be given in cases of suspected bladder perforation.
- BCG immunotherapy should not be given within the first 2 weeks of resection.
- Avoiding overdistension of the bladder and employing paralysis to limit the obturator reflex can reduce the chance of bladder perforation during resection.

KEY WEB LINKS

www.nccn.org
www.auanet.org

Multiple choice questions

1 Which of the following are not good indications for a patient with superficial disease to undergo cystectomy:

a Micropapillary features in a 60-year-old man with high-grade T1 bladder cancer
b Carcinoma *in situ* (CIS) recurrence after two failed cycles of BCG
c A third recurrence of papillary urothelial neoplasm of low malignant potential (PUNLMP) tumor in a 50-year-old man
d T1, high-grade papillary lesion in a diverticulum

2 Which intravesical therapy does not match its proposed mechanism (choose all that apply)

a Thiotepa—intercalating agent inhibiting topoisomerase II
b Mitomycin C—alkylating agent inhibiting DNA synthesis
c Valrubicin—alkylating agent inhibiting DNA synthesis
d BCG—immunotherapy stimulating a cytotoxic Th2 cell response

3 Which statement is false (choose all that apply)
  a CIS is associated with lymph node metastasis in up to 20% of cases.
  b Rate of progression to muscle invasive disease following two failed attempts at intravesical therapy with BCG is over 80%.
  c Both BCG and MMC reduce the rate of tumor recurrence and progression.
  d Urine cytology is highly sensitive for malignancy.

References

1 Jemal A, Ward E, Anderson RN, Murray T, Thun MJ. Widening of socioeconomic inequalities in U.S. death rates, 1993–2001. *PLoS One* 2008;3(5):e2181.
2 Lopez-Beltran A. Bladder cancer: clinical and pathological profile. *Scand J Urol Nephrol Suppl* 2008;(218): 95–109.
3 Freeman JA, Esrig D, Stein JP, et al. Radical cystectomy for high risk patients with superficial bladder cancer in the era of orthotopic urinary reconstruction. *Cancer* 1995;76(5):833–839.
4 Millan-Rodriguez F, Chechile-Toniolo G, Salvador-Bayarri J, Palou J, Algaba F, Vicente-Rodriguez J. Primary superficial bladder cancer risk groups according to progression, mortality and recurrence. *J Urol* 2000;164 (3 Pt 1):680–684.
5 Epstein JI, Amin MB, Reuter VR, Mostofi FK. The World Health Organization/International Society of Urological Pathology consensus classification of urothelial (transitional cell) neoplasms of the urinary bladder. Bladder Consensus Conference Committee. *Am J Surg Pathol* 1998;22(12):1435–1448.
6 Herr HW. Tumor progression and survival of patients with high grade, noninvasive papillary (TaG3) bladder tumors: 15-year outcome. *J Urol* 2000;163(1):60–61; discussion 61–62.
7 Richter J, Jiang F, Gorog JP, et al. Marked genetic differences between stage pTa and stage pT1 papillary bladder cancer detected by comparative genomic hybridization. *Cancer Res* 1997;57(14):2860–2864.
8 Degtyar P, Neulander E, Zirkin H, et al. Fluorescence in situ hybridization performed on exfoliated urothelial cells in patients with transitional cell carcinoma of the bladder. *Urology* 2004;63(2):398–401.
9 Khadra M, Richards JI, Robinson MM. Development and evaluation of a micropipette tip washing system. *J Immunol Methods* 2000;242(1–2):1–8.
10 Tissot WD, Diokno AC, Peters KM. A referral center's experience with transitional cell carcinoma misdiagnosed as interstitial cystitis. *J Urol* 2004;172(2):478–480.
11 Nabi G, Greene D, O'Donnell MO. Suspicious urinary cytology with negative evaluation for malignancy in the diagnostic investigation of haematuria: how to follow up? *J Clin Pathol* 2004;57(4):365–368.
12 Grossman HB, Messing E, Soloway M, et al. Detection of bladder cancer using a point-of-care proteomic assay. *JAMA* 2005;293(7):810–816.
13 Halling KC, King W, Sokolova IA, et al. A comparison of cytology and fluorescence in situ hybridization for the detection of urothelial carcinoma. *J Urol* 2000;164(5):1768–1775.
14 Mitra AP, Cote RJ. Molecular screening for bladder cancer: progress and potential. *Nat Rev Urol* 2010;7(1):11–20.
15 Jones JS. DNA-based molecular cytology for bladder cancer surveillance. *Urology* 2006;67(3 Suppl 1):35–45; discussion 7.
16 Denzinger S, Burger M, Walter B, et al. Clinically relevant reduction in risk of recurrence of superficial bladder cancer using 5-aminolevulinic acid-induced fluorescence diagnosis: 8-year results of prospective randomized study. *Urology* 2007;69(4):675–679.
17 Holzbeierlein JM, Smith JA, Jr. Surgical management of noninvasive bladder cancer (stages Ta/T1/CIS). *Urol Clin North Am* 2000;27(1):15–24, vii–viii.
18 Wang DS, Bird VG, Leonard VY, et al. Use of bipolar energy for transurethral resection of bladder tumors: pathologic considerations. *J Endourol* 2004;18(6):578–582.
19 Sylvester RJ, Oosterlinck W, van der Meijden AP. A single immediate postoperative instillation of chemotherapy decreases the risk of recurrence in patients with stage Ta T1 bladder cancer: a meta-analysis of published results of randomized clinical trials. *J Urol* 2004; 171(6 Pt 1):2186–2190, quiz 435.
20 Nieder AM, Brausi M, Lamm D, et al. Management of stage T1 tumors of the bladder: International Consensus Panel. *Urology* 2005;66(6 Suppl 1):108–125.
21 Dutta SC, Smith JA, Jr., Shappell SB, Coffey CS, Chang SS, Cookson MS. Clinical under staging of high risk nonmuscle invasive urothelial carcinoma treated with radical cystectomy. *J Urol* 2001;166(2):490–493.
22 Morales A, Eidinger D, Bruce AW. Intracavitary bacillus Calmette-Guerin in the treatment of superficial bladder tumors. *J Urol* 1976;116(2):180–183.
23 Bohle A, Brandau S. Immune mechanisms in bacillus Calmette-Guerin immunotherapy for superficial bladder cancer. *J Urol* 2003;170(3):964–969.
24 Lamm DL, Blumenstein BA, Crissman JD, et al. Maintenance bacillus Calmette-Guerin immunotherapy for recurrent TA, T1 and carcinoma in situ transitional cell carcinoma of the bladder: a randomized Southwest Oncology Group Study. *J Urol* 2000;163(4):1124–1129.
25 Hall MC, Chang SS, Dalbagni G, et al. Guideline for the management of nonmuscle invasive bladder

cancer (stages Ta, T1, and Tis): 2007 update. *J Urol* 2007;178(6):2314–2330.

26 Sylvester RJ, van der MA, Lamm DL. Intravesical bacillus Calmette-Guerin reduces the risk of progression in patients with superficial bladder cancer: a meta-analysis of the published results of randomized clinical trials. *J Urol* 2002;168(5):1964–1970.

27 Bassi P, Spinadin R, Carando R, Balta G, Pagano F. Modified induction course: a solution to side-effects? *Eur Urol* 2000;37(Suppl 1):31–32.

28 Durek C, Rusch-Gerdes S, Jocham D, Bohle A. Interference of modern antibacterials with bacillus Calmette-Guerin viability. *J Urol* 1999;162(6):1959–1962.

29 Sarosdy MF. Principles of intravesical chemotherapy and immunotherapy. *Urol Clin North Am* 1992;19(3): 509–519.

30 Morales A, Chin JL, Ramsey EW. Mycobacterial cell wall extract for treatment of carcinoma in situ of the bladder. *J Urol* 2001;166(5):1633–1637; discussion 7–8.

31 Bohle A, Bock PR. Intravesical bacille Calmette-Guerin versus mitomycin C in superficial bladder cancer: formal meta-analysis of comparative studies on tumor progression. *Urology* 2004;63(4):682–686; discussion 686–687.

32 Thrasher JB, Crawford ED. Complications of intravesical chemotherapy. *Urol Clin North Am* 1992;19(3): 529–539.

33 Kurth KH. Diagnosis and treatment of superficial transitional cell carcinoma of the bladder: facts and perspectives. *Eur Urol* 1997;31(Suppl 1):10–19.

34 Grossman HB, O'Donnell MA, Cookson MS, Greenberg RE, Keane TE. Bacillus calmette-guerin failures and beyond: contemporary management of non-muscle-invasive bladder cancer. *Rev Urol* 2008; 10(4):281–289.

35 Herr HW, Sogani PC. Does early cystectomy improve the survival of patients with high risk superficial bladder tumors? *J Urol* 2001;166(4):1296–1299.

36 Schrier BP, Hollander MP, van Rhijn BW, Kiemeney LA, Witjes JA. Prognosis of muscle-invasive bladder cancer: difference between primary and progressive tumours and implications for therapy. *Eur Urol* 2004;45(3): 292–296.

37 Peyromaure M, Weibing S, Sebe P, et al. Prognostic value of p53 overexpression in T1G3 bladder tumors treated with bacillus Calmette-Guerin therapy. *Urology* 2002;59(3):409–413.

38 O'Donnell MA, Lilli K, Leopold C. Interim results from a national multicenter phase II trial of combination bacillus Calmette-Guerin plus interferon alfa-2b for superficial bladder cancer. *J Urol* 2004;172(3):888–893.

Answers to multiple choice questions

1 c
2 a, c, and d
3 c and d

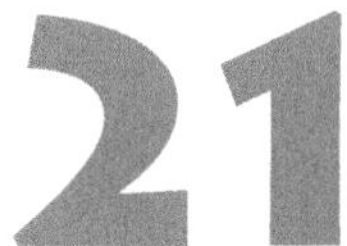

Invasive bladder cancer and urinary diversion

Ashley E. Ross and Trinity J. Bivalacqua

The James Buchanan Brady Urological Institute and Department of Urology, The Johns Hopkins School of Medicine, Baltimore, MD, USA

KEY POINTS

- Approximately 80% of patients presenting with muscle invasive bladder cancer initially present with muscle invasive disease.
- Deaths from bladder cancer are thought to be the result of distant metastases present at the time of locoregional therapy (with most occurring within 2 years after treatment but late recurrences being more common after perioperative systemic chemotherapy).
- Delay of surgery for longer than 12 weeks from the diagnosis is detrimental to the patient.
- Bilateral pelvic lymphadenectomy including external and internal iliac and obturator nodes is required for radical or partial cystectomy with the number of nodes removed and number of positive nodes both independently affecting survival.
- Radical cystectomy has a high perioperative complication rate which increases with advanced age.
- Options for urinary diversion include incontinent conduits, continent orthotopic neobladders, and catheterizable stomas.

CASE STUDY

A 72-year-old previous machinist with a long history of tobacco use presented with gross hematuria. Upper tract imaging with an abdominal and pelvis CT scan demonstrated no discernable renal or ureteral lesion but mild-to-moderate hydronephrosis was present on the left side and a left-sided lesion was seen on delayed phase as a filling defect in the bladder. No lymphadenopathy was noted on imaging. Examination under anesthesia was performed prior to endoscopic resection and a left-sided mass could be felt. Cystoscopy demonstrated a left trigonal lesion that abutted the ureteral orifice on that side. The tumor was resected with pathology later demonstrating muscle invasive urothelial carcinoma. Examination following resection still could identify a left-sided mass and the bladder was mobile. Chest CT was negative for pulmonary nodules or metastasis and liver enzymes, creatinine, and blood counts were all normal with the exception of mild anemia. He underwent neoadjuvant chemotherapy with gemcitabine and cisplatin and then presented for radical cystectomy. Preoperatively, he had expressed the desire for an orthotopic neobladder and it was discussed that this would be attempted, though if not oncologically sound he would be diverted by another method (he preferred a conduit diversion if that was the case). Intraoperatively, his bladder was mobile and there was no bulky lymphadenopathy. The bladder was removed with frozen sections taken from the urethra and bilateral ureters were performed. The left ureteral margin was positive for carcinoma *in situ* (CIS) and an additional section was submitted for frozen section, which was negative. The urethral margin was also positive for CIS and urethrectomy was then performed. Pelvic and iliac lymphadenectomy was then performed and samples were submitted to pathology. Final pathology would demonstrate transitional cell carcinoma invading into the extravesical mass with negative margins, one of the 45 removed lymph nodes was positive, pT3bN1Mx.

Handbook of Urology, First edition. J. Kellogg Parsons, John B. Eifler and Misop Han.
Published 2014 by John Wiley & Sons, Ltd.

An ileal conduit was then fashioned and ureters were implanted using a Bricker anastomosis. Postoperatively, his hospital stay was complicated by a protracted ileus, which was managed conservatively with bowel rest and parenteral nutrition and he left the hospital on POD 12 in good condition. At his 3-month follow-up, cytology from the conduit was negative, his creatinine was normal, and mild bilateral hydroureter was seen on ultrasound with no sign of frank recurrence.

Introduction

Muscle invasion refers to involvement of the muscularis propria (detrusor) muscle of the bladder by carcinoma. The presence of this level of invasion in most cases warrants aggressive therapy, the cornerstone of which is surgical extirpation. Despite aggressive locoregional control, however, approximately half of patients with muscle invasive bladder cancer will progress to metastatic disease. Thus, efforts toward multimodality therapy have been undertaken with the best current evidence supporting neoadjuvant therapy, particularly for those with extravesical disease [1]. Following removal of the bladder, the urinary stream is typically diverted to a conduit, neobladder, or catheterizable continent diversion depending on the patient's tumor characteristics, functional status, and preference. Radical cystectomy with reconstruction is associated with a high number of overall perioperative morbidities, the majority of which are related to the need for urinary diversion using bowel segments [2].

Staging and histology

Eighty percent of patients with invasive bladder cancer present with muscle invasive disease with the remainder having lesions that progressed from superficial disease. Among those that are candidates for cystectomy, pathologic tumor stage and nodal status are the primary variables affecting the risk of progression and survival [3]. Unlike superficial bladder cancer, muscle invasive bladder cancer, for obvious reasons, is not subdivided into high-grade and low-grade lesions. Instead, muscle invasive tumors are classified on the basis of their histology and stage. As with superficial bladder cancer, the majority of primary bladder cancers are of urothelial origin. Other subtypes include squamous cell cancers that predominate in countries where bilharziasis is endemic and in populations whose bladders are exposed to chronic inflammation from indwelling catheters and recurrent infections. Adenocarcinomas are uncommon but are found in exstrophy patients and may be associated with urachal diverticuli. Small cell tumors of the bladder are rare but can occur and are more likely to be associated with paraneoplastic syndromes through the production of ectopic hormones. Other unusual variants include lymphoepithelioma-like cancers that have a more favorable prognosis than transitional cell carcinoma and micropapillary disease which is very aggressive and frequently associated with lymphatic and vascular invasion.

Staging is based on a TNM schema, the details of which are summarized in the AJCC cancer staging manual [4]. Full staging includes a bimanual examination before and after endoscopic resection, upper tract imaging (preferably prior to tumor resection), and laboratory testing (which includes at a minimum a complete blood count and a comprehensive metabolic panel). T stage denotes the level of invasion of the primary tumor, with stage T2 indicating invasion into the muscularis propria, T3 indicating invasion into perivesical fat, and T4 denoting invasion of the prostatic stroma, seminal vesicles, uterus, vagina, pelvic wall, or abdominal wall. Presence of a tumor on bimanual examination following endoscopic resection indicates T3 disease with T4 disease suggested by involvement of other structures or fixation. Advanced T stage may also be suggested by hydronephrosis seen on upper tract imaging.

Though over-staging does occur, under-staging is far more common, particularly if muscularis propria is not present in an endoscopically resected specimen. Though selection bias likely plays a substantial role, most studies on patients who underwent cystectomy for T1 tumors demonstrate a large number of tumors found to be T2 at the time of surgery (roughly 40% in the series by Dutta et al. [5]). Because of this, most recommend re-resection of T1 lesions, particularly those which are high grade (see Chapter 20). In addition, to fully stage tumors prior to cystectomy, some advocate biopsy of the prostatic urethra in men and bladder neck in women (other urologists rely on frozen sections of the apical urethral margins to guide choices for diversion). In men, this can be performed by using a resectoscope loop to resect from the mid prostate to the mid distal verumontanum [6]. Negative prostatic urethral biopsies are associated with a negative apical urethral margin and can obviate the need for intraoperative frozen section [7]. In women, biopsy of the bladder neck acts as a surrogate. Of note, while the presence of carcinoma *in situ* (CIS) in the prostatic urethra or proximal female urethra may guide decisions regarding urinary tract reconstruction, the presence of CIS in the prostatic urethra or ducts does not lead to upstaging to T4 disease because outcome is determined by the primary cancer stage.

As mentioned, upper tract imaging not only can help describe the stage of the local tumor but also can evaluate for regional lymph node spread, synchronous urothelial cancers of the renal pelvis and potential metastasis. Current imaging is primarily performed by CT or MRI of the abdomen and pelvis. In addition, a chest CT should be included as a routine part of an evaluation of a patient with muscle invasive disease. Bone scintigraphy can be obtained when the patient has a new-onset bone pain or an elevated alkaline phosphatase.

Surgical therapy

Extirpative therapy is the cornerstone of the management of muscle invasive bladder cancer. Indeed, delay of cystectomy for longer than 12 weeks after the diagnosis of a muscle invasive lesion is associated with poorer outcomes [8]. In very general terms, surgery consists of three parts: radical cystectomy, pelvic and iliac lymphadenectomy, and urinary diversion.

Cystectomy

Surgery is traditionally performed in an open fashion through a lower midline incision that can be extended above the umbilicus if necessary for exposure. More recently efforts toward reducing the morbidity of cystectomy by using robot-assisted and laparoscopic techniques have been undertaken but there has been no long-term oncologic data as of yet to substantiate its use as a modality [9].

In the male, radical cystectomy should include the bladder and its surrounding perivesical fat and soft tissue, the prostate, and the seminal vesicles. Nerve sparing is appropriate in patients with no evidence of local extension intraoperatively and may improve continence in patients with a neobladder (this may be related to more meticulous dissection at the prostatic apex) [10]. In the female, anterior exoneration traditionally includes the bladder and perivesical tissue as well as the uterus, cervix, and anterior vagina. An exception to this is in sexually active women where vaginal preservation can be planned in some cases (those without posterior-based invasive cancer) as reports indicate that involvement of the uterus, cervix, and ovaries is uncommon and preservation of those structures may allow for more support particularly if a neobladder is planned [11, 12]. In both sexes, cystectomy should not be performed if the bladder is fixed to the pelvic sidewall or the tumor is involving the rectum, if there is extensive evidence of periureteral disease, or if lymph node metastases are unresectable due to bulk or extent (above the iliac vessels). Patients with grossly positive nodes should receive neoadjuvant or adjuvant systemic chemotherapy.

Intraoperatively, after cystectomy, evaluation of the urethra can be carried out by frozen section. Preoperatively, the urethra can also be evaluated by biopsy as mentioned above with the risk of urethral involvement being influenced by involvement of the prostate in men (with stromal invasion having a 30% likelihood of involvement) and involvement of tumor at the bladder neck in women [13]. Urethrectomy in men should be considered if there is cancer at the apical urethral margin on frozen section or if there is prostate stromal invasion or diffuse CIS within the prostatic ducts. All females should undergo urethrectomy except those with planned orthotopic diversion where urethral preservation of the distal two-thirds is necessary to achieve an adequate sphincter mechanism. This area is innervated by the pudendal nerve and is only infrequently involved by urothelial carcinoma [14, 15]. If the urethra is to be spared, the dissection should be limited to the soft tissue above endopelvic fascia in order to preserve sphincter innervation. Cancer at the bladder neck in women or in the urethral margin or a T4 tumor involving the anterior vagina are contraindications to urethral preservation.

The value of frozen sections at the ureteral margins is more controversial but they are commonly sent. Controversy arises from retrospective series demonstrating that margin status does not seem to independently alter the development of upper tract disease and that nephrectomy is not indicated for CIS [16]. Others report high sensitivity and specificity for ureteral frozen sections in predicting final margin status [17]. A general consensus is that if margins are sent, atypia or dysplasia does not require any change in management and that, if CIS is found, an attempt at achieving a negative margin should be made but without compromising ureteral length. Postoperatively upper tract recurrence can be monitored by imaging and voided cytology.

Lymphadenectomy

Positive lymph nodes are found in 25% of patients and are the most important prognostic factor in those patients [18]. In addition, the number of lymph nodes removed is an important factor influencing survival even in node-negative patients. In patients with nodal metastasis, the number of nodes removed and percentage of positive nodes are both independent predictors of recurrence and survival and many have chosen to report this as a combined variable of lymph node density [19]. Based on multi-institutional retrospective trials, we currently recommend that at least 25 lymph nodes be analyzed for proper staging as it likely identifies 75% of the positive nodes with examination of 45 nodes allowing for detection of 90% of disease [20]. At a minimum, 10 lymph nodes should be removed [21]. Because total lymph node counts are highly dependent on processing of tissue following removal, the most important factors at surgery are complete lymph node dissection and anatomic extent. An extended lymph node dissection should be performed bilaterally and should include the area from the aortic bifurcation superiorly, the genitofemoral nerve laterally, and Cooper's ligament inferiorly. In patients with T3 or T4 tumors and node-positive disease, nodes proximal to the common iliac bifurcation are positive in up to half of the cases [22].

Urinary diversion

Options for diversion include incontinent conduits and continent cutaneous diversions and orthotopic neobladders. Selection of diversion is based on patient and tumor characteristics.

Advantages of conduit diversions are that they are technically simple to perform and easy to manage. This ease of management gives them a high satisfaction rating. Bowel segments for conduit diversions are typically taken from the terminal ileum, but transverse colon can be used in cases of prior pelvic irradiation. Refluxing ureterointestinal anastomosis is created; particularly in ileal conduits where nonrefluxing anastomosis increases the stricture rate (an implant into the tinea of the colon is usually nonrefluxing). A Wallace reimplant, where the ureters are brought together to make a single lumen, further decreases the stricture rate but puts the patient at risk for bilateral obstruction. A rosebud end stoma is formed and usually placed in the right lower quadrant after examining the patient in lying, sitting, and standing positions.

Patients selected for continent diversions should have a life expectancy of >1 year, strong desire to be "bag free," good manual dexterity, normal or nearly normal renal function (CrCl $\geq$ 50 mL/min), and nearly normal bowel function. The right lower quadrant is the most common stoma site, however, the umbilicus can also be used, particularly in the obese patient where the distance to traverse will be made shorter. Continent cutaneous diversions can be created using ilium (Kock pouch) or right colon (Indiana, Florida, and Mainz). When colon is used, the continence mechanism relies on the ileocecal valve and loss of this valve may contribute to loose stools or diarrhea. Regardless of the diversion created, capacity is assured by detubularization, which disrupts the circular smooth muscle and thus decreases wall tension and folding. Continent diversions are usually created with nonrefluxing ureteral anastomoses. Orthotopic urinary diversions are made with similar principles in mind, using the sphincter as the continence mechanism. Expert consensus is that ureters can be implanted in a refluxing fashion. As mentioned above, candidates should not be at significant risk for developing cancer at the urethra. Orthotopic neobladders require manual dexterity as almost 20% of patients will require intermittent catheterization (women > men). Frank urinary retention in men, however, is uncommon and should alert the urologist to a possible recurrence. Nighttime incontinence is common, occurring in almost half of patients.

Complications

The complication rate following cystectomy and diversion is very high (64% having at least one complication within 90 days of surgery with 13% experiencing a high-grade complication and a 30-day mortality of 1.5%) [2]. In those older than 70 years, high-grade complications and mortality rates are increased. The majority of complications are related to bowel manipulation and infections. In the long term, an inevitable complication of urinary diversion is the reduction in absorptive capacity of the bowel with some patients (particularly those where the ileocecal valve is used) having loose stools and diarrhea. This can be managed first by stool-bulking agents such as Metamucil. Antimotility agents can also be tried. Further, as diarrhea can be related to bile salt irritation of the colon, treatment with cholestyramine can be used. Loss of ileum also leads to vitamin B12 deficiency which contributes to anemia and loss of myelin. While this typically takes at least 5 years to develop, it can occur earlier and it may be prudent to monitor levels annually after surgery. Absorption of ammonium and hydrogen chloride from the bowel segments can lead to hyperchloremic metabolic acidosis which contributes to osteoporosis (patients with renal insufficiency are at greater risk of this).

Neoadjuvant and adjuvant systemic chemotherapy

Up to half of the patients with muscle invasive disease develop metastasis, with death thought to occur from metastasis present at the time of cystectomy. After metastases develop, there are few long-term survivors though up to 70% are sensitive to chemotherapy suggesting that radical cystectomy and systemic therapy are needed to truly treat the majority of muscle invasive disease. Systemic chemotherapy can either be given before (neoadjuvant) or after (adjuvant) cystectomy. Advantages to neoadjuvant therapy are that the patients tend to have better performance before surgery and thus it is better tolerated. Furthermore, neoadjuvant therapy allows for true *in vivo* drug testing (allowing for better selection of therapies if tumors recur) and may down-stage some tumors making them easier to resect [23]. The major disadvantages are that neoadjuvant therapy may delay the time to cystectomy which may be particularly harmful to patients with tumors that are not responsive to the chemotherapy given. A theoretical disadvantage is that chemotherapy may make the surgery more difficult or predispose to complications postoperatively; this does not seem to be the case [1]. Corresponding to earlier randomized trials from the European Organization for Research and Treatment of Cancer (EORTC) and the Medical Research Council, the Southwest Oncology Group demonstrated a 5-year survival advantage after neoadjuvant chemotherapy for muscle invasive bladder cancer (methotrexate, vinblastine, adriamycin, and cisplatin [MVAC]) [1]. Here, there was a 25% reduction in the risk of death among those with neoadjuvant treatment with patients having advanced stage (≥T3) experiencing the greatest survival benefit. As these trials were limited by sample size, an advanced bladder cancer (ABC) metaanalysis was performed which also showed a survival advantage, albeit more modest (5%) with neoadjuvant therapy [24]. Because it is less toxic, most oncologists now prefer to use agents such as gemcitabine and cisplatin as oppose to MVAC [25]. Though critics of these studies state that the benefit for neoadjuvant therapy may be small and that there were no quality of life outcomes measured, neoadjuvant therapy has level 1 evidence supporting its use and we advocate doing so in the majority of patients presenting with muscle invasive disease.

Proponents of adjuvant chemotherapy state that it allows for immediate cystectomy and that it treats the tumor when the overall tumor burden has been lessened (after resection). Practically, however, given the high complication rate after cystectomy, it is not clear how many patients will be fit enough to receive adjuvant therapy [2, 26]. Unfortunately, trials testing adjuvant systemic chemotherapy suffered from poor accrual and design and no conclusion regarding its use can be made from any one trial and a meaningful metaanalysis cannot be performed [27]. Currently, adjuvant trials are still ongoing and hopefully results from EORTC 30994 will provide more insight. For now, however, best evidence for treatment supports neoadjuvant chemotherapy followed by radical cystectomy and complete lymph node dissection.

Bladder preservation protocols

Highly selected patients may be candidates for bladder preservation either by partial cystectomy or radical transurethral resection. Candidates for radical transurethral resection include those with tumors smaller than 3 cm, no CIS, clinical T2 disease, and disease not in the dome or posterior wall due to fear for bowel injury. Patients are re-resected at 3 months and if tumor is found, radical cystectomy or radiation is considered. Long-term survival in these selected patients is comparable to those undergoing radical cystectomy with about 25% of patients progressing to cystectomy [28]. Partial cystectomy candidates require that tumor be distant from trigone (ideal candidates are at the dome) and can be used in patient who have shown response to neoadjuvant chemotherapy [29]. No clinical trial has compared bladder preservation directly to cystectomy and most durable responses likely include bimodality or trimodality therapy. Because the study by Grossman showed that 60% of patients, believed to be in clinical stage T0, had persistent cancer, many authors recommend definitive therapy for muscle invasive bladder cancer [1].

Recurrence

Progression after definitive locoregional therapy usually occurs within the first 2 years in patients treated without systemic chemotherapy with the most common distant sites being the lung, liver, and bone. Central nervous system metastasis and peritoneal metastasis are more common after chemotherapy and tend to occur late. Patients should be monitored by routine physical examination, blood work, urine cytology, and imaging.

WHAT TO AVOID

- There should be no unnecessary delay between diagnosis and surgery (delay >12 weeks negatively affects outcome)
- Lymphadenectomy resulting in 10 or fewer nodes is inadequate
- Awareness of complications from urinary diversion may decrease their occurrence (i.e., electrolyte abnormalities, osteomalacia, B12 deficiency, urolithiasis)

KEY WEB LINKS

www.nccn.org

Multiple choice questions

1 Which of the following are true (select all that apply)?
   a In regards to neobladders, ureteral anastomosis should be made to be anti-refluxing in order to decrease the incidence of pyelonephritis
   b Patients report similar quality of life with all types of diversions
   c Ileal conduits pose a higher risk to the upper tracts than neobladders
   d A ureteroileal anastomosis using a Wallace technique reduces the frequency of anastomotic stricture

2 Prior to endoscopic resection, a mass is felt on examination along the left wall of the bladder. Resection is performed to completion. Repeat examination reveals a mobile, palpable mass of the left bladder wall. What is the clinical stage of this patient?
   a T1
   b T2
   c T3
   d T4

3 A 72-year-old gentleman with hydronephrosis and muscle invasive bladder cancer undergoes radical cystoprostatectomy with an ileal conduit after having neoadjuvant chemotherapy with MVAC (methotrexate, vinblastine, doxorubicin, and cisplatin). When compared to individuals who did not receive chemotherapy, he is more likely to experience recurrence in the...
   a Bone marrow
   b Brain
   c Liver
   d Lung

References

1 Grossman HB, Natale RB, Tangen CM, et al. Neoadjuvant chemotherapy plus cystectomy compared with cystectomy alone for locally advanced bladder cancer. *N Engl J Med* 2003;349(9):859–866.
2 Shabsigh A, Korets R, Vora KC, et al. Defining early morbidity of radical cystectomy for patients with bladder cancer using a standardized reporting methodology. *Eur Urol* 2009;55(1):164–174.
3 Manoharan M, Ayyathurai R, Soloway MS. Radical cystectomy for urothelial carcinoma of the bladder: an analysis of perioperative and survival outcome. *BJU Int* 2009;104(9):1227–1232.
4 Edge SB, Compton CC. The American Joint Committee on Cancer: the 7th edition of the AJCC cancer staging manual and the future of TNM. *Ann Surg Oncol* 2010;17(6):1471–1474.

5 Dutta SC, Smith JA, Jr., Shappell SB, Coffey CS, Chang SS, Cookson MS. Clinical under staging of high risk non-muscle invasive urothelial carcinoma treated with radical cystectomy. *J Urol* 2001;166(2):490–493.

6 Wood DP, Jr., Montie JE, Pontes JE, Levin HS. Identification of transitional cell carcinoma of the prostate in bladder cancer patients: a prospective study. *J Urol* 1989;142(1):83–85.

7 Lerner SP, Shen S. Pathologic assessment and clinical significance of prostatic involvement by transitional cell carcinoma and prostate cancer. *Urol Oncol* 2008;26(5):481–485.

8 Sanchez-Ortiz RF, Huang WC, Mick R, Van Arsdalen KN, Wein AJ, Malkowicz SB. An interval longer than 12 weeks between the diagnosis of muscle invasion and cystectomy is associated with worse outcome in bladder carcinoma. *J Urol* 2003;169(1):110–115; discussion 115.

9 Chade DC, Laudone VP, Bochner BH, Parra RO. Oncological outcomes after radical cystectomy for bladder cancer: open versus minimally invasive approaches. *J Urol* 2010;183(3):862–869.

10 Kessler TM, Burkhard FC, Perimenis P, et al. Attempted nerve sparing surgery and age have a significant effect on urinary continence and erectile function after radical cystoprostatectomy and ileal orthotopic bladder substitution. *J Urol* 2004;172(4 Pt 1):1323–1327.

11 Chang SS, Cole E, Cookson MS, Peterson M, Smith JA, Jr. Preservation of the anterior vaginal wall during female radical cystectomy with orthotopic urinary diversion: technique and results. *J Urol* 2002;168 (4 Pt 1):1442–1445.

12 Ali-El-Dein B, Gomha M, Ghoneim MA. Critical evaluation of the problem of chronic urinary retention after orthotopic bladder substitution in women. *J Urol* 2002;168(2):587–592.

13 Hardeman SW, Soloway MS. Urethral recurrence following radical cystectomy. *J Urol* 1990;144(3):666–669.

14 Stenzl A, Colleselli K, Poisel S, Feichtinger H, Pontasch H, Bartsch G. Rationale and technique of nerve sparing radical cystectomy before an orthotopic neobladder procedure in women. *J Urol* 1995;154(6):2044–2049.

15 Stenzl A, Draxl H, Posch B, Colleselli K, Falk M, Bartsch G. The risk of urethral tumors in female bladder cancer: can the urethra be used for orthotopic reconstruction of the lower urinary tract? *J Urol* 1995;153(3 Pt 2):950–955.

16 Schumacher MC, Scholz M, Weise ES, Fleischmann A, Thalmann GN, Studer UE. Is there an indication for frozen section examination of the ureteral margins during cystectomy for transitional cell carcinoma of the bladder? *J Urol* 2006;176(6 Pt 1):2409–2413; discussion 2413.

17 Osman Y, El-Tabey N, Abdel-Latif M, Mosbah A, Moustafa N, Shaaban A. The value of frozen-section analysis of ureteric margins on surgical decision-making in patients undergoing radical cystectomy for bladder cancer. *BJU Int* 2007;99(1):81–84.

18 Stein JP, Lieskovsky G, Cote R et al. Radical cystectomy in the treatment of invasive bladder cancer: long-term results in 1,054 patients. *J Clin Oncol* 2001;19(3):666–675.

19 Quek ML, Flanigan RC. The role of lymph node density in bladder cancer prognostication. *World J Urol* 2009;27(1):27–32.

20 Capitanio U, Suardi N, Shariat SF, et al. Assessing the minimum number of lymph nodes needed at radical cystectomy in patients with bladder cancer. *BJU Int* 2009;103(10):1359–1362.

21 Wright JL, Lin DW, Porter MP. The association between extent of lymphadenectomy and survival among patients with lymph node metastases undergoing radical cystectomy. *Cancer* 2008;112(11):2401–2408.

22 Vazina A, Dugi D, Shariat SF, Evans J, Link R, Lerner SP. Stage specific lymph node metastasis mapping in radical cystectomy specimens. *J Urol* 2004;171(5):1830–1834.

23 Calabro F, Sternberg CN. Neoadjuvant and adjuvant chemotherapy in muscle-invasive bladder cancer. *Eur Urol* 2009;55(2):348–358.

24 Advanced Bladder Cancer (ABC) Meta-analysis Collaboration. Neoadjuvant chemotherapy in invasive bladder cancer: update of a systematic review and meta-analysis of individual patient data advanced bladder cancer (ABC) meta-analysis collaboration. *Eur Urol* 2005;48(2):202–205; discussion 5-6.

25 Dash A, Pettus JA 4th, Herr HW, et al. A role for neoadjuvant gemcitabine plus cisplatin in muscle-invasive urothelial carcinoma of the bladder: a retrospective experience. *Cancer* 2008;113(9):2471–2477.

26 Donat SM. Integrating perioperative chemotherapy into the treatment of muscle-invasive bladder cancer: strategy versus reality. *J Natl Compr Canc Netw* 2009;7(1):40–47.

27 Sternberg CN, Collette L. What has been learned from meta-analyses of neoadjuvant and adjuvant chemotherapy in bladder cancer? *BJU Int* 2006;98(3):487–489.

28 Herr HW. Transurethral resection of muscle-invasive bladder cancer: 10-year outcome. *J Clin Oncol* 2001;19(1):89–93.

29 Koga F, Kihara K, Fujii Y, et al. Favourable outcomes of patients with clinical stage T3N0M0 bladder cancer treated with induction low-dose chemo-radiotherapy plus partial or radical cystectomy vs immediate radical cystectomy: a single-institutional retrospective comparative study. *BJU Int* 2009;104(2):189–194.

Answers to multiple choice questions

1 b, c, d
2 c
3 b

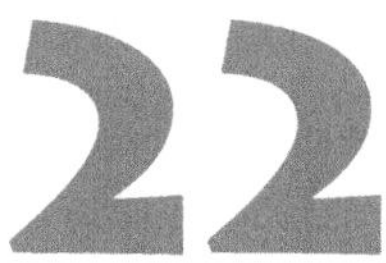

22 Penile and urethral cancer

Nicholas C. Field and Matthew Eric Hyndman
University of Calgary, Calgary, Alberta, Canada

KEY POINTS

- Penile cancer risk increases significantly with increasing age, poor hygiene, and the presence of a foreskin.
- Clinical examination of the inguinal lymph nodes is critical, as nodal involvement is a poor prognostic feature. Patients with T2 or higher grade tumors and lymphovascular invasion are at high risk of nodal involvement and probably should have a lymph node dissection.
- Penile lesions are often infected and cause significant surrounding inflammation. Despite this, 50% of palpable nodes will be malignant.
- Complications are relatively common after an inguinal lymph node dissection (ILD) and proper meticulous surgical technique is important to decrease postoperative morbidity.
- Urethral cancer is rare and may present as urinary obstruction or as an infectious lesion with a fistula and abscess.

CASE STUDY

A 63-year-old man presents to his primary care physician with progressing phimosis, discharge, and a somewhat painful enlarging glans. He is an uncircumcised single man who immigrated from the southern hemisphere with a long history of cigarette smoking, chewing tobacco, and snuff use. Past medical history includes diabetes, reflux, and a remote history of treated sexually transmitted disease and IV drug use. Antibiotics were initially helpful but have subsequently failed. He was eventually referred to his local urologist who was unable to retract his foreskin to directly examine his glans. Further examination revealed a firm glans with possible extension into the shaft of his penis. Inguinal nodes were nonpalpable. Imaging did not reveal evidence of distant disease. He was consented for a penile biopsy and possible partial penectomy. During the surgery, a partial penectomy was performed and final pathology revealed Grade 2 squamous cell carcinoma invading the corpora cavernosum with lymphovascular invasion and 2 cm clear margins. The option of performing a bilateral IND was discussed with the patient and he elected to proceed. A bilateral superficial resection was performed with no evidence of disease during the surgery but final pathology showed unilateral nodal involvement within one node on the right. Unfortunately he postoperatively developed a lymphocele shortly after his drain was removed which ultimately resolved with percutaneous drainage. He has now been disease-free for 6 months.

Handbook of Urology, First edition. J. Kellogg Parsons, John B. Eifler and Misop Han.
Published 2014 by John Wiley & Sons, Ltd.

Epidemiology

Squamous cell carcinoma of the penis and primary urethral cancer are relatively rare compared to other GU malignancies in developed nations. There is a much higher incidence in countries such as Uganda and Brazil [1] and very low rates in Israel. It is most commonly diagnosed in, but not exclusively a disease of, the elderly. Poorer socioeconomic status has been shown to confer increased risk and also possibly contribute to a delay in treatment. Early diagnosis, grading, and staging can lead to effective treatments with multimodal therapy; however, late-stage disease ultimately has a poor prognosis.

There are a number of well-established risk factors for penile cancer. The presence of a foreskin has been reported to cause a 3-fold increased risk [2, 3] of developing penile cancer and phimosis increases this to 16–65 fold [4, 5]. It has been speculated that inflammation and smegma contribute to the increased risk. Interestingly, other studies have shown that only early circumcision in the neonatal period is protective, which argues against chronic inflammation as the underlying mechanism [6, 7]. Smoking, chewing tobacco, number of sexual partners, and HPV 16/18 are also risk factors for squamous cell carcinoma to the penis.

Clinical presentation

Benign lesions such as inclusion cysts, lipomas, and neuromas may arise but usually they have been present for extended periods of time with little or no clinical change. A number of premalignant lesions which require treatment and close follow-up are listed in Table 22.1. Differentiating between benign, premalignant, and malignant lesions can be challenging and up to 25% of dysplastic premalignant lesions are incorrectly diagnosed [2]; therefore, a very low threshold to biopsy a lesion in question is advisable.

Penile carcinoma usually presents with a lump or nodule on the glans and prepuce and less commonly on the coronal sulcus and shaft [8]. Delays in seeking medical attention is a problem and can lead to patients presenting with large fungating ulcerative lesions often with evidence of metastatic disease through direct extension and/or inguinal nodes' involvement. Despite local invasion, pain is not proportional to clinical examination unless a secondary infection arises. Clinical examination should include careful inspection of the glans, foreskin, shaft, scrotum, and perineal region. A rectal examination and meticulous palpation of the inguinal nodes is also essential.

Investigations

Focused laboratory investigations directed to investigate anemia, infection, urinary obstruction, and hypercalcemia should be undertaken in addition to standard bloodwork. Direct extension and obstruction of the urethra needs to be considered and hypercalcemia secondary to paraneoplastic syndrome has been reported with penile cancer.

Distant metastasis does occur but usually presents later in the course of the disease after palpable inguinal metastasis. Therefore, initial staging with radiological

Table 22.1 Premalignant lesions which have been shown to evolve into squamous cell carcinoma, their associated pathology, and recommended treatments

Premalignant lesion	Pathology	Recommended treatment
Cutaneous horn	Hyperkeratosis, associated with HPV 16	Surgical excision and close observation
Pseudoepitheliomatous micaceous and keratotic balanitis	Hyperkeratotic and micaceous growth	Surgical excision and close observation
Lichen sclerosis (BXO)	Atrophic epidermis and loss of rete pegs	Topical steroid cream and surgical excision
Leukoplakia	Hyperkeratosis and leukoplakia	Surgical excision circumcision
Condyloma accuminata	HPV infection	Imiquimod cream (5%)
Verrucous carcinoma	Broad round rete pegs/HPV 6 and 11	Surgical excision. Radiotherapy is associated with malignant degeneration

imaging has limited utility in patients with nonpalpable disease. Ultrasound and cross-sectional imaging have both been investigated and have been shown to help modestly with staging of the primary lesion. They may be more useful in obese patients in whom an inguinal node examination is difficult. Imaging can be helpful in patients with palpable inguinal nodes to further delineate the extent of distant disease.

Staging and grading

Penile cancer grading is based on cellular anaplasia; Grade 1 well differentiated, Grade 2 moderately differentiated, and Grade 3 poorly differentiated. Some grading systems include a fourth category defined as undifferentiated [9]. Increasing grade is associated with increasing probability of nodal involvement and therefore prognosis [10, 11]. In addition to grade and stage, lymphovascular invasion is prognostic and may be important in guiding the decision to perform a lymph node dissection. Patients with T2 or higher grade tumors and lymphovascular invasion are at high risk of nodal involvement and probably should have a lymph node dissection [12, 13]. Other investigators have similarly shown that lymphovascular invasion, high grade tumors and nodes are the strongest predictors of metastatic disease [14]. The AJCC TNM staging system has recently been revised and is outlined in Table 22.2.

Table 22.2 AJCC 2010 TNM penile cancer staging

Primary tumor (T)	
TX	Primary tumor cannot be assessed
T0	No evidence of primary tumor
Tis	Carcinoma *in situ*
Ta	Noninvasive verrucous carcinoma
T1a	Tumor invades subepithelial connective tissue without lymph vascular invasion and is not poorly differentiated (i.e., Grade 3–4)
T1b	Tumor invades subepithelial connective tissue with lymph vascular invasion or is poorly differentiated
T2	Tumor invades corpus spongiosum or cavernosum
T3	Tumor invades urethra
T4	Tumor invades other adjacent structures
Regional lymph nodes (N) clinical stage definition	
cNX	Regional lymph nodes cannot be assessed
cN0	No palpable or visibly enlarged inguinal lymph nodes
cN1	Palpable mobile unilateral inguinal lymph node
cN2	Palpable mobile multiple or bilateral inguinal lymph nodes
cN3	Palpable fixed inguinal nodal mass or pelvic lymphadenopathy unilateral or bilateral
Regional lymph node: pathologic stage definition	
pNX	Regional lymph nodes cannot be assessed
pN0	No regional lymph node metastasis
pN1	Metastasis in a single inguinal lymph node
pN2	Metastases in multiple or bilateral inguinal lymph nodes
pN3	Extranodal extension of lymph node metastasis or pelvic lymph node(s) unilateral or bilateral
Distant metastasis (M)	
M0	No distant metastasis
M1	Distant metastasis

Primary lesion

Treatment of the primary lesion is dependent on the clinical stage and location. A more conservative treatment should be reserved for smaller lesions, whereas more aggressive surgical approaches should be directed to larger lesions. Irrespective of the approach, the goal of all treatments is to achieve negative surgical or destructive margins. In general, Tis, Ta, and T1a (lower grade) tumors can be treated with surgical excision, laser ablation, or Mohs microsurgery. T1b high grade and T2 tumors involving the glans should be resected. T2 tumors into the corpora should be surgically resected with a partial amputation if feasible [15]. Patients with T3 disease require a total penectomy and perineal urethrostomy. Finally, T4 disease can be approached surgically in select patients who respond to neoadjuvant chemotherapy [16].

Radiotherapy as external beam and/or brachytherapy is an alternative to surgical excision with reasonable local control rates, but it should be limited to lesions smaller than 4 cm. Salvage surgery may be required with recurrence [17–19]. Complications include urethral stenosis, glans necrosis, and fibrosis of the corpora [19].

Inguinal lymph nodes

Lymphatic drainage of the penis is bilateral and recent drainage studies have revealed that sentinel nodes are somewhat variable but are primarily located in the superior and central inguinal zones, with the majority being in the medial superior zone [20]. Complications from inguinal node dissections (INDs) such as skin edge necrosis, lymphedema, wound infection, seroma formation, and DVT are relatively common even though complication rates have decreased since the modification of the surgical template. These complications have led to the development of sentinel node biopsy which has seen significant improvements recently with reported sensitivities and specificities of 100% and 95%, respectively [21, 22]. Preoperative injection of Tc99 and blue dye is performed followed by surgical mapping and the standard surgical inguinal node template is completed if the sentinel nodes are positive. Nevertheless, there is some controversy as to which, and how, patients with nonpalpable nodes should undergo a node dissection. Approximately 20% of nonpalpable nodes are later found to contain tumor. More recent evidence suggests that early lymphadenectomy results in a 2-fold improvement in 5-year survival compared to delayed lymphadenectomy [23]. Classification systems incorporating patients into low (pTis, pTaG1-2, pT1G1), intermediate (T1G2), and high risk (T2 any G3) groups are helpful and may be used as a guide. The probability of having nodal involvement with these abovementioned categories was 7.7%, 28.6%, and 75%, respectively [24]. Surveillance of nonpalpable nodes can be performed in patients with low risk tumor, Tis, Ta, and T1G1. Intermediate risk patients, as outlined above, are dependent on lymphovascular invasion, and if present are likely to benefit from removal of the inguinal nodes. High risk patients benefit from a bilateral node dissection.

The timing of surgical intervention has also been investigated, where early intervention in some studies is associated with improved survival compared to delayed lymphadenectomy [23, 25]. Further, Theodoric et al. found a high relapse rate in patients undergoing surveillance with initially node-negative disease [26]. This data suggests that if a node dissection is going to be performed in node-negative patients, then it should be performed early rather than be delayed.

Palpable inguinal nodes

Almost half of patients with penile cancer present with palpable nodes [27] and ~50% of palpable nodes are inflammatory. Therefore a trial of antibiotics may be warranted, followed by re-examination. If the nodes remain palpable after antibiotic treatment or are obviously metastatic then aggressive intervention is likely needed. Surgical templates include the superficial and deep inguinal nodes bilaterally even with the presence of unilateral disease, given the lateral crossover of lymphatics and a 60% chance of bilateral disease. Neoadjuvant chemotherapy has recently been investigated in a few small studies with promising results and therefore it could be considered in select cases [28, 29].

Surgical technique of inguinal node dissection

The surgical inguinal lymph node dissection (ILD) for patients with clinically negative inguinal nodes was modified by Catalona [30, 31] to decrease postoperative complications. A shorter incision, limiting the lateral dissection to the femoral artery and preservation of the saphenous vein, decreased complications and prevented the need for sartorius muscle transposition. A full standard dissection (laterally the sartorius muscle, inferiorly the base of the femoral triangle, and medially to the adductor longus muscle) should be carried out if nodes are palpable or if the frozen section is positive during a modified template.

Pelvic lymph node dissection

Survival with penile SCC metastasized to the pelvic node involvement is poor, with an average 5-year survival of ~10% [32]. Nevertheless, some argue that a pelvic lymph node dissection (PLND) should be part of the surgical algorithm as it may have some benefit and palliation. Pelvic lymph nodes should only be considered for removal if there is inguinal involvement. More than two positive inguinal nodes have been shown to be predictive of pelvic lymph node involvement [23, 33] and therefore can be used to guide the decision to perform a PLND. Further, if there is clear metastasis in the pelvis and abdomen then a PLND should not be undertaken; however, a palliative IND has been argued to be beneficial [32, 34].

Complications of lymph node dissection

Complications after an IND dissection are common. Skin necrosis, flap necrosis, lymphocele, seroma, lymphedema, DVT, and cellulitis are all known to occur [32]. Prevention of the complications is primarily dependent on preservation of the skin flap vascular supply and careful handling of flap tissue. Postoperative drainage is recommended and grafting and muscle flaps can be used especially in extensive disease.

Summary

Penile cancer is a relatively rare GU malignancy in the developed world. Key points in its management include a low threshold for biopsy and excision of suspicious lesions as misdiagnosis is common. Low-stage lesions (CIS, T1) can be managed with local excision and somewhat conservatively; however, radical operative approaches are necessary as the stage of the presenting lesion increases. Lymphadenectomy, depending on the presenting lesion, should be performed; however, the extent and whether to include a pelvic node dissection is controversial. Sentinel node biopsy techniques seem to be improving and are reported to be reproducible, but currently should be performed in surgical centers with technical expertise.

Urethral cancer

Less than 1% of all malignancies in male patients are primary urethral cancer [35]. Urethral cancer is greater in men than in women with the overall annual incidence rate being 4.3 per million for men and 1.5 per million for women [36]. From 1973–2002, the incidence of all histological types of primary urethral cancer has been trending downward [36]. Inflammation of the urethra due to sexually transmitted infections, urethritis, or urethral stricture is thought to increase the risk of developing urethral cancer.

Anatomy and pathology

The urethra has three distinct segments. The prostatic and bulbomembranous segments are lined with transitional epithelium, whereas the penile segment is lined with pseudocolumnar stratified epithelium. Typically, transitional cell carcinoma and adenocarcinomas arise in the proximal segment of the urethra, whereas squamous cell carcinoma arises in both the proximal and the distal urethra. The major route of spread is by drainage into regional lymph nodes. The lymphatic drainage bed varies depending on the segment of the urethra. The penile urethra drains into the superficial and deep inguinal nodes, whereas the bulbomembranous and prostatic urethra segments drain into the internal and external iliac nodes [37].

Clinical presentation

Urethral cancers can present with symptoms ranging from urinary tract obstruction, dysuria, purulent discharge, and hematuria. Hematuria is typically present on initiation of micturition. The presence of a periurethral abscesses or fistula should raise the suspicion of urethral carcinoma and a biopsy is often warranted.

Initial evaluation

Initial evaluation of a patient suspected of having urethral cancer should include a meticulous physical examination of the urethra, surrounding structures, and lymph nodes, as well as a history that questions risk factors associated with urethral strictures and causes of urethral inflammation. Direct visualization with cystoscopy and a biopsy of the suspected lesions are likewise critical components of the initial investigation. Patients with fistulas or urethral abscesses should also be considered to potentially have malignant lesions. Imaging of the abdomen and pelvis should be performed with either MRI or enhanced CT.

Treatment

Well-defined treatment algorithms are poorly defined given that primary urethral cancer is so rare. Nevertheless, clinical staging (Table 22.3), grade, and location of the tumor have been found to be the predominant factors in determining clinical

Table 22.3 AJCC 2010 TNM urethral cancer staging

Primary tumor (T)	
TX	Primary tumor cannot be assessed
T0	No evidence of primary tumor
Tis	Carcinoma *in situ*
Ta	Noninvasive papillary, polypoid, or verrucous carcinoma
T1	Tumor invades subepithelial connective tissue
T2	Tumor invades any of the following: corpus spongiosum, prostate, periurethral muscle
T3	Tumor invades any of the following: corpus cavernosum, beyond prostatic capsule, anterior vagina, bladder neck
T4	Tumor invades other adjacent organs
Urothelial (transitional cell) carcinoma of the prostate	
Tis pu	Carcinoma *in situ*, involvement of the prostatic urethra
Tis pd	Carcinoma *in situ*, involvement of the prostatic ducts
T1	Tumor invades urethral subepithelial connective tissue
T2	Tumor invades any of the following: prostatic stroma, corpus spongiosum, periurethral muscle
T3	Tumor invades any of the following: corpus cavernosum, beyond prostatic capsule, bladder neck (extraprostatic extension)
T4	Tumor invades other adjacent organs (invasion of the bladder)
Regional lymph nodes (N)	
NX	Regional lymph nodes cannot be assessed
N0	No regional lymph node metastasis
N1	Metastasis in a single lymph node 2 cm or less in greatest dimension
N2	Metastasis in a single node more than 2 cm in greatest dimension, or in multiple nodes
Distant metastasis (M)	
M0	No distant metastasis
M1	Distant metastasis

management and patient survival [38]. For low-stage tumors (Ta-2, N0, M0) that involve only the distal urethra, surgical excision, or radiotherapy are viable treatment options. [37]. Overall, for patients with low-stage disease (Ta-2, N0, M0), treatment outcomes are improved regardless of the method of treatment [38]. Multimodal therapy (neoadjuvant chemotherapy and radiation therapy, either with or without surgery) has been shown to be beneficial in later-stage tumors [38]. Predictors of increased likelihood of death, as well as death from disease, include advanced age, higher grade, higher T stage, systemic metastasis, other histology (non-TCC, non-SCC, nonadenocarcinoma) versus TCC, and no surgery versus radical resection [35]. Other than stage and grade, predictors of mortality are nodal metastasis and adenocarcinoma as compared with TCC [35]. In men with T2-4 nonmetastatic urethral cancer, significantly higher cancer-specific survival was noted with excision or radical surgery alone compared with radiation alone or with neither surgery nor radiation [35].

Summary

Urethral cancer is a rare but morbid disease. Treatment is primarily dependent on location and stage at presentation. High-stage lesions should be treated with multimodal therapy.

WHAT TO AVOID

- Penile lesions are often misdiagnosed; therefore, surgeons must have a low threshold for biopsies of suspicious lesions.
- Urethral lesions/strictures associated with fistulas or abscesses should be biopsied and have a high suspicion for urethral cancer.

KEY WEB LINKS

National Comprehensive Cancer Network
http://www.nccn.org/professionals/physician_gls/f_guidelines.asp

European Urological Association
http://www.uroweb.org/guidelines/online-guidelines/

Multiple choice questions

1 Prognosis of squamous cell carcinoma of the penis is most dependent on:
  a Grade
  b Smoking history
  c Lymph node involvement
  d Lymphovascular invasion

2 All are premalignant lesions for squamous cell carcinoma of the penis except:
  a Verrucous carcinoma
  b BXO
  c Leukoplakia
  d Pseudoepitheliomatous keratotic and micaceous balanitis
  e Herpes

References

1 Landis SH, Murray T, Bolden S, Wingo PA. Cancer statistics, 1999. *CA Cancer J Clin* 1999;49(1):8–31, 1. Epub 1999/04/14.

2 Deem S, Keane T, Bhavsar R, El-Zawahary A, Savage S. Contemporary diagnosis and management of squamous cell carcinoma (SCC) of the penis. *BJU Int* 2011;108(9):1378–1392. Epub 2011/10/26.

3 Licklider S. Jewish penile carcinoma. *J Urol* 1961;86:98. Epub 1961/07/01.

4 Hellberg D, Valentin J, Eklund T, Nilsson S. Penile cancer: is there an epidemiological role for smoking and sexual behaviour? *Br Med J* 1987;295(6609):1306–1308. Epub 1987/11/21.

5 Bleeker MC, Heideman DA, Snijders PJ, Horenblas S, Dillner J, Meijer CJ. Penile cancer: epidemiology, pathogenesis and prevention. *World J Urol* 2009;27(2): 141–150. Epub 2008/07/09.

6 Maden C, Sherman KJ, Beckmann AM, et al. History of circumcision, medical conditions, and sexual activity and risk of penile cancer. *J Natl Cancer Inst* 1993;85(1): 19–24. Epub 1993/01/06.

7 Schoen EJ, Oehrli M, Colby C, Machin G. The highly protective effect of newborn circumcision against invasive penile cancer. *Pediatrics* 2000;105(3):E36. Epub 2000/03/04.

8 Sufrin G, Huben R. Benign and malignant lesions of the penis. In: Gillenwater JY, Howards SS, Duckett JW, editors. *Adult and Pediatric Urology*. 2nd ed. St. Louis, MO: Mosby-Year Book; 1991.

9 Velazquez EF, Ayala G, Liu H, et al. Histologic grade and perineural invasion are more important than tumor

thickness as predictor of nodal metastasis in penile squamous cell carcinoma invading 5 to 10 mm. *Am J Surg Pathol* 2008;32(7):974–979. Epub 2008/05/08.

10 Solsona E, Iborra I, Rubio J, Casanova JL, Ricos JV, Calabuig C. Prospective validation of the association of local tumor stage and grade as a predictive factor for occult lymph node micrometastasis in patients with penile carcinoma and clinically negative inguinal lymph nodes. *J Urol* 2001;165(5):1506–1509. Epub 2001/05/09.

11 Ficarra V, Zattoni F, Cunico SC, et al. Lymphatic and vascular embolizations are independent predictive variables of inguinal lymph node involvement in patients with squamous cell carcinoma of the penis: Gruppo Uro-Oncologico del Nord Est (Northeast Uro-Oncological Group) Penile Cancer data base data. *Cancer* 2005;103(12):2507–2516. Epub 2005/04/28.

12 Horenblas S. Lymphadenectomy for squamous cell carcinoma of the penis. Part 1: diagnosis of lymph node metastasis. *BJU Int* 2001;88(5):467–472. Epub 2001/10/09.

13 Slaton JW, Morgenstern N, Levy DA, et al. Tumor stage, vascular invasion and the percentage of poorly differentiated cancer: independent prognosticators for inguinal lymph node metastasis in penile squamous cancer. *J Urol* 2001;165(4):1138–1142. Epub 2001/03/21.

14 Bhagat SK, Gopalakrishnan G, Kekre NS, et al. Factors predicting inguinal node metastasis in squamous cell cancer of penis. *World J Urol* 2010;28(1):93–98. Epub 2009/06/03.

15 Gotsadze D, Matveev B, Zak B, Mamaladze V. Is conservative organ-sparing treatment of penile carcinoma justified? *Eur Urol* 2000;38(3):306–312. Epub 2000/08/15.

16 Ornellas AA, Kinchin EW, Nobrega BL, Wisnescky A, Koifman N, Quirino R. Surgical treatment of invasive squamous cell carcinoma of the penis: Brazilian National Cancer Institute long-term experience. *J Surg Oncol* 2008;97(6):487–495. Epub 2008/04/22.

17 de Crevoisier R, Slimane K, Sanfilippo N, et al. Long-term results of brachytherapy for carcinoma of the penis confined to the glans (N- or NX). *Int J Radiat Oncol Biol Phys* 2009;74(4):1150–1156. Epub 2009/04/28.

18 Azrif M, Logue JP, Swindell R, Cowan RA, Wylie JP, Livsey JE. External-beam radiotherapy in T1-2 N0 penile carcinoma. *Clin Oncol* 2006;18(4):320–325. Epub 2006/05/18.

19 Zouhair A, Coucke PA, Jeanneret W, et al. Radiation therapy alone or combined surgery and radiation therapy in squamous-cell carcinoma of the penis? *Eur J Cancer* 2001;37(2):198–203. Epub 2001/02/13.

20 Leijte JA, Valdes Olmos RA, Nieweg OE, Horenblas S. Anatomical mapping of lymphatic drainage in penile carcinoma with SPECT-CT: implications for the extent of inguinal lymph node dissection. *Eur Urol* 2008;54(4):885–890. Epub 2008/05/27.

21 Lont AP, Horenblas S, Tanis PJ, Gallee MP, van Tinteren H, Nieweg OE. Management of clinically node negative penile carcinoma: improved survival after the introduction of dynamic sentinel node biopsy. *J Urol* 2003;170(3):783–786. Epub 2003/08/13.

22 Wawroschek F, Vogt H, Bachter D, Weckermann D, Hamm M, Harzmann R. First experience with gamma probe guided sentinel lymph node surgery in penile cancer. *Urol Res* 2000;28(4):246–249. Epub 2000/09/30.

23 McDougal WS. Carcinoma of the penis: improved survival by early regional lymphadenectomy based on the histological grade and depth of invasion of the primary lesion. *J Urol* 1995;154(4):1364–1366. Epub 1995/10/01.

24 Hungerhuber E, Schlenker B, Karl A, et al. Risk stratification in penile carcinoma: 25-year experience with surgical inguinal lymph node staging. *Urology* 2006;68(3):621–625. Epub 2006/09/19.

25 Johnson DE, Lo RK. Management of regional lymph nodes in penile carcinoma. Five-year results following therapeutic groin dissections. *Urology* 1984;24(4): 308–311. Epub 1984/10/01.

26 Theodorescu D, Russo P, Zhang ZF, Morash C, Fair WR. Outcomes of initial surveillance of invasive squamous cell carcinoma of the penis and negative nodes. *J Urol* 1996;155(5):1626–1631. Epub 1996/05/01.

27 Horenblas S, Van Tinteren H, Delemarre JF, Moonen LM, Lustig V, Kroger R. Squamous cell carcinoma of the penis: accuracy of tumor, nodes and metastasis classification system, and role of lymphangiography, computerized tomography scan and fine needle aspiration cytology. *J Urol* 1991;146(5):1279–1283. Epub 1991/11/01.

28 Bermejo C, Busby JE, Spiess PE, Heller L, Pagliaro LC, Pettaway CA. Neoadjuvant chemotherapy followed by aggressive surgical consolidation for metastatic penile squamous cell carcinoma. *J Urol* 2007;177(4): 1335–1338. Epub 2007/03/27.

29 Pagliaro LC, Williams DL, Daliani D, et al. Neoadjuvant paclitaxel, ifosfamide, and cisplatin chemotherapy for metastatic penile cancer: a phase II study. *J Clin Oncol* 2010;28(24):3851–3857. Epub 2010/07/14.

30 Catalona WJ. Modified inguinal lymphadenectomy for carcinoma of the penis with preservation of saphenous veins: technique and preliminary results. *J Urol* 1988;140(2):306–310. Epub 1988/08/01.

31 Colberg JW, Andriole GL, Catalona WJ. Long-term follow-up of men undergoing modified inguinal lymphadenectomy for carcinoma of the penis. *Brit J Urol* 1997;79(1):54–57. Epub 1997/01/01.

32 Heyns CF, Fleshner N, Sangar V, Schlenker B, Yuvaraja TB, van Poppel H. Management of the lymph nodes in penile cancer. *Urology* 2010;76(2 Suppl 1):S43–S57. Epub 2010/08/19.
33 Horenblas S, van Tinteren H, Delemarre JF, Moonen LM, Lustig V, van Waardenburg EW. Squamous cell carcinoma of the penis. III. Treatment of regional lymph nodes. *J Urol* 1993;149(3):492–497. Epub 1993/03/01.
34 Abi-Aad AS, deKernion JB. Controversies in ilioinguinal lymphadenectomy for cancer of the penis. *Urol Clin North Am* 1992;19(2):319–324. Epub 1992/05/01.
35 Rabbani F. Prognostic factors in male urethral cancer. *Cancer* 2010;117(11):2426–2434. Epub 2010/12/16.
36 Swartz MA, Porter MP, Lin DW, Weiss NS. Incidence of primary urethral carcinoma in the United States. *Urology* 2006;68(6):1164–1168. Epub 2006/12/05.
37 Koontz BF, Lee WR. Carcinoma of the urethra: radiation oncology. *Urol Clin North Am* 2010;37(3):459–466. Epub 2010/08/03.
38 Eng TY, Naguib M, Galang T, Fuller CD. Retrospective study of the treatment of urethral cancer. *Am J Clin Oncol* 2003;26(6):558–562. Epub 2003/12/10.

Answers to multiple choice questions

1 c
2 e

23 Ureteral and renal pelvic tumors

Elias Hyams and Brian Matlaga

The James Buchanan Brady Urological Institute and Department of Urology, The Johns Hopkins School of Medicine, Baltimore, MD, USA

KEY POINTS

- Upper tract urothelial cancer is relatively rare, and constitutes 10% of renal malignancies and 5% of urothelial cancers overall.
- Diagnosis of this entity has been rising over the last several decades likely due to improved axial imaging techniques, advances in endoscopic technology, and improved survival from bladder cancer leading to higher rates of metachronous upper tract recurrence.
- Patients with transitional cell carcinoma (TCC) of the upper tract generally present with gross or microscopic hematuria (80%).
- Diagnostic evaluation should include axial abdominal imaging including CT or MR urography, chest imaging, urine cytology, cystoscopy, full bloodwork including assessment of renal function and liver function tests, and endoscopic evaluation with biopsy.
- The gold standard treatment for high-grade, invasive, and/or bulky upper tract lesions is radical nephroureterectomy with bladder cuff excision; this can be performed by open or minimally invasive techniques.
- Nephron-sparing surgery, either segmental ureterectomy or endoscopic ablation, should be considered for low-risk disease and/or when there is a compelling reason for renal preservation (e.g., chronic kidney disease, solitary kidney); however, these patients should be counseled regarding the risks of recurrence and the need for vigilant lifelong surveillance.
- Platinum-based chemotherapy has a role in treating high-risk upper tract TCC in both neoadjuvant and adjuvant settings; however, the purported benefits of these approaches are extrapolated from the bladder cancer experience.

CASE STUDY 1

A 75-year-old man presents to the urologist with microscopic hematuria, referred by his primary care physician. His medical history is remarkable for hypertension and coronary artery disease. He reports a 30 pack-year smoking history though he quit 8 years ago. His physical examination is unremarkable. A recent serum creatinine is 1.2 and liver function tests are normal. As part of his hematuria evaluation, he has a CT urogram performed that reveals a 1.5 cm filling defect in the right renal pelvis, suspicious for a soft tissue neoplasm. An office cystoscopy is performed, which reveals a normal bladder without lesions. A voided urine cytology is atypical but cannot exclude high-grade urothelial cancer.

The patient undergoes ureteroscopy with biopsy of the renal lesion; this reveals a large necrotic neoplasm in the right renal pelvis. Selective cytology is taken as barbotage over the tumor. Several biopsies of the lesion are taken and sent for pathology. A ureteral stent is placed to prevent perioperative renal colic.

The cytology and biopsy from the operating room show a high-grade urothelial neoplasm. The patient has a full metastatic evaluation, including a chest X-ray and repeat bloodwork that show no evidence of metastatic disease. The patient is scheduled for a laparoscopic radical nephroureterectomy with bladder cuff excision. The nephrectomy is performed with standard laparoscopic techniques.

Handbook of Urology, First edition. J. Kellogg Parsons, John B. Eifler and Misop Han.
Published 2014 by John Wiley & Sons, Ltd.

A lymphadenectomy is performed including renal hilar and paracaval nodes, which are not grossly enlarged. A Gibson incision is made in the right lower quadrant for dissection of the distal ureter and bladder cuff. The surgery is uncomplicated and the patient is discharged in 3 days with a Foley catheter in place. He returns at 1 week for a cystogram showing a healed bladder, and the Foley catheter is removed. His final pathology shows pT3N0Mx high-grade urothelial cancer. His postoperative serum creatinine is 1.5. He is sent for a consultation with medical oncology for consideration of adjuvant chemotherapy; however, decision is made to follow him expectantly with imaging, bloodwork, and cystoscopy.

CASE STUDY 2

A 59-year-old woman with a history of diabetes mellitus and chronic kidney disease underwent a CT scan in the emergency department (ED) for the evaluation of abdominal pain; the scan detected a lesion in her left kidney. She is referred to the urology clinic for follow-up. She reports acute abdominal cramping that resolved soon after arriving in the ED. A thorough workup in the ED included the scan above, as well as bloodwork that revealed a creatinine of 2.1, stable from prior values, and normal liver function tests. A chest X-ray was normal in the ED. The CT scan showed a possible 1 mass within the left upper pole calyx, and was done with oral contrast only based on elevated creatinine.

In clinic, a physical examination is unremarkable. A urine cytology is sent and shows no abnormal cells, only red blood cells and inflammation. A urinalysis shows 10 rbc/hpf without signs of infection. The patient is scheduled for an MR urogram based on her renal dysfunction and concern regarding nephrotoxicity of iodinated contrast. The MR urogram shows an 8 mm filling defect in the left upper pole, as well as a 5 mm defect within the renal pelvis. The patient is then scheduled for endoscopic evaluation in the operating room.

Cystoscopy in the operating room reveals no bladder tumors. Ureteroscopy is performed revealing a small papillary tumor within the upper pole and renal pelvis, as noted on MRI. Urine cytology is selectively aspirated and biopsies are obtained. These reveal a low-grade papillary neoplasm. Treatment options are discussed with the patient, including endoscopic ablative therapy versus nephroureterectomy. Given concern regarding worsened renal dysfunction with extirpative surgery, and her apparently limited low-grade disease, she opts for endoscopic ablation. She is brought back to the operating room where flexible ureteroscopic Holmium laser ablation is performed of her lesions. She tolerates this well and has a stent placed that is removed in clinic 1 week later.

Three months later, she has repeat endoscopy that shows a small papillary regrowth near the site of prior ablation. This is biopsied and re-ablated. Biopsy again shows low-grade neoplasm. Cytology at that time shows mildly atypical cells. She is scheduled for repeat endoscopic evaluation with contralateral retrograde pyelogram 3 months later.

Introduction

Upper tract urothelial tumors are relatively rare, comprising ~10% of all renal tumors and 5% of urothelial tumors [1]. These tumors occur more commonly in the renal collecting system (75%) but also occur within the ureter (25%). The histology of these lesions is transitional cell carcinoma (TCC) in >90% of patients; this chapter will focus primarily on details of this process, as other upper tract tumors occur quite infrequently. The pathophysiology and treatment paradigms for upper tract TCC mirror those in bladder cancer, as urothelial cancer is considered a "field defect" that places the entire urinary tract at risk. In this chapter, we review the epidemiology and pathophysiology of upper tract TCC, as well as the standard diagnostic evaluation and treatment options that include both extirpative and ablative surgical techniques.

Pathology

Upper tract urothelial tumors are TCC in the vast majority of cases (>90%). As in the bladder, upper tract TCC can be papillary or sessile, as well as uni- or multifocal. Invasion is thought to occur more rapidly in the upper tract, however, because of the thinner muscular layer of the urothelium. In fact, 60% of upper tract lesions are invasive at diagnosis compared with

15% of bladder tumors [2]. There is a micropapillary subtype of TCC that is infrequently seen but is associated with a poor outcome.

Other histopathologies for upper tract tumors include squamous cell carcinoma (SCC) (9%), adenocarcinoma, sarcoma, and inverted papilloma (1%). Risk factors for SCC are thought to include chronic inflammation, infection, and cyclophosphamide exposure. These tumors occur more commonly in the renal pelvis, and have a higher likelihood of invasive disease at initial diagnosis. Adenocarcinoma is associated with inflammation, stone disease, and long-term obstruction, and generally presents at an advanced stage. Sarcomas occur infrequently and may include leiomyosarcoma, plasmacytoma, and angiosarcoma [3]. Additional benign tumors of the upper tract include inverted papilloma, fibroepithelial polyps, and neurofibroma.

Epidemiology

Recent studies have demonstrated a rise in the incidence of upper tract TCC in the last 30 years, with peak incidence occurring in patients 75–79 years old (10 per 100,000) [4, 5]. Rising incidence has been thought to result from refinements in cross-sectional abdominal imaging techniques, as well as from improvements in upper tract endoscopic technology. Also, improvements in bladder cancer survival have likely led to an increased susceptibility to metachronous upper tract recurrence [4]. Upper tract TCC occurs three to four times more commonly in males compared with females, and Caucasians are affected approximately twice as frequently as African Americans. Geographically, the highest incidence of upper tract TCC occurs in Balkan countries, where urothelial cancer comprises 40% of all renal cancers [3].

Tobacco smoking is considered the most significant risk factor for upper tract TCC. Increased coffee consumption, analgesic abuse (i.e., phenacetin), arsenic exposure, and certain occupational exposures including aromatic amines have also been reported to be risk factors. Aristolochic acid and certain Chinese herbs have proposed causative roles for upper tract TCC. A high incidence of this disease has been seen in Taiwan, and an association with blackfoot disease has been described.

Balkan nephropathy is a degenerative interstitial nephropathy that has been reported to occur with increased frequency in the Balkan nations, that is, Southeastern Europe, and is associated with an increased incidence of upper tract TCC. Tumors in these patients are typically low grade, and are more commonly multiple and bilateral. There is thought to be an environmental etiology that has not been precisely identified. Upper tract tumors related to Balkan nephropathy, analgesic abuse, and arsenic exposure are thought to have an increased tendency toward multiple and bilateral recurrences [3].

Pathophysiology

TCC in the upper tract is thought to evolve from hyperplasia to dysplasia, to carcinoma *in situ* (CIS) and then to invasive cancer [3]. This pathophysiology is thought to mirror cell progression in the lower urinary tract. It is hypothesized that there is a "field defect" in urothelial cancer such that all urothelial cells are theoretically at risk as they may spawn from the same progenitor cell. High-grade tumors are more likely to invade underlying tissues, and to be associated with CIS elsewhere on the urothelium. The risk of invasion may be higher in the upper tract compared with the bladder, as the renal pelvis and ureter have a thinner muscle layer that may increase risk of invasive disease. Some have hypothesized that the ureter may be at particular risk for tumor extension as the kidney has parenchyma to act as a barrier to local progression [3]. However, when adjusted for tumor stage, tumor location (renal pelvis vs. ureter) does not appear to independently impact prognosis [2, 6]. Ureteral tumors occur more frequently in the distal ureter (80%) compared with the mid (25%) and the proximal ureter (5%) [3]. Bilateral upper tract disease occurs in 1.6–6% of sporadic cases [3].

Upper tract TCC can spread via direct invasion, lymphovascular invasion, and/or epithelial advancement by seeding or direct spread. Lymphatic spread depends on the location and stage of the primary tumor, but can involve para-aortic, paracaval, and ipsilateral common iliac and pelvic lymph nodes. Hematogenous metastasis can involve the liver, lung, bones, and regional lymph nodes [3].

Upper tract TCC occurs after bladder cancer treatment in up to 7% of patients [7, 8]. Patients with CIS of the bladder are more likely to have upper tract recurrence [3]. Additional risk factors for upper tract recurrence include high-grade, nonmuscle invasive disease, and trigonal or periureteral disease [9]. Patients with upper tract TCC have a 15–75% risk of developing metachronous bladder cancer within 5 years; downstream seeding of tumor cells is thought to contribute to this high rate [3].

The molecular and genetic biology of upper tract TCC is thought to be similar to disease in the bladder. Overexpression of certain tumor suppressor genes have been implicated, including TP53, RB, gene foci on chromosome 9 [3]. Certain genetic syndromes are associated with upper tract TCC; in particular, Lynch syndrome II is associated with colonic tumors and extracolonic neoplasms including upper tract carcinoma. This syndrome is caused by mutations in DNA mismatch repair genes.

Diagnosis

Hematuria (gross or microscopic) is the most common presenting sign of upper tract urothelial cancer (80%). Pain may occur in up to 30% of cases, and symptoms of advanced disease may include weight loss, anorexia, and fatigue. Up to 40% of patients develop upper tract obstruction from tumor or blood clots [3]. Incidental diagnosis during imaging occurs in up to 15% of patients.

Initial evaluation for suspected upper tract TCC includes a history and physical examination, cross-sectional abdominal imaging, chest imaging, cystoscopy, urine cytology, and full bloodwork including a complete blood count, basic metabolic panel, and liver function tests.

Contemporary axial imaging for assessment of upper tract cancer includes computed tomography (CT) or magnetic resonance (MR) urography. Scans are obtained with delayed phases to detect enhancing lesions and filling defects within the renal pelvis and ureters. These modalities have superior detection for upper tract lesions compared with conventional excretory urography or ultrasound [10]. Pooled sensitivity and specificity of CT urography may exceed 96% for upper tract lesions [11]. Findings suggestive of upper tract disease include radiolucent filling defects on urographic phases, mass lesions with enhancement, and/or obstruction or incomplete filling of the upper tract. Differentiating primary renal neoplasms from urothelial cancer is generally straightforward, as urothelial cancers arise from the collecting system and may have a more infiltrative appearance, while renal neoplasms are more encapsulated and within the parenchyma. However, in selected cases, discriminating between these lesions can be challenging and ureteroscopic evaluation may be needed for differentiation prior to pursuing treatment. Axial abdominal imaging also provides staging information regarding local extent, lymphadenopathy, and visceral metastatic disease, and delineates the anatomy and function of the contralateral kidney. Patients who have contraindications to intravenous contrast, either iodinated or gadolinium, can alternatively undergo retrograde pyelography. Chest imaging, either plain radiography or CT, should be performed to ensure the absence of lung metastasis. Additional imaging may be warranted based on clinical presentation or laboratory data, for example, a nuclear bone scan for the presence of bone pain or high-serum LDH.

Cystoscopy should be performed in patients with suspected upper tract TCC as these patients are at risk for synchronous bladder lesions. This may require staging and definitive management as well that can be coordinated with treatment of upper tract disease. Urine cytology from the bladder should be obtained, though sensitivity may vary based on tumor grade [12]. Patients may be encountered with positive bladder urine cytology but a normal bladder and prostatic urethra endoscopically, and normal upper tract imaging; in these patients, selective upper tract cytology should be obtained with consideration of ureteroscopy to rule out upper tract CIS.

Diagnosis of a filling defect or suspicious urothelial process mandates a ureteroscopic evaluation. Indeed, small, sessile lesions or CIS may not be evident on urographic imaging. Upper tract endoscopy has advanced technologically in the last several decades to enable routine access to the upper tract. Smaller and more flexible endoscopes allow for assessment of the entire collecting system, with improved resolution from digital technology. Diagnostic accuracy can improve up to 90% with endoscopic evaluation from 75% with excretory or retrograde urography [3].

If a tumor is discovered, biopsy should be performed with a basket, grasper, or brush device through the ureteroscope. If there is high suspicion for superficial disease with limited focality, ablative treatment can be performed at that time (see the discussion in the Management section below). Otherwise, definitive management should await biopsy results, as these may determine whether extirpative or ablative treatment is recommended. Ureteroscopy with biopsy enables staging with good sensitivity for tumor grade (78%) [13, 14].

See Table 23.1 for the TNM clinical staging system for upper tract TCC [15].

Table 23.1 American Joint Committee on Cancer (AJCC) tumor, node, metastasis clinical classification for renal pelvis and ureteral tumors

T	
Tx	Primary tumor cannot be assessed
T0	No evidence of primary tumor
Ta	Noninvasive papillary carcinoma
Tis	Carcinoma *in situ*
T1	Tumor invades subepithelial connective tissue
T2	Tumor invades the muscularis
T3	Renal pelvis: tumor invades beyond muscularis into peripelvic fat or renal parenchyma
	Ureter: tumor invades beyond muscularis into periureteric fat
T4	Tumor invades adjacent organs or through the kidney into perinephric fat
N	
Nx	Regional lymph nodes cannot be assessed
N0	No regional lymph node metastasis
N1	Metastasis in a single lymph node ≤2 cm in greatest dimension
N2	Metastasis in a single lymph node >2 cm but ≤5 cm in greatest dimension, or multiple lymph nodes (all ≤5 cm)
N3	Metastasis in a lymph node >5 cm in greatest dimension
M	
Mx	Distant metastasis cannot be assessed
M0	No distant metastasis
M1	Distant metastasis

Source: American Joint Committee on Cancer. *AJCC Cancer Staging Manual*. New York: Springer; 2010; 646.

Management

Treatment options for upper tract TCC include both extirpative and ablative techniques. The extirpative techniques include open versus laparoscopic radical nephroureterectomy and open versus laparoscopic segmental ureterectomy; the ablative techniques include retrograde versus antegrade/percutaneous tumor ablation. The gold standard treatment for invasive, high-grade, and/or bulky disease is radical nephroureterectomy with bladder cuff excision. Nephron-sparing approaches (i.e., segmental ureterectomy or endoscopic ablation) can be considered for noninvasive, low-grade disease, and/or those with impaired renal function or medical contraindications to extirpative surgery. Unfortunately, the low incidence of upper tract TCC and lack of level 1 evidence regarding treatment options has made it difficult to draw definitive conclusions about relative treatment efficacy [16].

Neoadjuvant chemotherapy has recently entered the treatment paradigm for upper tract TCC, similar to its role in bladder cancer [17]. Patients with advanced disease (>T2) may obtain a survival advantage from neoadjuvant therapy, typically platinum-based agents analogous to those utilized in the lower tract experience. Neoadjuvant therapy may enable high-risk patients to receive chemotherapy that might be contraindicated after nephroureterectomy based on deterioration of renal function [18]. Given the low incidence of this disease, however, benefits for upper tract patients are extrapolated from the lower tract literature, and there is no level 1 evidence of a survival benefit in this population.

Extirpative surgery

Historically, partial nephrectomy has been considered for selected invasive tumors with an imperative indication for renal preservation (e.g., solitary kidney). However, this is not the standard of care, and high recurrence rates have been reported [3]. Even for solitary kidneys with high-risk lesions, it is presently thought that radical nephroureterectomy with dialysis is the preferred option to maximize survival [3].

The gold standard treatment for high-grade, invasive (≥T2) lesions is radical nephroureterectomy with bladder cuff excision [19]. This can be performed by either open or minimally invasive techniques with comparable outcomes [20]. Also, bulky or multifocal low-grade disease may be best treated with nephroureterectomy. Excision of the distal ureter and bladder cuff are mandatory, as there is a high rate of recurrence if this is not done (7–30%) [12].

Open radical nephroureterectomy can be performed through various incisions including a long midline incision, a subcostal incision in addition to a Gibson, lower midline, or Pfannenstiel incision for bladder cuff removal, or a single thoracoabdominal incision. The specimen should include the kidney, Gerota's fascia, perinephric fat with or without the ipsilateral adrenal gland, ureter, and bladder cuff. The adrenal may be spared if there are no radiographic abnormalities and it is grossly normal during dissection.

Laparoscopic/robotic surgery can be performed as well through standard nephrectomy techniques. The approach can be transperitoneal, retroperitoneal, and hand assisted. Lower perioperative morbidity is achieved through the minimally invasive approach, including shorter hospital stay, less postoperative pain, and expedited overall recovery [21]. Long-term cancer control with laparoscopic nephroureterectomy has been shown to be equivalent to open surgery [22, 23]. However, distal ureteral and bladder cuff dissection typically require additional ports to triangulate toward the distal ureter and pelvis. Laparoscopic nephrectomy with open bladder cuff excision, through a Gibson, midline, or Pfannenstiel incision, is a viable approach, as the lower incision allows for both straightforward bladder dissection and extraction of the specimen. There are numerous techniques for managing the distal ureter and bladder cuff in a minimally invasive fashion. These include transurethral resection of the ureteral orifice, intussusception (stripping) technique, transvesical ligation and detachment, and a total laparoscopic/robotic technique [3]. Importantly, TCC has the potential to seed surfaces that it contacts, thus maintaining a "closed system" is mandatory [3]. This includes controlling the ureter with ties or clips during dissection, as well as placing the specimen within a specimen bag prior to extraction.

Regional lymphadenectomy should be performed with radical nephroureterectomy when feasible. For tumors of the renal pelvis and proximal or mid ureter, removal of ipsilateral renal hilar nodes as well as para-aortic or paracaval nodes are generally recommended [3]. If patients have grossly positive and/or fixed nodes, dissection should be limited or not performed per surgeon discretion. These patients have a high risk of systemic disease and are unlikely to be cured by lymphadenectomy. Indeed, most patients with positive lymph nodes develop early metastasis [3]. However, if lymphadenectomy can be performed expeditiously, it can provide valuable staging information and may have therapeutic value in selected patients [3].

Segmental ureterectomy with ureteroureterostomy or ureteral reimplantation can be considered for low-grade disease that is not amenable to endoscopic treatment. This procedure can also be performed open or via minimally invasive techniques. Wide dissection of the area with tumor should be performed. A regional lymphadenectomy should be performed. A tension-free repair should be completed with ureteral stenting and closed-suction drainage of the pelvis. Psoas hitch or Boari flap may be required if a tension-free reimplantation cannot be performed. There has been some evidence that locally advanced or high-grade lesions can be safely treated with segmental ureterectomy without compromise of cancer-specific outcomes; this may enable preservation of renal function so that adjuvant chemotherapy can be administered [24]. This approach, however, is controversial.

Adjuvant chemotherapy can be considered following extirpative surgery, as distant relapse is the primary impediment to survival in high-risk TCC patients. Guidelines suggest adjuvant chemotherapy for patients with stage pT2 or higher and nodal metastasis [25]. While adjuvant chemotherapy has been shown to improve recurrence-free survival in certain series, there is no level 1 evidence and a significant impact on overall survival has not been shown [2].

Ablative surgery

Low-grade, noninvasive lesions may be suitable for endoscopic tumor ablation. This approach enables local tumor control with preservation of the ipsilateral renal unit, which may reduce the risk of renal dysfunction [26] and provide renal redundancy should there be contralateral metachronous recurrence. Retrospective data suggest that for low-grade lesions, there is similar cancer-specific and overall survival for ablation versus extirpative treatment, with the caveat that there is a high rate of recurrence (30–71%) necessitating endoscopic retreatment [27]. Disease does typically remain low grade, but there is a risk of progression and lifelong surveillance is needed [28, 29]. Up to one-third of the patients may ultimately require extirpative treatment, though recent series report rates in the range of 13% [28, 30]. While there are no large series of extirpative surgery following prior endoscopic management, studies suggest that delaying nephroureterectomy does not impact survival [31, 32].

Ureteroscopy is the preferred approach for tumor ablation because it maintains the integrity of the urinary tract, decreasing risk of tumor seeding, and has lower morbidity than percutaneous approaches. Rigid ureteroscopy can be used for evaluation of the mid-distal ureter, while flexible ureteroscopy is required for the proximal ureter and collecting system. Although flexible scopes have greater maneuverability, smaller channels may limit irrigant flow and the size of working instruments. Certain portions of the collecting system may be challenging to access even with flexible instrumentation, for example, the lower pole. Also, retrograde access may be more challenging in patients with prior urinary diversion, necessitating percutaneous access in certain patients.

When a lesion is viewed on retrograde endoscopy, a saline "barbotage" or washing of that area can be obtained and sent for fluid cytology. A forceps or basket is then used to obtain tissue from the lesion. This can be sent for analysis and treatment deferred if there is suspicion for high-grade disease that would necessitate extirpative therapy. However, if low-grade disease is suspected and the disease burden is low, one can proceed with tumor ablation. For removal of bulky tissue, a rigid ureteral resectoscope can be used, with biopsy forceps employed for gross tumor removal. The base of the lesion is then ablated with laser or thermal energy. Holmium laser energy is frequently used for this purpose based on its limited tissue penetration (<0.5 mm) and hemostatic effects, though Bugbee cautery can be used as well. Ureteral stents can be placed at the discretion of the surgeon. A low rate of complications has been reported from these procedures, including ureteral perforation or stricture formation.

Retrograde instillation of topical chemotherapy can be considered (e.g., mitomycin, BCG), though no studies have demonstrated a significant difference in recurrence or survival with this practice [29]. Treatment of the upper tract can be performed by placing a ureteral stent and then instilling the agent into the bladder via Foley catheter in the supine position. This allows for the intravesical therapy to reflux to the upper tract. For instance, BCG can be instilled in the setting of upper tract CIS akin to treatment approaches in the bladder. As with adjuvant treatment in the bladder, there are risks of BCG toxicity and sepsis that need to be considered and weighed against potential benefits. However, while further investigation of adjuvant therapy for upper tract disease is needed, it is nonetheless a valid treatment option for selected patients.

There have been concerns regarding understaging of cancer on endoscopic evaluation, leading to potential risks of undertreatment and disease progression. However, recent studies have shown a high accuracy of ureteroscopic diagnosis (up to 94%) as well as a high concordance of pathological grading (up to 92%) and a high correlation between grade and stage [3]. As these patients are at risk for disease in the contralateral upper tract, may require chemotherapy in the future, and in general may benefit from avoidance of chronic kidney disease, preservation of the ipsilateral kidney has been increasingly prioritized for low-risk tumors, leading to increasing reliance on endoscopic ablative approaches. Given the lack of rigorous survival data, however, patients should be counseled regarding alternative treatment approaches and the need for vigilant surveillance. Management decisions should integrate all available data, including radiographic appearance, endoscopic findings, biopsy/cytology results, and patient preferences [14, 33].

Percutaneous ablative treatment of upper tract lesions can be considered for bulky, low-grade disease when renal preservation is prioritized or for upper tract disease when retrograde access is challenging or prohibited, for example, by prior urinary diversion. Percutaneous surgery can enable larger tract access to the kidney for higher volume tumors, for which larger instruments can be utilized including renoscopy/cold cup biopsy, tumor resection with a resectoscope, or use of laser energy. A nephrostomy tube can be left in place for administration of topical adjuvant therapy or for "second look" evaluations in cases of large volume tumors. Percutaneous approaches, however, are associated with increased morbidity compared with retrograde techniques, and incur a greater potential for tumor seeding, thus are not commonly performed.

Prognosis

Stage and grade are the two most important predictors of survival from upper tract TCC, though stage is the single most important determinant [3, 34]. These factors are most important for prognosis regardless of treatment technique [3]. While the 5-year cancer-specific survival for pT1–2 lesions is ~90%, this rate falls to 70% for patients with pT3–4 disease, and to 34–41% with nodal metastasis [35]. Lymphovascular invasion is also a poor prognostic factor [12].

After surgical therapy, recurrence of upper tract TCC occurs at a median 12–26 months postoperatively [12]. Sites of recurrence include the bladder in up to 40% of cases, and the contralateral upper tract in up to 6% [2, 12]. Metachronous ipsilateral disease generally occurs distal to the primary lesion, in 33–55% of cases [3]. Ipsilateral recurrences, as well as metachronous bladder tumors, are thought to be caused by distal seeding as well as multifocal field effects.

Competing causes of mortality are important in this population, accounting for >1/3 of observed deaths [34]. Age has been shown to correlate strongly with overall survival from upper tract TCC [4, 36] and is the strongest predictor of noncancer-related death in these patients [34]. Interestingly, advancing age has also been shown to confer a worse disease-specific survival, even after adjustment for stage, grade, and treatment type [37].

Biomarkers to predict progression or recurrence have been studied for upper tract TCC. Ki-67 has been shown to independently predict advanced stage and progression of upper tract TCC; alterations/loss of p63 expression have been associated with advanced tumor stage and worse prognosis; and p53 overexpression has been shown to correlate with increased mortality. Formal validation of these and other markers are needed before they gain a useful clinical role.

Surveillance

Guidelines for surveillance following treatment of upper tract TCC have been enumerated by both the National Comprehensive Cancer Network (NCCN) and the European Association of Urology (NCCN, Roupret). After treatment, patients should be evaluated every 3 months with history and physical examination, urinalysis, voided urine cytology, and office cystoscopy for at least 1 year. The interval for evaluation can be increased thereafter, typically every 6 months for an additional year, and then annually thereafter. Upper tract surveillance should be performed with CT or MR urography at 6–12-month intervals. This enables assessment of the ipsilateral upper tract (when preserved) as well as the contralateral unit. Radiographic surveillance also allows for detection of occult visceral metastasis. Chest imaging in the form of plain radiography or CT should be performed on an annual basis. After local ablative treatments, repeat endoscopy at 3-month intervals should be performed for 1 year as well, with increasing intervals thereafter. Bloodwork including liver function tests and assessment of renal function are needed on a routine basis. Additional testing like bone scintigraphy depending on symptoms may be considered. Lifelong follow-up is required for these patients.

WHAT TO AVOID

- It is critical to surgically excise the entire ureter and a bladder cuff during nephroureterectomy for upper tract urothelial cancer.
- Surveillance of the upper urinary tract should be performed after prior treatment for bladder carcinoma to ensure no metachronous upper tract recurrence.
- Patients with suspicious voided urine cytology but a negative cystoscopic examination should have random biopsies of the bladder and prostatic urothelium, as well as selective cytology and retrograde pyelograms of the upper tracts to ensure the absence of upper tract urothelial cancer.
- Endoscopic treatment of high-grade and/or invasive upper tract urothelial cancer is contraindicated and should be used only for low-grade superficial disease based on cytology and tissue biopsy results.

KEY WEB LINKS

National Comprehensive Cancer Network
http://www.nccn.org/professionals/physician_gls/f_guidelines.asp

European Urological Association
http://eu-acme.org/europeanurology/upload_articles/Morgan%20Rouprêt,.pdf

Multiple choice questions

1 Risk factors for upper tract urothelial carcinoma include all of the following except:
- a Phenacetin abuse
- b Chronic infection
- c Tobacco use
- d Bladder CIS
- e Aristolochic acid

2 Which of the following is a true statement?
- a Pain is frequently associated with the presentation of upper tract urothelial cancer.
- b Bladder recurrence after treatment of upper tract disease is uncommon.
- c Molecular markers have an important clinical role in the diagnosis of upper tract urothelial cancer.
- d High-grade upper tract cancer can be safely treated with endoscopic ablative techniques.
- e None of the above.

References

1 Jemal A, Siegel R, Ward E, Hao Y, Xu J, Thun MJ. Cancer statistics, 2009. *CA Cancer J Clin* 2009;59(4):225–249.

2 Roupret M, Zigeuner R, Palou J, et al. European guidelines for the diagnosis and management of upper urinary tract urothelial cell carcinomas: 2011 update. *Eur Urol* 2011;59:584–594.

3 Sagalowsky AI, Jarrett TW, Flanigan RC. Urothelial tumors of the upper urinary tract and ureter. In: *Campbell-Walsh Urology*. 10th ed. Philadelphia, PA: Elsevier; 2011 pp.1516–1553.

4 Raman JD, Messer J, Sielatycki JA, Hollenbeak CS. Incidence and survival of patients with carcinoma of the ureter and renal pelvis in the USA, 1973–2005. *BJU Int* 2010;107:1059–1064.

5 Munoz JJ, Ellison LM. Upper tract urothelial neoplasms: incidence and survival during the last 2 decades. *J Urol* 2000;164(5):1523–1525.

6 Milojevic B, Djokic M, Sipetic-Grujicic S et al. Upper urinary tract transitional cell carcinoma: location is not correlated with prognosis. *BJU Int* 2012;109:1037–1042

7 Ayyathurai R, Soloway MS. Monitoring of the upper urinary tract in patients with bladder cancer. *Ind J Urology* 2011;27(2):238–244.

8 Volkmer BG, Schnoeller T, Kuefer R, Gust K, Finter F, Hautmann RE. Upper urinary tract recurrence after radical cystectomy for bladder cancer–who is at risk? *J Urol* 2009;182(6):2632–2637.

9 Wright JL, Hotaling J, Porter MP. Predictors of upper tract urothelial cell carcinoma after primary bladder cancer: a population based analysis. *J Urol* 2009;181(3):1035–1039.

10 Vikram R, Sandler CM, Ng CS. Imaging and staging of transitional cell carcinoma: part 2, upper urinary tract. *AMR Am J Roentgenol* 2009;192(6):1488–1493.

11 Chlapoutakis K, Theocharopoulos N, Yarmenitis S, Damilakis J. Performance of computed tomographic urography in diagnosis of upper urinary tract urothelial carcinoma, in patients presenting with hematuria: systematic review and meta-analysis. *Eur J Radiol* 2008;73(2):334–338.

12 Sun M, Abdo A, Abdollah F, et al. Management of upper urinary tract urothelial carcinoma. *Expert Rev Anticancer Ther* 2010;10(12):1955–1965.

13 Blute ML, Segura JW, Patterson DE, Benson RC, Jr, Zincke H. Impact of endourology on diagnosis and management of upper urinary tract urothelial cancer. *J Urol* 1989;141(6):1298–1301.

14 Guarnizo E, Pavlovich CP, Seiba M, Carlson DL, Vaughan ED, Jr, Sosa RE. Ureteroscopic biopsy of upper tract urothelial carcinoma: improved diagnostic accuracy and histopathological considerations using a multi-biopsy approach. *J Urol* 2000;163(1):52–55.

15 American Joint Committee on Cancer. *AJCC Cancer Staging Manual*. NY: Springer; 2010;646.

16 Rai BP, Shelley M, Coles B, Biyani CS, El-Mokadem I, Nabi G. Survival management for upper urinary tract transitional cell carcinoma (Review). *Cochrane Database Syst Rev* 2011;4:CD007349.

17 Grossman HB, Natale RB, Tangen CM, et al. Neoadjuvant chemotherapy plus cystectomy compared with cystectomy alone for locally advanced bladder cancer. *N Engl J Med* 2003;349(9):859–866.

18 Kaag MG, O'Malley RL, O'Malley P, et al. Changes in renal function following nephroureterectomy may affect the use of perioperative chemotherapy. *Eur Urol* 2010;58(4):581–587.

19 Margulis V, Shariat SF, Matin SF, et al. Outcomes of radical nephroureterectomy: a series from the upper tract urothelial carcinoma collaboration. *Cancer* 2009;115:1224–1233.

20 Capitanio U, Shariat SF, Isbarn H, et al. Comparison of oncologic outcomes for open and laparoscopic nephroureterectomy: a multi-institutional analysis of 1249 cases. *Eur Urol* 2009;56(1):1–9.

21 Rassweiler J, Schulze M, Marrero R, Frede T, Palou Redorta J, Bassi P. Laparoscopic nephroureterectomy for upper urinary tract transitional cell carcinoma: is it better than open surgery? *Eur Urol* 2004;46:690–697.

22 Berger A, Haber GP, Kamoi K, et al. Laparoscopic radical nephroureterectomy for upper tract transitional cell

carcinoma: oncological outcomes at 7 years. *J Urol* 2008;180(3):849–854.

23 Waldert M, Remzi M, Klingler HC, Mueller L, Marberger M. The oncological results of laparoscopic nephroureterectomy for upper urinary tract transitional cell cancer are equal to those of open nephroureterectomy. *BJU Int* 2009;103(1):66–70.

24 Jeldres C, Lughezzani G, Sun M, et al. Segmental ureterectomy can safely be performed in patients with transitional cell carcinoma of the ureter. *J Urol* 2010;183(4):1324–1329.

25 National Comprehensive Cancer Network (NCCN). Bladder cancer – including upper tract tumors and urothelial carcinoma of the prostate. *National Clinical practice Guidelines in oncology v2*.2010;2010:1–51.

26 Pak RW, Moskowitz EJ, Bagley DH. What is the cost of maintaining a kidney in upper-tract transitional-cell carcinoma? An objective analysis of cost and survival. *J Endo* 2009;23(3):341–346.

27 Gadzinski AJ, Roberts WW, Faerber GJ, Wolf JS, Jr. Long-term outcomes of nephroureterectomy versus endoscopic management for upper tract urothelial carcinoma. *J Urol* 2010;183:2148–2153.

28 Thompson RH, Krambeck AE, Lohse CM, Elliott DS, Patterson DE, Blute ML. Endoscopic management of upper tract transitional cell carcinoma in patients with normal contralateral kidneys. *Urol* 2008;71(4):713–717.

29 Iwaszko MR, Krambeck AE. Conservative management of upper tract transitional cell carcinoma. *Indian J Urol* 2008;24(2):159–163.

30 Gurbuz C, Youssef RF, Shariat SF, et al. The impact of previous ureteroscopic tumor ablation on oncologic outcomes after radical nephroureterectomy for upper urinary tract urothelial carcinoma. *J Endo* 2011;25:775–779.

31 Lucas SM, Svatek RS, Olgin G, et al. Conservative management in selected patients with upper tract urothelial carcinoma compares favourably with early radical surgery. *BJU Int* 2008;102:172–176.

32 Boorjian S, Ng C, Munver R, et al. Impact of delay to nephroureterectomy for patients undergoing ureteroscopic biopsy and laser tumor ablation of upper tract transitional cell carcinoma. *Urology* 2005;66:283–287.

33 Raymundo EM, Lipkin ME, Banez LB, et al. Third prize: the role of endoscopic nephron-sparing surgery in the management of upper tract urothelial carcinoma. *J Endourol* 2011;25(3):377–384.

34 Inman BA, Tran VT, Fradet Y, Lacombe L. Carcinoma of the upper urinary tract: predictors of survival and competing causes of mortality. *Cancer* 2009;115(13): 2853–2862.

35 Jeldres C, Sun M, Lughezzani G, et al. Highly predictive survival nomogram after upper urinary tract urothelial carcinoma. *Cancer* 2010;116(16):3774–3784.

36 Shariat SF, Godoy G, Lotan Y, et al. Advanced patient age is associated with inferior cancer-specific survival after radical nephroureterectomy. *BJU Int* 2010;105(12):1672–1677.

37 Yap SA, Schupp CW, Chamie K, Evans CP, Koppie TM. Effect of age on transitional cell carcinoma of the upper urinary tract: presentation, treatment, and outcomes. *Urology* 2011;78(1):87–92.

Answers to multiple choice questions

1 b
2 e

24 Angiomyolipoma, oncocytoma, and retroperitoneal fibrosis

Phillip M. Pierorazio

The James Buchanan Brady Urological Institute and Department of Urology, The Johns Hopkins School of Medicine, Baltimore, MD, USA

KEY POINTS

- Angiomyolipoma (AML) is a benign lesion of the kidney characterized by the proliferation of blood vessels, adipose tissue, and smooth muscle.
  - AML represents <10% of all renal tumors.
  - AML is associated with tuberous sclerosis.
  - Most contain fat and diagnosis is confirmed by the presence of fat on axial imaging.
  - Treatment is observation if <4 cm and asymptomatic or selective embolization and/or extirpative surgery if symptomatic (bleeding) or ≥4 cm.
- Oncocytoma is a benign lesion of the kidney composed of cells with granular, eosinophilic cytoplasm due to a large abundance of mitochondria.
  - Oncocytoma represents 3–7% of all renal tumors.
  - Cytogenetic abnormalities include loss of chromosome 1p and Y, loss of heterozygosity at 14q and rearrangements at 11q13.
  - Classic radiographic and gross histologic finding includes a central scar.
- Retroperitoneal fibrosis is a rare disease in which fibrosis encases retroperitoneal structures (including the ureter) and leads to urinary obstruction.
  - The most common etiology is idiopathic (also known as Ormond's disease); other causes include inflammatory disease, medication, malignancy, radiation, abdominal aortic aneurysms, and subsequent repairs.
  - Initial management includes relief of the urinary obstruction and biopsy of encasing tissue.
  - Subsequent treatment options include corticosteroids, tamoxifen, and ureterolysis.

CASE STUDY 1: AML

A 46-year-old woman with no past medical history comes to the emergency room complaining of right upper quadrant pain. During workup for cholecystitis, she is noted to have a 3.5 cm mass in the right kidney. The mass is heterogeneous and a section demonstrates negative Hounsfield units, indicating the presence of fat and an AML. She returns to your office at 6 and 12 months following the diagnosis and the mass measures 3.7 cm; she has no symptoms. She returns annually for surveillance imaging and over the next 5 years, the mass grows to 4.5 cm in maximum diameter. She remains symptom free.

A few months later, she is involved in a motor vehicle accident and complains of right flank pain, radiating into her groin. CT scan in the emergency room demonstrates a retroperitoneal hematoma and her hemoglobin trends from 12.6 to 10.8 to 8.5 over the next few hours. She remains hemodynamically stable but the hematoma is increasing on imaging. While providing resuscitative fluids and close hemodynamic monitoring, interventional radiology is consulted and the patient is brought to the angiography suite. Under fluoroscopic guidance, a bleeding source is identified in the area of the right renal mass. The bleeding vessel is selectively embolized and the patient's hemoglobin stabilizes. The following day she develops fever (39.2°C); she is treated with Tylenol. Repeat CT scan demonstrates stability of the hematoma and infarction of the renal mass. She is discharged without further sequelae.

Handbook of Urology, First edition. J. Kellogg Parsons, John B. Eifler and Misop Han.
Published 2014 by John Wiley & Sons, Ltd.

CASE STUDY 2: RPF

A 65-year-old man is transferred to the medical intensive care unit from an outside hospital for acute renal failure and oliguria. He weighs 245 pounds (BMI 33.2) and has a history of cardiac and peripheral vascular disease; he underwent aortic aneurysm repair 2 years ago. He takes daily aspirin and is on a number of antihypertensive medications including hydrochlorothiazide, a β-blocker, and an ACE inhibitor. His serum creatinine is 4.2 (baseline 1.3) and when a Foley catheter is placed only 30 cc of urine is returned despite not voiding in the past several hours. His serum electrolytes are within normal limits, his ESR is noted to be elevated and an acute renal failure workup is initiated. Ultrasound reveals bilateral hydronephrosis and subsequent CT scan demonstrates medial deviation of both ureters and a dense collection of tissue in the retroperitoneum and surrounding both ureters. Due to anesthetic risks, he is taken to the interventional radiology suite and bilateral nephroureteral stents are placed without issue under local anesthesia and sedation. Percutaneous biopsy of the retroperitoneal mass reveals collagen deposits with nonspecific chronic inflammation. Over the next few days, his urine output improves, his creatinine decreases to 1.5, and he is discharged.

As an outpatient he is started on a 2-month course of corticosteroids. At the end of 2 months, he remains dependent on nephrostomy tube drainage to maintain his urine output. After 1 month, he undergoes laparoscopic ureterolysis with omental interposition without complications. After 6 weeks, his nephroureteral stents are removed without issue.

Benign renal masses constitute a heterogeneous grouping of masses that derive from the renal cortical tissue or closely associated mesenchymal derivates. As the incidence of renal masses has increased due to the increased use of axial imaging, so has the incidence of benign renal masses [1, 2]. In some series, specifically those regarding small renal masses (<4 cm), benign lesions may constitute upward of 30% of surgically removed tumors [3]. Benign tumors may include cysts, renal cortical adenomas, metanephric adenomas, cystic nephromas, mixed epithelial stromal tumors, and a variety of tumors of mesenchymal origin including leiomyomas, fibromas, lipomas, and hemangiomas. This chapter will focus on the benign entities of angiomyolipoma (AML), oncocytoma, and retroperitoneal fibrosis (RPF).

General considerations in the diagnosis and evaluation of benign renal masses

While certain demographic information, radiographic appearance, and percutaneous biopsy may provide information as to the histology of a renal mass, definitive diagnosis of benign or malignant disease is usually established only upon extirpative treatment of the mass. Clinical features indicative of benign etiology include smaller size, female sex, and older age [3–5], with younger women being nearly twice as likely as age-matched men to have benign masses [6, 7]. The only definitive radiographic indicators of benign etiology include the presence of fat in AML and thin-walled, water-density simple cysts. While biopsy may provide information regarding histology, upward of 20% of biopsies are nondiagnostic and the presence of oncocytic cells may coexist with renal cell carcinoma (RCC) [8]. Therefore, most renal cortical tumors should be assumed to be malignant and undergo appropriate evaluation and management (discussed in Chapter 25).

Angiomyolipoma

Epidemiology and etiology

AML is a benign, neoplastic lesion of the kidney characterized by the proliferation of thick-walled blood vessels, adipose tissue, and smooth muscle [9]. AML is present in <0.3% of the general population and represents <10% of renal tumors [10]. AML is predominantly found in females, strongly expresses estrogen and androgen receptors and is rare before puberty—indicating a likely hormonal influence [11]. The majority of AML are sporadic; however, 20–30% occur in patients with tuberous sclerosis (TS) and 50–80% of patients with TS develop AML [10, 12]. TS is an autosomal dominant disease characterized by the triad of mental retardation, epilepsy, and adenoma sebaceum. TS patients with AML tend to present earlier in life (mean age 30 years), have less predominance of the female sex, are often multifocal, bilateral, and symptomatic; and more likely to develop RCC later in life [10].

Diagnosis

The typical sporadic presentation is a solitary, incidental lesion in a middle-aged woman. AML is the most common renal lesion to be associated with spontaneous bleeding and can present with a retroperitoneal hematoma, associated flank pain, hematuria, palpable mass, and hypovolemic shock in these patients [13]. This clinical constellation is known as the Wunderlich syndrome and is present in 10% of historical series [14]. The risk of spontaneous bleeding is related to size with 82% and 51% of patients with AML > 4 cm presenting with symptoms and spontaneous bleeding, respectively [14].

AML can be confidently diagnosed on cross-sectional imaging by the presence of fat within the lesion. CT is the most useful modality, with -20 HU or less indicative of fat [15]. However, upward of 14% of AML may be "fat-poor," lacking appreciable amounts of adipose [16, 17]. Ultrasound may demonstrate a highly echogenic lesion with shadowing; angiography demonstrates aneurysmal dilation in 50% of AML; and MRI (with fat-suppression) can be useful in distinguishing AML [16]. Other entities that may mimic AML on imaging include liposarcoma and clear-cell RCC. Liposarcoma tends to extrinsically compress renal parenchyma; and RCC containing fat, while extremely rare, usually contains calcifications in addition to fat while an AML will never have calcifications [16, 18, 19].

Histology and pathology

AML appear grossly as a yellowish, gray tumor lacking a capsule. AML may have cellular atypia and hemorrhage, making the distinction from sarcoma (i.e., fibrosarcoma, leiomyosarcoma, and liposarcoma) difficult in some cases where relative amounts of adipose, vascular, and smooth muscle are present. A couple of histologic entities are available to distinguish AML from other entities: (1) necrosis is never present in AML and (2) staining with HMB-45, a monoclonal antibody against melanoma-associated protein, is characteristic of AML [10, 19].

Management

Smaller (<4 cm), asymptomatic tumors can be safely monitored with repeat serial imaging every 6–12 months [20]. For patients with large or symptomatic tumors, nephron-sparing treatments are preferred. Selective embolization is the preferred first-line treatment, demonstrating long-term success despite a substantial proportion of patients requiring repeat embolization [21, 22]. In patients with acute or life-threatening bleeding, selective embolization is preferred as surgery often results in nephrectomy. Partial nephrectomy (PN) or thermal ablation can be used to treat stable AML in patients requiring intervention. The preservation of renal parenchyma and function are of paramount importance in patients with this benign diagnosis, especially in patients with TS (high risk of recurrence) or existing renal insufficiency.

Oncocytoma

Epidemiology and etiology

Renal oncocytoma is one of the most common of benign renal masses, accounting for 3–7% of kidney tumors [23]. While oncocytoma may appear as an enhancing, malignant mass on axial imaging, it is a clinically distinct entity from RCC with unique cell of origin and cytogenetic abnormalities [24, 25]. Rare case reports of metastatic oncocytoma may represent malignant degeneration, coexistence of RCC, or pseudometastases [26].

Oncocytomas are more common in older patients with small, incidentally discovered renal masses [6, 27]. Generally, they are more common in men than women (2:1 ratio), present in the fourth to sixth decade of life and can present bilaterally, multifocally, or metachronously in 6–13% of cases [12]. Oncocytomatosis refers to the clinical entity of multifocal oncocytoma and may be associated with the Birt–Hogg–Dubé syndrome [28].

Diagnosis

In general, it is exceedingly difficult to distinguish oncocytoma from RCC based on clinical or radiographic testing. However, a number of characteristic radiographic findings are common in oncocytoma. On CT, oncocytoma may demonstrate a central stellate scar; on angiography, a spoke wheel pattern of feeding arteries may be present; and on MRI, a well-defined capsule, central stellate scar, and a distinctive pattern on T1 and T2 images may indicate oncocytoma [8, 29]. Renal biopsy has a limited role in the diagnosis of oncocytoma, particularly because it can be difficult to distinguish from granular clear-cell or chromophobe RCC and may co-exist with RCC in 7–32% of cases [8].

Histology and pathology

Oncocytomas appear grossly as tan, homogenous tumors with a well-formed pseudocapsule and typically have a central stellate scar. Microscopically, cells are derived from distal tubules, are rounded, and are highly eosinophilic due to an abundance of mitochondria. Cells are typically arranged in a nested pattern and can demonstrate perinephric extension, pleomorphism, prominent nucleoli, and atypia, making the distinction between RCC difficult [30, 31]. Chromosomal analysis may be helpful in distinguishing oncocytoma and RCC: chromosomal abnormalities associated with RCC are not present in oncocytoma, and oncocytoma will commonly present with loss of chromosome 1p, loss of Y or 14q, and rearrangements of 11q13 [24, 25]. Hale's colloidal iron stain has traditionally been used to identify oncocytoma, however, can have nonspecific staining patterns leading to difficult interpretation [32]. More recently, cytokeratin profiles (i.e., vimentin, glutathione-*S*-transferase α, and epithelial cell adhesion molecule) have been used to distinguish oncocytoma from RCC [33].

Management

Most often oncocytomas are clinically assumed to be RCC and have the same management strategies available including active surveillance (AS), radical nephrectomy (for large tumors of uncertain etiology), and nephron-sparing surgeries (NSS) including PN and thermal ablation. Oncocytomas under AS have demonstrated rapid growth and therefore this parameter does not have the best performance in predicting oncocytoma or outcome after intervention [34, 35]. When the diagnosis of oncocytoma is known or highly suspected, NSS should be employed due to the benign nature of these lesions. PN is preferred to thermal ablation as a definitive diagnosis can be made from the analysis of the tumor rather than biopsy specimens.

Retroperitoneal fibrosis

Retroperitoneal fibrosis (RPF) is a benign condition in which the proliferation of fibrotic and inflammatory tissue obstructs retroperitoneal structures including one or both ureters. While RPF is not a renal parenchymal mass lesion, like AML or oncocytoma, it represents a benign proliferation of tissue that may require evaluation and management by urology.

Epidemiology and etiology

In large, cross-sectional studies, RPF is relatively rare, presenting in 0.1 to 1 per 100,000 to 200,000 people [36, 37]. It is more common in men than women (2–3:1) and typically presents in the sixth to seventh decade, although has been found in pediatric and elderly populations [38, 39]. While an inheritance pattern has not been documented, RPF is linked to a number of autoimmune disorders and the HLA-DRB1*03 allele [40].

The etiology of RPF is not well understood and a number of hypotheses exist. Possible etiologies include a vasculitis of the small vessels associated with the aorta [41], immunologic dysregulation manifested by antibody production against fibroblasts or a B-cell disorder [42, 43], or reactive inflammation in response to environmental toxins. As such, a number of medications, chemicals, radiation treatment, local, and systemic diseases are associated with the development of RPF (Table 24.1) [42, 44]. However, a specific etiology is identified in only 30% of RPF cases [45]. Malignancy is associated with 8–10% of RPF cases and should always be considered during initial workup [46].

Diagnosis

RPF is an insidious disease; patients are often asymptomatic or present in an advanced stage when symptoms of ureteral or vascular obstruction occur [46]. Nonspecific signs and symptoms may be related to the underlying etiology; back, abdominal, or flank pain; constitutional symptoms (weight loss, anorexia, and malaise); low-grade fever; hypertension; or lower extremity edema. Acute phase reactants (erythrocyte sedimentation rate and c-reactive protein) may be elevated in 80–100% of patients and serum creatinine, hypergammaglobulinemia, anemia, and autoimmune

Table 24.1 Conditions associated with retroperitoneal fibrosis.

Autoimmune disorders	**Medications (cont.)**
Amyloidosis	Hydralazine
Ankylosing spondylitis	Lysergic acid diethylamide (LSD)
Glomerulonephritis	Methyldopa
Pancreatitis	Methysergide
Primary biliary cirrhosis	Pergolide
Psoriasis	Phenacetin
Rheumatoid arthritis	Reserpine
Sclerosing cholangitis	**Retroperitoneal disease, trauma, or surgery**
Thyroid disease	Aortic or iliac artery aneurysm; repair thereof
Uveitis	Ascending lymphangitis
Vasculitis, small- or medium-sized vessels	Collagen vascular disease
Chemicals	Endometriosis
Avitene	Hemorrhage
Asbestosis	Henoch–Schonlein purpura with hemorrhage
Methyl methacrylate	Inflammatory response to advanced atherosclerosis
Talcum powder	Ruptured viscera
Infections	**Retroperitoneal Malignancy**
Chronic urinary tract infection	Lymphoma
Gonorrhea	Renal cell carcinoma
Syphilis	Testicular
Tuberculosis	Urothelial carcinoma
Medications	Metastases
Amphetamines	Any radiation or chemotherapy thereof
β-Blockers	**Systemic disease**
Bromocriptine	Inflammatory bowel disease
Ergotamine alkaloids	Sarcoidosis
Haloperidol	Erdheim–Chester disease

factors (antinuclear antibody, rheumatoid factor, etc.) may be abnormal but, in general, are not specific for RPF [42, 47].

Typical findings on imaging include hydronephrosis, medial deviation of the ureter(s), and a smooth, well-demarcated retroperitoneal mass that surrounds the aorta, inferior vena cava (IVC), iliac vessels, and ureters. CT and MRI are excellent modalities for establishing a diagnosis although ultrasound and intravenous pyelography can be used as adjuncts [46, 48, 49].

Histology and pathology

RPF appears as a fibrous, white plaque that encases the major retroperitoneal vessels and structures. Most commonly it involves the aorta, IVC, major branches of both vessels, and the ureters. The plaque usually extends cranially from the renal hilum to the pelvic brim caudally, although has been demonstrated to extend into the pelvis or the mediastinum. Histologically the plaque is composed of fibrotic cellular material (myofibroblasts and type-1 collagen) and a chronic inflammatory infiltrate (lymphocytes, macrophages, plasma cells, and eosinophils) [43].

Management

Biopsy is required for the diagnosis of RPF and to exclude malignancy. Core biopsy is preferred to fine-needle aspiration; open or laparoscopic biopsy can be performed during ureterolysis if indicated. If histologic findings are consistent with RPF, all potentially inciting agents or exposures should be discontinued (Table 24.1). However, if obstructive uropathy is present, primary therapy should be directed at relieving the obstruction and maintaining renal function before initiating a biopsy for diagnosis or medical treatment. Retrograde ureteral stents are often easily passed in patients with RPF; however, percutaneous nephrostomy tubes can be placed if stenting is not possible or unsuccessful.

Once the urinary obstruction is relieved and a tissue diagnosis is obtained, medical therapy is the preferred initial treatment. Primary treatment is directed at assumed autoimmune and inflammatory etiologies of RPF, initially with a prolonged course of corticosteroids. Using prednisolone or prednisone, a number of dosing regimens are demonstrated to be initially effective in 67–89% of patients with follow-up extending from 15 to 55 months [50–52]. Azathioprine, colchicines, cyclophosphamide, mycophenolate mofetil, and tamoxifen have been used to treat patients with severe RPF or RPF refractory to steroids [51, 53–56]. Importantly, no randomized, prospective studies exist addressing the utility of varying medical treatments or the initial use of medical versus surgical treatment for RPF.

In patients refractory or unable to undergo medical treatment, ureterolysis can be performed to relieve ureteral obstruction. Ureterolysis can be performed via an open, laparoscopic or robot-assisted laparoscopic approach [57, 58]. Principles of ureterolysis include biopsy of the fibrotic lesion, initiation of dissection in an area free of disease, avoidance of devascularization of the ureter, lateralization of the ureter, stenting for 6–8 weeks, and enclosure within peritoneum or omentum to preserve ureteral vascularity and prevent recurrence [59]. In addition, bilateral ureterolysis should be performed in all cases (even if only a unilateral process is evident during evaluation) as the disease can progress to involve both sides and reoperative surgery can be technically challenging. Successful treatment has been reported in 66–100% of surgical series with variable follow-up extending over many years [57, 60, 61]. Therefore, long-term follow-up is required with serial axial imaging and renal functional studies for an indefinite period of time.

KEY WEB LINKS

Tuberous Sclerosis
www.tuberous-sclerosis.com

Retroperitoneal Fibrosis
http://www.ncbi.nlm.nih.gov/pubmedhealth/PMH0001497/

WHAT TO AVOID

- The presence of a small amount of fat on axial imaging is indicative of AML; however, 14% of AML do not contain fat. Additionally, AML never has calcifications; a fat-containing mass with calcification is usually indicative of RCC with fat.
- Oncocytoma shares many characteristics with chromophobe renal cell carcinoma (chRCC), distinguishing characteristics include
  - Cytoplasm of oncocytoma is eosinophilic in comparison to the granular and pale cytoplasm of chRCC.
  - Electron microscopy reveals mitochondria in oncocytoma and microvesicles in chRCC.
  - Hale's colloidal iron stain insinuates the cellular rim of oncocytic cells and the cytoplasm of chRCC.
- Renal biopsy has limited value in distinguishing oncocytoma and RCC as 7–32% of oncocytoma may occur with RCC and RCC may contain nests of oncocytic cells.
- In 15% of RPF cases, fibrosis may extend beyond the retroperitoneum. Fibrosis typically surrounds the aorta first and extends circumferentially outward. The ureters are usually the first organ to be functionally compromised.

Multiple choice questions

1 A 47-year-old woman presents to an emergency room with acute right flank pain, nausea, and vomiting. Laboratory values reveal hemoglobin of 6.5 g/dL and creatinine 1.2 mg/dL (baseline 1.0). CT scan is performed and demonstrates a heterogeneous, 8 cm

right renal mass with an associated perinephric hematoma. There are low-density areas (Hounsfield units of −30) within the mass. After transfusion, the next step is:

a Observation
b Discharge
c PN
d Angiographic embolization
e Radical nephrectomy

2 Effective management strategies for RPF include all of the following except:

a Ureteral stenting
b Antibiotics
c Ureterolysis
d Steroids (prednisone, prednisolone)
e Immunomodulatory drugs (cyclophosphamide, mycophenolate mofetil, or tamoxifen)

References

1 Cancer Facts and Figures. The American Cancer Society, 2010.
2 Patard JJ. Incidental renal tumours. *Curr Opin Urol* 2009;19(5):454–458.
3 Kutikov A, Fossett LK, Ramchandani P, et al. Incidence of benign pathologic findings at partial nephrectomy for solitary renal mass presumed to be renal cell carcinoma on preoperative imaging. *Urology* 2006;68(4):737–740.
4 Kouba E, Smith A, McRackan D, Wallen EM, Pruthi RS. Watchful waiting for solid renal masses: insight into the natural history and results of delayed intervention. *J Urol* 2007;177(2):466–470; discussion 470.
5 Pierorazio PM, Murphy AM, Benson MC, McKiernan JM. Gender discrepancies in the diagnosis of renal cortical tumors. *World J Urol* 2007;25(1):81–85.
6 Cao Y, Paner GP, Perry KT, Flanigan RC, Campbell SC, Picken MM. Renal neoplasms in younger adults: analysis of 112 tumors from a single institution according to the new 2004 World Health Organization classification and 2002 American Joint Committee on Cancer Staging System. *Arch Pathol Lab Med* 2005;129(4):487–491.
7 Snyder ME, Bach A, Kattan MW, Raj GV, Reuter VE, Russo P. Incidence of benign lesions for clinically localized renal masses smaller than 7 cm in radiological diameter: influence of sex. *J Urol* 2006;176(6 Pt 1):2391–2395; discussion 2395–2396.
8 Licht MR. Renal adenoma and oncocytoma. *Semin Urol Oncol* 1995;13(4):262–266.
9 Bissler JJ, Kingswood JC. Renal angiomyolipomata. *Kidney Int* 2004;66(3):924–934.
10 Eble JN. Angiomyolipoma of kidney. *Semin Diagn Pathol* 1998;15(1):21–40.
11 Boorjian SA, Sheinin Y, Crispen PL, Lohse CM, Kwon ED, Leibovich BC. Hormone receptor expression in renal angiomyolipoma: clinicopathologic correlation. *Urology* 2008;72(4):927–932.
12 Minor LD, Picken MM, Campbell SC. Benign renal tumors. *AUA Update* 2003;22:170–175.
13 Zhang JQ, Fielding JR, Zou KH. Etiology of spontaneous perirenal hemorrhage: a meta-analysis. *J Urol* 2002;167(4):1593–1596.
14 Oesterling JE, Fishman EK, Goldman SM, Marshall FF. The management of renal angiomyolipoma. *J Urol* 1986;135(6):1121–1124.
15 Simpfendorfer C, Herts BR, Motta-Ramirez GA, et al. Angiomyolipoma with minimal fat on MDCT: can counts of negative-attenuation pixels aid diagnosis? *AJR Am J Roentgenol* 2009;192(2):438–443.
16 Lemaitre L, Claudon M, Dubrulle F, Mazeman E. Imaging of angiomyolipomas. *Semin Ultrasound CT MR* 1997;18(2):100–114.
17 Milner J, McNeil B, Alioto J, et al. Fat poor renal angiomyolipoma: patient, computerized tomography and histological findings. *J Urol* 2006;176(3):905–909.
18 Clark PE, Novick AC. Exophytic noninvasive growth pattern of renal angiomyolipomas: implications for nephron sparing surgery. *J Urol* 2001;165(2):513–514.
19 Wang LJ, Wong YC, Chen CJ, See LC. Computerized tomography characteristics that differentiate angiomyolipomas from liposarcomas in the perinephric space. *J Urol* 2002;167(2 Pt 1):490–493.
20 De Luca S, Terrone C, Rossetti SR. Management of renal angiomyolipoma: a report of 53 cases. *BJU Int* 1999;83(3):215–218.
21 Nelson CP, Sanda MG. Contemporary diagnosis and management of renal angiomyolipoma. *J Urol* 2002;168(4 Pt 1):1315–1325.
22 Harabayashi T, Shinohara N, Katano H, Nonomura K, Shimizu T, Koyanagi T. Management of renal angiomyolipomas associated with tuberous sclerosis complex. *J Urol* 2004;171(1):102–105.
23 Morra MN, Das S. Renal oncocytoma: a review of histogenesis, histopathology, diagnosis and treatment. *J Urol* 1993;150(2 Pt 1):295–302.
24 Lindgren V, Paner GP, Omeroglu A, et al. Cytogenetic analysis of a series of 13 renal oncocytomas. *J Urol* 2004;171(2 Pt 1):602–604.
25 Paner GP, Lindgren V, Jacobson K, et al. High incidence of chromosome 1 abnormalities in a series of 27 renal oncocytomas: cytogenetic and fluorescence in situ hybridization studies. *Arch Pathol Lab Med* 2007;131(1):81–85.
26 Oxley JD, Sullivan J, Mitchelmore A, Gillatt DA. Metastatic renal oncocytoma. *J Clin Pathol* 2007;60(6):720–722.

27 Skolarus TA, Serrano MF, Berger DA, et al. The distribution of histological subtypes of renal tumors by decade of life using the 2004 WHO classification. *J Urol* 2008;179(2):439–443; discussion 443–4.

28 Al-Saleem T, Cairns P, Dulaimi EA, Feder M, Testa JR, Uzzo RG. The genetics of renal oncocytosis: a possible model for neoplastic progression. *Cancer Genet Cytogenet* 2004;152(1):23–28.

29 Harmon WJ, King BF, Lieber MM. Renal oncocytoma: magnetic resonance imaging characteristics. *J Urol* 1996;155(3):863–867.

30 Amin MB, Crotty TB, Tickoo SK, Farrow GM. Renal oncocytoma: a reappraisal of morphologic features with clinicopathologic findings in 80 cases. *Am J Surg Pathol* 1997;21(1):1–12.

31 Perez-Ordonez B, Hamed G, Campbell S, et al. Renal oncocytoma: a clinicopathologic study of 70 cases. *Am J Surg Pathol* 1997;21(8):871–883.

32 Leroy X, Moukassa D, Copin MC, Saint F, Mazeman E, Gosselin B. Utility of cytokeratin 7 for distinguishing chromophobe renal cell carcinoma from renal oncocytoma. *Eur Urol* 2000;37(4):484–487.

33 Liu L, Qian J, Singh H, Meiers I, Zhou X, Bostwick DG. Immunohistochemical analysis of chromophobe renal cell carcinoma, renal oncocytoma, and clear cell carcinoma: an optimal and practical panel for differential diagnosis. *Arch Pathol Lab Med* 2007;131(8):1290–1297.

34 Kawaguchi S, Fernandes KA, Finelli A, Robinette M, Fleshner N, Jewett MA. Most renal oncocytomas appear to grow: observations of tumor kinetics with active surveillance. *J Urol* 2011;186(4):1218–1222.

35 Siu W, Hafez KS, Johnston WK, 3rd, Wolf JS, Jr. Growth rates of renal cell carcinoma and oncocytoma under surveillance are similar. *Urol Oncol* 2007;25(2):115–119.

36 Uibu T, Oksa P, Auvinen A, et al. Asbestos exposure as a risk factor for retroperitoneal fibrosis. *Lancet* 2004;363(9419):1422–1426.

37 Debruyne FM, Bogman MJ, Ypma AF. Retroperitoneal fibrosis in the scrotum. *Eur Urol* 1982;8(1):45–48.

38 Wu J, Catalano E, Coppola D. Retroperitoneal fibrosis (Ormond's disease): clinical pathologic study of eight cases. *Cancer Control* 2002;9(5):432–437.

39 Miller OF, Smith LJ, Ferrara EX, McAleer IM, Kaplan GW. Presentation of idiopathic retroperitoneal fibrosis in the pediatric population. *J Pediatr Surg* 2003;38(11):1685–1688.

40 Martorana D, Vaglio A, Greco P, et al. Chronic periaortitis and HLA-DRB1*03: another clue to an autoimmune origin. *Arthritis Rheum* 2006;55(1):126–130.

41 Baker LR. Auto-allergic periaortitis (idiopathic retroperitoneal fibrosis). *BJU Int* 2003;92(7):663–665.

42 Vaglio A, Salvarani C, Buzio C. Retroperitoneal fibrosis. *Lancet* 2006;367(9506):241–251.

43 Corradi D, Maestri R, Palmisano A, et al. Idiopathic retroperitoneal fibrosis: clinicopathologic features and differential diagnosis. *Kidney Int* 2007;72(6):742–753.

44 Nakada, SY and Hsu THS. Chapter 41: Management of upper urinary tract. In: Kavoussi LR, Novick AC, Partin AW, Peters CA, Wein AJ, editors. *Campbell-Walsh Urology*. 10th ed. Vol. 2. Philadelphia, PA: Elsevier Saunders; 2012. pp. 1108–1112.

45 Koep L, Zuidema GD. The clinical significance of retroperitoneal fibrosis. *Surgery* 1977;81(3):250–257.

46 Amis ES, Jr. Retroperitoneal fibrosis. *AJR Am J Roentgenol* 1991;157(2):321–329.

47 Monev S. Idiopathic retroperitoneal fibrosis: prompt diagnosis preserves organ function. *Cleve Clin J Med* 2002;69(2):160–166.

48 Mulligan SA, Holley HC, Koehler RE, et al. CT and MR imaging in the evaluation of retroperitoneal fibrosis. *J Comput Assist Tomogr* 1989;13(2):277–281.

49 Vivas I, Nicolas AI, Velazquez P, Elduayen B, Fernandez-Villa T, Martinez-Cuesta A: Retroperitoneal fibrosis: typical and atypical manifestations. *Br J Radiol* 2000;73(866):214–222.

50 Kardar AH, Kattan S, Lindstedt E, Hanash K. Steroid therapy for idiopathic retroperitoneal fibrosis: dose and duration. *J Urol* 2002;168(2):550–555.

51 van Bommel EF, Siemes C, Hak LE, van der Veer SJ, Hendriksz TR. Long-term renal and patient outcome in idiopathic retroperitoneal fibrosis treated with prednisone. *Am J Kidney Dis* 2007;49(5):615–625.

52 Fry AC, Singh S, Gunda SS, et al. Successful use of steroids and ureteric stents in 24 patients with idiopathic retroperitoneal fibrosis: a retrospective study. *Nephron Clin Pract* 2008;108(3):c213–c220.

53 Marcolongo R, Tavolini IM, Laveder F, et al. Immunosuppressive therapy for idiopathic retroperitoneal fibrosis: a retrospective analysis of 26 cases. *Am J Med* 2004;116(3):194–197.

54 Swartz RD, Lake AM, Roberts WW, Faerber GJ, Wolf JS, Jr. Idiopathic retroperitoneal fibrosis: a role for mycophenolate mofetil. *Clin Nephrol* 2008;69(4): 260–268.

55 Adler S, Lodermeyer S, Gaa J, Heemann U. Successful mycophenolate mofetil therapy in nine patients with idiopathic retroperitoneal fibrosis. *Rheumatology (Oxford)* 2008;47(10):1535–1538.

56 Scheel PJ, Jr., Piccini J, Rahman MH, Lawler L, Jarrett T. Combined prednisone and mycophenolate mofetil treatment for retroperitoneal fibrosis. *J Urol* 2007;178(1):140–143; discussion 143–144.

57 Duchene DA, Winfield HN, Cadeddu JA, et al. Multi-institutional survey of laparoscopic ureterolysis for retroperitoneal fibrosis. *Urology* 2007;69(6): 1017–1021.

58 Stifelman MD, Shah O, Mufarrij P, Lipkin M. Minimally invasive management of retroperitoneal fibrosis. *Urology* 2008;71(2):201–204.

59 Varkarakis IM, Jarrett TW. Retroperitoneal fibrosis. *AUA Update Series* 2005;24:18-23.

60 Elashry OM, Nakada SY, Wolf JS, Jr., Figenshau RS, McDougall EM, Clayman RV. Ureterolysis for extrinsic ureteral obstruction: a comparison of laparoscopic and open surgical techniques. *J Urol* 1996;156(4):1403–1410.

61 Alexopoulos E, Memmos D, Bakatselos S, et al. Idiopathic retroperitoneal fibrosis: a long-term follow-up study. *Eur Urol* 1987;13(5):313–317.

Answers to multiple choice questions

1 d A large, bleeding renal mass may be a renal cell carcinoma (RCC). However, negative Hounsfield units on CT is indicative of angiomyolipoma (AML). For patients with large or symptomatic tumors, nephron-sparing treatments are preferred. Selective embolization is the preferred first-line treatment. In patients with acute or life-threatening bleeding, selective embolization is preferred as surgery often results in nephrectomy. Partial nephrectomy (PN) or thermal ablation can be used to treat stable AML in patients requiring intervention.

2 b Antibiotics. Retroperitoneal fibrosis (RPF) has not been demonstrated to have an infectious etiology and antibiotics are not effective in altering the progress of this progressive disorder.

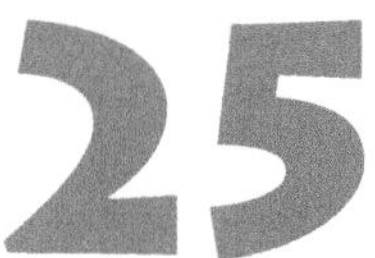

Malignant Renal parenchymal tumors

Phillip M. Pierorazio

The James Buchanan Brady Urological Institute and Department of Urology, The Johns Hopkins School of Medicine, Baltimore, MD, USA

KEY POINTS

- Renal masses can be benign, malignant, or inflammatory; renal cell carcinoma (RCC) is the most common renal tumor (80–85% of all renal tumors).
- The incidence of RCC has increased by 3–4% per year since 1970s due to the increased use of axial imaging; approximately 58,000 and 13,000 are diagnosed and die of RCC annually, respectively.
- RCC is more common in the aged (older than 50 years), men, African Americans, smokers, the obese, and those with familial syndromes; less common in those who consume moderate levels of alcohol, fresh fruits, vegetables, and fatty fish; and is not related to NSAID use or occupational factors.
- RCC is a disease of altered cellular metabolism; established gene mutations of RCC (Von Hippel–Lindau [VHL], c-MET, etc.) affect pathways of metabolic stress or nutrient stimulation including those of oxygen, iron, and energy metabolism.
- Initial evaluation should include physical examination, laboratory studies including complete blood count, basic metabolic panel and liver function tests; axial imaging of the abdomen with contrast to accurately stage the tumor and chest X-ray to evaluate the lungs.
- Prognosis is based on tumor characteristics (pathologic stage, size, nuclear grade, histologic subtype), and patient characteristics (performance status).
- Staging is based on the TNM system (AJCC, 2009).
- Histologic subtypes include
  - a Clear cell (70–80%)—clear cells due to abundant glycogen and lipid content, vascular tumors, 75% have VHL mutation.
  - b Papillary (10–15%)—hypovascular with attenuated enhancement pattern on CT, more common in patients with chronic renal failure.
  - c Chromophobe (4–5%).
  - d Collecting duct—rare, presents at advanced stage (40% metastatic), poor prognosis (5% survival at 5 years).
  - e Medullary—rare, associated with sickle cell trait, presents at an advanced stage, poor prognosis.
- Adverse tumor characteristics include sarcomatoid differentiation and necrosis.
- Treatment options for clinically localized RCC include radical nephrectomy, partial nephrectomy, energy ablation (cryoablation and radiofrequency ablation), and active surveillance.

CASE STUDY: SMALL RENAL MASS

A 75-year-old man with hypertension, hyperlipidemia, and a smoking history suffers a myocardial infarction (MI) and undergoes urgent coronary artery stenting. During his preoperative workup, a CT scan demonstrates a 2.5 cm enhancing mass in the upper pole of his left kidney. After 4 months, recovering from his MI and coronary artery stent, he meets with a urologist. Repeat CT of the image demonstrates no significant changes in the size or quality of the mass and renal function demonstrates a glomerular filtration rate (GFR) of 49 mL/min/1.73 m^2 (creatinine 1.4 ng/mL). Due to his significant comorbidities, he elects to undergo a period of active surveillance (AS). Over the following year, the mass is imaged by ultrasound twice more and demonstrates a size increase to 3.1 cm (growth rate 0.6 cm/yr). He elects percutaneous renal biopsy (PRB) and histology demonstrates a low-grade, clear-cell type RCC. Percutaneous renal cryoablation is performed. At 1 year following ablation, the patient is disease free and his GFR remains stable.

Handbook of Urology, First edition. J. Kellogg Parsons, John B. Eifler and Misop Han.
Published 2014 by John Wiley & Sons, Ltd.

CASE STUDY: METASTATIC RCC

A 64-year-old man presents to his internist with new onset hematuria. On review of systems, he complains of cough and an unplanned 10-pound weight loss over the past few months. He is otherwise healthy, is not taking any medications, and is not limited in any daily activities, playing golf several times per week. CT scan reveals a 13 cm mass in the right kidney and two small pulmonary nodules in the left lung (largest 1.8 cm). Biopsy of the lung nodules reveals metastatic RCC. He elects cytoreductive nephrectomy and simultaneous resection of both lung nodules. Pathology reveals a 12.9 cm clear-cell RCC, grade 3 with perinephric extension (pT3a) but no adrenal, renal vein, or lymph node involvement. He is started on interferon-alpha treatment. After 1 year, he is noted to have new pulmonary nodules on surveillance CT scan. He is started on sunitinib and over the 6 months his pulmonary nodules remain stable on CT. After 8 months on initiating sunitinib treatment, new pulmonary nodules, bone, and brain lesions are noted on CT scan. Within a few weeks, he develops intractable pain, elects hospice care, and dies shortly after.

According to the American Cancer Society, over 58,000 cases of renal cancer were diagnosed in 2010 [1]. The majority of cancers (92%) are renal parenchymal tumors; the remainder includes renal pelvic (urothelial) and Wilms' tumors. This chapter will discuss malignant renal parenchymal tumors, focusing specifically on renal cell carcinoma (RCC).

Epidemiology

The incidence of RCC has surged over the past few decades, from 28,000 in 1997 to 58,000 in 2010, and is believed to be due to the increased use of axial imaging [1]. This increasing incidence has been accompanied by a dramatic stage migration—small renal masses (SRMs, ≤4 cm in greatest dimension) account for the largest proportion of the incident rise in RCC and nearly 40% of all renal tumors diagnosed [2, 3]. During the same time period, the number of deaths from kidney cancer has remained stable (11,000–13,000 from 1997 to 2010), decreasing only modestly in the past few years [1]. Therefore, RCC is considered one of the most lethal urological malignancies with a 65% disease-specific survival at 5 years [4].

RCC is a disease of older adults, most patients are diagnosed after 50 years of age and many new diagnoses occur in elderly patients [4]. RCC is more common in men than women (ratio 3:2) and has a 10–20% higher incidence in African Americans than Caucasians [4, 5]. Most cases are sporadic with familial or inherited forms of RCC in 2–3% of patients [4].

Risk factors

The most common risk factors for developing RCC are obesity and tobacco use, representing 40% and 20% of cases, respectively [4–7]. Hypertension and acquired renal cystic disease are also implicated as risk factors for RCC [4, 5, 8]. Moderate alcohol use [9], fruit and vegetable [10], and fatty fish intake [11] reduce the risk of RCC. Nonsteroidal anti-inflammatory medications or occupational exposures are not related to the development of RCC [4, 12].

While the minority of cases are familial, a number of inherited syndromes are associated with RCC. All familial syndromes associated with RCC are rare and demonstrate an autosomal dominant inheritance pattern. Von Hippel–Lindau (VHL) disease is caused by a defect in the *VHL* gene (chromosome 3p25-26) and causes clear-cell RCC, hemangioblastomas of the central nervous system, retinal angiomas, and pheochromocytoma. Hereditary papillary RCC (HPRCC) is caused by a mutation in the *c-MET* proto-oncogene (7q31) and leads to type 1 papillary RCC tumors. Hereditary leiomyomatosis and RCC (HLRCC) is caused by a defect in fumarate hydratase (1q42) and leads to aggressive, type 2 papillary RCC tumors; cutaneous and uterine leiomyomas. Birt–Hogg–Dubé (BHD), through a defect in the *BHD1* gene, leads to a defect in the protein, folliculin, and bilateral and multifocal chromophobe RCC, oncocytomas, and hybrid tumors of both histologies. The remainder of the BHD manifestations includes cutaneous fibrofolliculomas, lung cysts, and spontaneous pneumothorax. While these genetic syndromes are rare, the study of these patients and tumors provide insight into the molecular genetics of RCC and indicate that the development of malignancy within the kidney results from the dysregulation of a number of cellular metabolic pathways [13].

Diagnosis and evaluation

RCC can present with a wide range of symptoms and signs. However, >60% of patients now present incidentally and the classic triad of hematuria, flank pain, and abdominal mass occurs in <10% of patients [14, 15]. RCC-specific symptoms may result from local tumor invasion (hematuria, flank pain, and perirenal hematoma), distant metastases (cough, bone pain, and constitutional symptoms), or inferior vena cava (IVC) invasion (right-sided varicocele or lower extremity edema). A number of systemic syndromes are associated with RCC including elevated erythrocyte sedimentation rate (55.6%), hypertension (37.5%), anemia (36.3%), and cachexia (34.5%). Less common manifestations include pyrexia, abnormal liver function tests, hypercalcemia, polycythemia, neuromyopathy, and amyloidosis. In total, paraneoplastic syndromes have been identified in upward of 20% of patients with RCC [16]. Stauffer syndrome is an RCC-specific paraneoplastic syndrome, occurring in 3–20% of patients, and characterized by hepatic dysfunction (elevated alkaline phosphatase, prothrombin time, bilirubin, and transaminase levels; and hypoalbuminemia) and constitutional symptoms. Stauffer syndrome manifestations are reversed with radical nephrectomy (RN) and removal of the primary tumor [17].

Proper imaging is essential to the evaluation, characterization, and staging of RCC. Ultrasound, computed tomography (CT) and magnetic resonance imaging (MRI) can be used to evaluate renal masses; each has strengths and weaknesses for evaluating renal tumors. Ultrasound is cheap, relatively fast, does not expose that patient to radiation, and is excellent for the evaluation and surveillance of simple renal cysts. The Bosniak classification system describes the malignant potential of renal cysts and guides the management of these lesions (Table 25.1) [18, 19]. Renal masses, other than simple cysts, should be evaluated by CT, ideally with intravenous contrast in multiple phases. While CT utilizes ionizing radiation, it is fast and offers excellent characterization of the renal mass, accurately determines the stage by visualizing the remainder of the abdomen (including the adrenals, liver, and IVC) and provides information regarding morphology and function of the kidneys. MRI avoids exposure to radiation, can characterize a renal mass as solid or cystic, demonstrates many of the anatomic relationships and is particularly useful for determining soft tissue boundaries in locally invasive disease, potential venous involvement, and in patients who cannot receive intravenous CT contrast material. Nephrogenic systemic fibrosis (NSF) is a rare complication associated specifically with gadolinium contrast used for MRI. NSF, although rare, leads to significant disability and mortality through progressive fibrosis of the skin and other organs in patients with preexisting renal disease [20].

Table 25.1 Bosniak classification system of renal cysts [18, 19]

Bosniak	Radiography	Risk of Malignancy	Management
I	Water density Homogenous No septa, calcifications No enhancement	None	Only if symptomatic
II	Thin septa Thin calcification No enhancement Hyperdense	0–5%	Surveillance
IIF (1993)	Septa may have nodular thickening, calcifications No enhancement Can be intrarenal	0–10%	Surveillance
III	Thick septa Thick calcification Heterogeneity No enhancement	50%	Excision
IV	Thick walls Heterogeneity Enhancement	75–90%	Excision

In general, no imaging modality can accurately identify benign from malignant lesions or subtypes of RCC. However, using CT scan, tumors that enhance by >15 Hounsfield units (HU) should be considered RCC until proven otherwise. Tumors demonstrating negative HU indicate fat and are indicative of angiomyolipoma (AML). In addition, papillary RCC may demonstrate a distinct, unique pattern of hypoenhancement in contrast to clear-cell RCC which rapidly enhances and washes out during multiphasic CT imaging [21, 22]. Adenopathy ≥2 cm indicates an increased likelihood of metastatic diseases. MRI or CT may be used to accurately stage renal vein or IVC invasion [23–25].

Routine metastatic evaluation should include the assessment of performance status, chest radiography, basic metabolic panel (BMP), and liver function tests. Performance status reflects overall patient health, life expectancy, and may guide management. A BMP evaluates renal function while chest radiography and liver function tests evaluate visceral metastases. Chest CT should be reserved only for patients with pulmonary symptoms or an abnormal chest X-ray [26]. Bone scan is indicated only in patients with an elevated alkaline phosphatase, bone pain, or precipitous decline in performance status [27]. Similarly, head imaging is not routinely recommended as patients with brain metastases typically present with symptoms related to a brain lesion.

Percutaneous renal biopsy (PRB) is indicated in patients in whom suspicion of renal abscess is high, when the renal lesion may represent a metastasis from another primary malignancy or lymphoma. PRB may be useful in patients who may be managed by either active surveillance (AS) or primary intervention. In general, PRB should be avoided in young, healthy patients who are good surgical candidates given the small, but real risk of complications (bleeding, pneumothorax), a nondiagnostic rate of approximately 20% and poor reliability in determining tumor grade [28–30].

Histology and tumor grade

All RCC are by definition, adenocarcinoma, derived from renal epithelial tubular cells. The World Health Organization (WHO), in 2004, classified RCC according to distinct subtypes, each with a distinct genetic basis and clinical features [31]. Clear-cell RCC, previously known as "conventional" RCC, is the most common histologic subtype (70–80%). On gross examination, they are yellow, vascular tumors. In total, 70% have *VHL* gene mutations associated with loss of chromosome 3p. Papillary RCC is the second most common subtype (10–15%); are often hypovascular (accounting for characteristic hypoenhancement on CT), commonly found in patients with end-stage renal disease and acquired renal cystic disease, and are multicentric in ≤40% of cases. Type 1 papillary RCC is more common and in general, has a better prognosis than clear cell RCC. Type 2 papillary RCC, while rare and associated with HLRCC, is often aggressive tumors that present in an advanced stage. Chromophobe RCC (3–5%) derives from the collecting duct and (in the absence of sarcomatoid features or metastases) carries a good prognosis in comparison to clear-cell RCC. Collecting duct carcinoma (<1%), or carcinoma of the collecting ducts of Bellini, often presents in patients younger than 50 years old and are high-grade, advanced stage tumors that carry a poor prognosis regardless of treatment. Renal medullary carcinoma is also a rare subtype of RCC, almost exclusively associated with sickle-cell trait, occurs in young, African American patients, presents in an advanced stage, and carries a poor prognosis.

Tumor grading is based on the Fuhrman classification system and is based on nuclear size, shape, and the presence of nucleoli (Table 25.2). Fuhrman 1–2 tumors are well differentiated and considered low grade; Fuhrman 3–4 tumors are poorly differentiated and considered high grade. Any histologic subtype of RCC can have sarcomatoid differentiation. By definition, sarcomatoid differentiation indicates a high-grade tumor, equivalent to a Fuhrman grade 4, is diagnosed by the presence of spindle-cell histology, and is associated with an infiltrative growth pattern, aggressive local and metastatic behavior, and a poor prognosis in general [32, 33].

Table 25.2 Fuhrman grading system for renal cell carcinoma [54, 55]

Grade	Size (μm)	Contour	Nucleoli
I	10	Round, smooth, uniform	No
II	15	Minor irregularity	No
III	20	Major irregularity	Yes
IV	≥20	Multi-lobulated, pleomorphic, or spindle-shaped	Yes

Staging and prognosis

Staging is based on the TNM system and was updated by the American Joint Committee on Cancer (AJCC) in 2009 (Table 25.3). Tumor size (T-stage) is one of the most important determinants of outcome for patients with RCC. Increasing tumor size indicates a higher likelihood of clear-cell histology, high-grade tumor, and metastatic disease [34–37]. Within the T-stage, T1a (≤4 cm) tumors carry an excellent prognosis following treatment and very rarely demonstrate metastases. Important distinctions have also been made at the 7 and 10 cm cut points, both for oncologic prognosis and management decisions as smaller tumors are often more amenable to nephron-sparing treatments [38].

While stage is the strongest predictor of outcome, a number of important factors contribute to prognosis. As discussed, histologic subtype carries prognostic information with clear-cell RCC being associated with a worse prognosis when compared to papillary or chromophobe RCC; [32, 39] and the rare collecting

Table 25.3 AJCC TNM staging for renal cell carcinoma [56]

T: Primary tumor		5-yr survival (%)
Tx: Primary tumor cannot be assessed		
T0: No evidence of primary tumor		
T1: Tumor ≤ 7.0 cm in greatest diameter, confined to kidney	T1a: <4.0 cm	90–100
	T1b: 4–7.0 cm	80–90
T2: Tumor > 7.0 cm in greatest diameter, confined to kidney (Gerota's fascia)	T2a: >7.0–10.0 cm	65–80
	T2b: >10.0 cm	50–70
T3: Tumor extends into major veins or perinephric tissues but not into the ipsilateral adrenal or beyond Gerota's fascia	T3a: Tumor invades perinephric structures (not Gerota's fascia) or grossly extends into a renal vein or segmental (muscle containing) branches	50—70
	T3b: Tumor extends into IVC below diaphragm	30–50
	T3c: Tumor extends into IVC above diaphragm invades the wall of the IVC	20–40
T4: Tumor invades beyond Gerota's fascia		0–30
N: Regional lymph nodes		
NX: Regional nodes cannot be assessed		
N0: No regional node metastasis		
N1: Metastasis in regional lymph nodes		0–20
M: Distant metastasis		
MX: Distant metastasis cannot be assessed		
M0: No distant metastasis		
M1: Distant metastasis		0–10
Stage		
I	T1N0M0	70–90
II	T2N0M0	50–80
III	T1 or T2, N1M0	20–70
	T3, N0 or N1, M0	
IV	T4, Any N, M0	0–30
	Any T, Any N, M1	

duct subtypes having the worse prognosis. Fuhrman grade is an independent predictor of cancer-specific survival (CSS) and includes consideration of tumors with sarcomatoid features [33, 40, 41]. Tumor necrosis is associated with large, high-grade, high-stage, clear-cell, and papillary tumors [42–44]. Microvascular invasion and renal collecting system invasion, while occurring in less than 10% of patients, are poor prognostic indicators for patients with clinically localized RCC [44, 45]. Clinical patient features including performance status and the presence of symptoms have been demonstrated to predict survival [45, 46]. Finally, in patients with metastatic disease, lung metastases have proven to be favorable while bone, brain, liver, and multiple metastases are poor prognostic indicators [47, 48].

Treatment

A number of treatment options for RCC exist and are tailored to stage. For patients with clinically localized disease, management options include AS, RN, partial nephrectomy (PN), and energy ablative (EA) treatments (cryotherapy and radiofrequency ablation).

AS involves a period of serial imaging for patients with small renal masses, usually <4 cm, and considerable medical comorbidities or reluctance to undergo surgery. Rates of progression to metastatic disease are <2% in retrospective series and prospective studies demonstrate promising short-term results [49, 50]. The American Urological Association (AUA) recommends all patients undergoing AS to understand the small but real risk of cancer progression, loss of a window of opportunity for nephron-sparing surgery (NSS), lack of curative treatments for metastatic RCC, limitations of renal biopsy, and deficiencies in the current literature [38].

RN is the surgical removal of the kidney, the investing Gerota's fascia, the contents within Gerota's fascia, and is considered the gold standard for kidney surgery due to excellent oncologic outcomes. However, given considerations of chronic kidney disease and associated cardiovascular morbidity and mortality, RN has fallen out of favor for small renal tumors. However, due to equivalent oncological outcomes and improved recovery when compared to open surgery, laparoscopic RN has become the standard for uncomplicated tumors, <7 cm, not amenable to NSS, and has been safely demonstrated in larger tumors [38]. Surgical principles of RN include early ligation of the renal vessels, removal of the ipsilateral adrenal gland, and regional lymph node dissection. Adrenalectomy is not always necessary when tumors are situated in the lower pole or in the absence of radiographic involvement [51]. Similarly, lymph node dissection in the absence of lymphadenopathy is controversial as a randomized study does not demonstrate a benefit to lymphadenectomy [51, 52]. Laparoscopic RN can be performed through a transperitoneal or retroperitoneal approach while open RN can be performed through flank, subcostal, or thoracoabdominal approach. For patients with locally advanced tumors or tumors invading the IVC, a midline incision can be made to access the great vessels or extended to include a sternotomy in the case of a thrombus extending above the diaphragm or an atrial thrombus.

Historically, the absolute indications for PN include patients with a solitary kidney, bilateral tumors, or baseline renal insufficiency. According to the AUA, PN is the standard-of-care for clinical T1 tumors amenable to NSS [38]. The basic principles of PN include excellent exposure and vascular control, excision of the tumor with a margin of normal renal parenchyma, and reconstruction of the kidney to minimize the risk of hemorrhage or fistula. PN can be performed via an open or laparoscopic approach. Serious adverse events following open PN are among the lowest of all NSS. The benefits of the laparoscopic approach should be weighed against higher risk of complications and longer ischemia times reported in the literature [38].

EA can be performed via an open, laparoscopic, or percutaneous approach. While EA may be a valid treatment for older patients or those with substantial comorbidities, the long-term oncologic efficacy of EA is unknown and local recurrence rates are higher than other NSS. While a promising treatment of RCC, ongoing concerns with EA include local recurrence rates, radiographic parameters of success, and difficulty with salvage.

Survival is generally poor for patients with metastatic RCC and no standard approach to treatment exists. Some patients may benefit from cytoreductive nephrectomy and systemic immunotherapy [48]. Novel systemic, targeted immunotherapies have proven to extend survival in some patients with metastatic disease [53].

WHAT TO AVOID

- Renal tumors are generally asymptomatic; the classic triad of hematuria, flank pain, and abdominal mass occurs in <10% of patients.
- Percutaneous biopsy is indicated in those patients in whom there is concern for renal abscess (fever, recurrent UTI, and flank pain), suspicion of metastases in a patient with a non-renal primary malignancy or lymphoma.
- RCC is a chemo- and radiation-resistant malignancy. However, RCC is an immunogenic malignancy and treatment options for metastatic RCC include cytoreductive nephrectomy with concomitant removal of solitary synchronous or metachronous metastases with systemic immunotherapy (interleukin 2 or interferon alpha) or targeted molecular agents (sunitinib, sorafenib, etc.).

KEY WEB LINKS

National Cancer Institute
http://www.cancer.gov/cancertopics/types/kidney

Cancer Treatment Centers of America
http://www.cancercenter.com/ (for patients)

Multiple choice questions

1 A healthy, 58-year-old man without a medical history is found to have an incidental 4 cm mass in his left kidney following ER evaluation for a motor vehicle accident. The mass is peripheral and mostly exophytic. It demonstrates fluid density on CT but has several solid components that enhance with IV contrast. His left kidney and renal function are normal. The most suitable management strategy recommended by the AUA is

a PN
b AS
c Cryoablation
d Renal biopsy
e RN

2 Standard evaluation of a patient with a large (>7 cm) renal mass includes all of the following except:

a High-quality axial image with contrast
b CT scan of the chest
c Liver function tests
d BMP
e Chest X-ray

References

1 Cancer Facts and Figures. The American Cancer Society 2010.
2 Hollingsworth JM, Miller DC, Daignault S, Hollenbeck BK. Rising incidence of small renal masses: a need to reassess treatment effect. *J Natl Cancer Inst* 2006;98(18):1331–1334.
3 Nguyen MM, Gill IS, Ellison LM. The evolving presentation of renal carcinoma in the United States: trends from the Surveillance, Epidemiology, and End Results program. *J Urol* 2006;176(6 Pt 1):2397–2400; discussion 400.
4 Lipworth L, Tarone RE, McLaughlin JK. The epidemiology of renal cell carcinoma. *J Urol* 2006;176(6 Pt 1):2353–2358.
5 Chow WH, Gridley G, Fraumeni JF, Jr., Jarvholm B. Obesity, hypertension, and the risk of kidney cancer in men. *N Engl J Med* 2000;343(18):1305–1311.
6 Bjorge T, Tretli S, Engeland A. Relation of height and body mass index to renal cell carcinoma in two million Norwegian men and women. *Am J Epidemiol* 2004;160(12):1168–1176.
7 Yu MC, Mack TM, Hanisch R, Cicioni C, Henderson BE. Cigarette smoking, obesity, diuretic use, and coffee consumption as risk factors for renal cell carcinoma. *J Natl Cancer Inst* 1986;77(2):351–356.
8 Shapiro JA, Williams MA, Weiss NS, Stergachis A, LaCroix AZ, Barlow WE. Hypertension, antihypertensive medication use, and risk of renal cell carcinoma. *Am J Epidemiol* 1999;149(6):521–530.
9 Greving JP, Lee JE, Wolk A, Lukkien C, Lindblad P, Bergstrom A. Alcoholic beverages and risk of renal cell cancer. *Br J Cancer* 2007;97(3):429–433.
10 Lee JE, Giovannucci E, Smith-Warner SA, Spiegelman D, Willett WC, Curhan GC. Intakes of fruits, vegetables, vitamins A, C, and E, and carotenoids and risk of renal cell cancer. *Cancer Epidemiol Biomarkers Prev* 2006;15(12):2445–2452.
11 Wolk A, Larsson SC, Johansson JE, Ekman P. Long-term fatty fish consumption and renal cell carcinoma incidence in women. *JAMA* 2006;296(11):1371–1376.
12 McCredie M, Pommer W, McLaughlin JK, et al. International renal-cell cancer study. II. Analgesics. *Int J Cancer* 1995;60(3):345–349.
13 Linehan WM, Srinivasan R, Schmidt LS. The genetic basis of kidney cancer: a metabolic disease. *Nat Rev Urol* 2010;7(5):277–285.
14 Jayson M, Sanders H. Increased incidence of serendipitously discovered renal cell carcinoma. *Urology* 1998;51(2):203–205.
15 Pantuck AJ, Zisman A, Rauch MK, Belldegrun A. Incidental renal tumors. *Urology* 2000;56(2):190–196.

16 Gold PJ, Fefer A, Thompson JA. Paraneoplastic manifestations of renal cell carcinoma. *Semin Urol Oncol* 1996;14(4):216–222.
17 Young RC. Metastatic renal-cell carcinoma: what causes occasional dramatic regressions? *N Engl J Med* 1998;338(18):1305–1306.
18 Bosniak MA. The use of the Bosniak classification system for renal cysts and cystic tumors. *J Urol* 1997;157(5):1852–1853.
19 Israel GM, Bosniak MA. An update of the Bosniak renal cyst classification system. *Urology* 2005;66(3):484–488.
20 Bach AM, Zhang J. Contemporary radiologic imaging of renal cortical tumors. *Urol Clin North Am* 2008;35(4):593–604; vi.
21 Sheir KZ, El-Azab M, Mosbah A, El-Baz M, Shaaban AA. Differentiation of renal cell carcinoma subtypes by multislice computerized tomography. *J Urol* 2005;174(2):451–455; discussion 455.
22 Kim JK, Kim TK, Ahn HJ, Kim CS, Kim KR, Cho KS. Differentiation of subtypes of renal cell carcinoma on helical CT scans. *AJR Am J Roentgenol* 2002;178(6):1499–1506.
23 Studer UE, Scherz S, Scheidegger J, et al. Enlargement of regional lymph nodes in renal cell carcinoma is often not due to metastases. *J Urol* 1990;144(2 Pt 1):243–245.
24 Guzzo TJ, Pierorazio PM, Schaeffer EM, Fishman EK, Allaf ME. The accuracy of multidetector computerized tomography for evaluating tumor thrombus in patients with renal cell carcinoma. *J Urol* 2009;181(2):486–490; discussion 91.
25 Ng CS, Wood CG, Silverman PM, Tannir NM, Tamboli P, Sandler CM. Renal cell carcinoma: diagnosis, staging, and surveillance. *AJR Am J Roentgenol* 2008;191(4):1220–1232.
26 Lim DJ, Carter MF. Computerized tomography in the preoperative staging for pulmonary metastases in patients with renal cell carcinoma. *J Urol* 1993;150(4):1112–1114.
27 Seaman E, Goluboff ET, Ross S, Sawczuk IS. Association of radionuclide bone scan and serum alkaline phosphatase in patients with metastatic renal cell carcinoma. *Urology* 1996;48(5):692–695.
28 Leveridge MJ, Finelli A, Kachura JR, et al. Outcomes of small renal mass needle core biopsy, nondiagnostic percutaneous biopsy, and the role of repeat biopsy. *Eur Urol* 2011;60(3):578–584.
29 Blumenfeld AJ, Guru K, Fuchs GJ, Kim HL. Percutaneous biopsy of renal cell carcinoma underestimates nuclear grade. *Urology* 2010;76(3):610–613.
30 Lane BR, Samplaski MK, Herts BR, Zhou M, Novick AC, Campbell SC. Renal mass biopsy–a renaissance? *J Urol* 2008;179(1):20–27.
31 Eble JN, Sauter G, Epstein JI, Sesterhenn IA. *Pathology and Genetics of Tumours of the Urinary System and Male Genital Organs.* Lyon, France: IARC Press; 2004.
32 Cheville JC, Lohse CM, Zincke H, Weaver AL, Blute ML. Comparisons of outcome and prognostic features among histologic subtypes of renal cell carcinoma. *Am J Surg Pathol* 2003;27(5):612–624.
33 Zhou M, Rubin MA. Molecular markers for renal cell carcinoma: impact on diagnosis and treatment. *Semin Urol Oncol* 2001;19(2):80–87.
34 Thompson RH, Hill JR, Babayev Y, et al. Metastatic renal cell carcinoma risk according to tumor size. *J Urol* 2009;182(1):41–45.
35 Thompson RH, Kurta JM, Kaag M, et al. Tumor size is associated with malignant potential in renal cell carcinoma cases. *J Urol* 2009;181(5):2033–2036.
36 Rothman J, Egleston B, Wong YN, Iffrig K, Lebovitch S, Uzzo RG. Histopathological characteristics of localized renal cell carcinoma correlate with tumor size: a SEER analysis. *J Urol* 2009;181(1):29–33; discussion 33–34.
37 Nguyen MM, Gill IS. Effect of renal cancer size on the prevalence of metastasis at diagnosis and mortality. *J Urol* 2009;181(3):1020–1027; discussion 1027.
38 Campbell SC, Novick AC, Belldegrun A, et al. Guideline for management of the clinical T1 renal mass. *J Urol* 2009;182(4):1271–1279.
39 Beck SD, Patel MI, Snyder ME, et al. Effect of papillary and chromophobe cell type on disease-free survival after nephrectomy for renal cell carcinoma. *Ann Surg Oncol* 2004;11(1):71–77.
40 Pantuck AJ, Zisman A, Belldegrun A. Biology of renal cell carcinoma: changing concepts in classification and staging. *Semin Urol Oncol* 2001;19(2):72–79.
41 Lohse CM, Cheville JC. A review of prognostic pathologic features and algorithms for patients treated surgically for renal cell carcinoma. *Clin Lab Med* 2005;25(2):433–464.
42 Sengupta S, Lohse CM, Leibovich BC, et al. Histologic coagulative tumor necrosis as a prognostic indicator of renal cell carcinoma aggressiveness. *Cancer* 2005;104(3):511–520.
43 Klatte T, Said JW, de Martino M, et al. Presence of tumor necrosis is not a significant predictor of survival in clear cell renal cell carcinoma: higher prognostic accuracy of extent based rather than presence/absence classification. *J Urol* 2009;181(4):1558–1564; discussion 63–64.
44 Sorbellini M, Kattan MW, Snyder ME, et al. A postoperative prognostic nomogram predicting recurrence for patients with conventional clear cell renal cell carcinoma. *J Urol* 2005;173(1):48–51.
45 Lane BR, Kattan MW. Prognostic models and algorithms in renal cell carcinoma. *Urol Clin North Am* 2008;35(4):613–625; vii.

46 Lee CT, Katz J, Fearn PA, Russo P. Mode of presentation of renal cell carcinoma provides prognostic information. *Urol Oncol* 2002;7(4):135–140.

47 Vogelzang NJ, Priest ER, Borden L. Spontaneous regression of histologically proved pulmonary metastases from renal cell carcinoma: a case with 5-year followup. *J Urol* 1992;148(4):1247–1248.

48 Flanigan RC, Mickisch G, Sylvester R, Tangen C, Van Poppel H, Crawford ED. Cytoreductive nephrectomy in patients with metastatic renal cancer: a combined analysis. *J Urol* 2004;171(3):1071–1076.

49 Smaldone MC, Kutikov A, Egleston BL, et al. Small renal masses progressing to metastases under active surveillance: a systematic review and pooled analysis. *Cancer* 2012;118(4):997–1006.

50 Mason RJ, Abdolell M, Trottier G, et al. Growth kinetics of renal masses: analysis of a prospective cohort of patients undergoing active surveillance. *Eur Urol* 2011;59(5):863–867.

51 O'Malley RL, Godoy G, Kanofsky JA, Taneja SS. The necessity of adrenalectomy at the time of radical nephrectomy: a systematic review. *J Urol* 2009;181(5):2009–2017.

52 Blom JH, van Poppel H, Marechal JM, et al. Radical nephrectomy with and without lymph-node dissection: final results of European Organization for Research and Treatment of Cancer (EORTC) randomized phase 3 trial 30881. *Eur Urol* 2009;55(1):28–34.

53 Hutson TE. Targeted therapies for the treatment of metastatic renal cell carcinoma: clinical evidence. *Oncologist* 2011;16(Suppl 2):14–22.

54 Fuhrman SA, Lasky LC, Limas C. Prognostic significance of morphologic parameters in renal cell carcinoma. *Am J Surg Pathol* 1982;6(7):655–663.

55 Zhou M: Pathology of renal cell carcinomas. In: Rini BI, Campbell SC, editors. *Renal Cell Carcinoma*. Shelton, CT: People's Medical Publishing House; 2009.

56 Kidney. In: Edge SB, Byrd DR, Compton CC, editors. *AJCC Cancer Staging Manual*. 7th ed. New York: Springer; 2010. pp. 479–489.

Answers to multiple choice questions

1 a This lesion can be classified as a Bosniak IV lesion and requires treatment in a healthy, young patient. According to the 2009 AUA Guidelines for the Management of the Clinical Stage 1 Renal Mass, partial nephrectomy (PN) is the standard treatment for cT1a lesions amenable to nephron-sparing surgery (NSS). This lesion is peripheral and exophytic, and likely amenable to an NSS approach. While thermal ablation and active surveillance (AS) are options, they are less favorable choices in a young, healthy patient. Renal biopsy is not indicated in this patient.

2 b CT scan of the chest. Routine metastatic evaluation for patients with large or advanced tumors should include the assessment of performance status, chest radiography, basic metabolic panel (BMP), and liver function tests. Performance status reflects overall patient health, life expectancy, and may guide management. A BMP evaluates the renal function, chest radiography and liver function tests evaluate visceral metastases. Chest CT should be reserved only for patients with pulmonary symptoms or an abnormal chest X-ray. Bone scan is indicated only in patients with an elevated alkaline phosphatase, bone pain, or precipitous decline in the performance status. Similarly, head imaging is not routinely recommended as patients with brain metastases typically present with symptoms related to a brain lesion.

26 Adrenal disorders

Jeffrey K. Mullins

The James Buchanan Brady Urological Institute and Department of Urology, The Johns Hopkins School of Medicine, Baltimore, MD, USA

KEY POINTS

- The adrenal cortex is subdivided into the zona glomerulosa, zona fasciculata, and zona reticularis. These zones secrete aldosterone, cortisol, and sex steroids, respectively.
- The adrenal medulla secretes catecholamines which serve a variety of functions throughout the body.
- Cushing's syndrome is due to excessive glucocorticoids and is most commonly caused by exogenous administration of synthetic glucocorticoids.
- ACTH-dependent Cushing's syndrome is due to a pituitary adenoma or ACTH-secreting tumor, both of which are managed surgically.
- ACTH-independent Cushing's syndrome is due to adrenal hyperplasia or adrenal adenoma. Treatment depends on severity of syndromes and disease laterality.
- Primary hyperaldosteronism is due to excessive secretion of aldosterone.
- The majority of cases of primary hyperaldosteronism is due to adrenal hyperplasia or adrenal adenomas.
- Treatment of primary aldosteronism depends on the etiology. Adenomas are typically resected while bilateral hyperplasia is managed with aldosterone receptor agonists.
- Pheochromocytomas are catecholamine-secreting lesions of the adrenal medulla.
- Classic symptoms of a pheochromocytoma include headache, episodic hypertension, and tachycardia.
- Surgical resection is the mainstay of treatment of pheochromocytomas.
- Adrenal insufficiency is treated with replacement of glucocorticoids and mineralocorticoids.
- Adrenal cortical carcinoma is characterized by large lesions (>4–6 cm) that typically present at an advanced stage and carry a poor prognosis.
- Metastatic deposits are common lesions in the adrenal. Melanoma, lung cancer, and renal cell carcinoma are common cancers that metastasize to the adrenal.

CASE STUDY 1

A 50-year-old female presents to her primary care physician with a chief complaint of fatigue and weight gain. Her past medical and surgical histories are unremarkable. She does have a 25 pack per year smoking history. On physical examination her blood pressure is 175/96. She has central obesity with peripheral wasting of her extremities. Additionally, she has purple striae on her abdomen, and has numerous bruises on her arms. She denies trauma or abuse. Laboratory evaluation was significant for a fasting blood sugar of 170.

This patient has the classic appearance of Cushing's syndrome as well as systemic symptoms associated with the syndrome (hypertension/glucose intolerance). As part of her work-up she first undergoes a late-night salivary cortisol level. Her elevated level of 25.6 nmol/L establishes the diagnosis of Cushing's syndrome. In order to determine the etiology of her Cushing's syndrome, she has an ACTH level drawn which is markedly elevated. Furthermore, a high-dose dexamethasone suppression test fails to suppress cortisol levels. She next undergoes a CT scan of the chest/abdomen/pelvis which demonstrates a spiculated mass in the left lung. After a negative metastatic work-up, she underwent left lower lung lobectomy. Pathology was consistent with small cell carcinoma of the lung. After surgery, her symptoms associated with her Cushing's syndrome subsided. This woman had Cushing's syndrome secondary to ectopic ACTH secretion from a small cell lung cancer.

Handbook of Urology, First edition. J. Kellogg Parsons, John B. Eifler and Misop Han. © 2014 by John Wiley & Sons, Ltd. Published 2014 by John Wiley & Sons, Ltd.

CASE STUDY 2

A 53-year-old male is being evaluated by his PCP for persistent hypertension. He was first diagnosed with hypertension 6 months ago. Prior to this he was normotensive. His past medical history is notable for gastroesophageal reflux disease and hyperlipidemia. He has had no previous surgery. He has no allergies. Current medications include hydrochlorothiazide, metoprolol, and captopril. Today, his blood pressure is 195/100. Furthermore, on laboratory evaluation his creatinine was found to be 1.7. Upon further questioning, the patient does describe a recent history of headaches and occasional flushing.

This patient has significant hypertension refractory to multiple medications with evidence of end organ damage (Cr: 1.7). Given this scenario, his PCP begins working him up for other causes of hypertension. As part of this evaluation, a CT scan is performed which demonstrates a 5 cm right adrenal mass which avidly enhances with contrast and has a slow washout. At this time the patient is referred to his urologist for further evaluation. His urologist obtains plasma-free metanephrines, 24-hour urinary catecholamines, and 24-hour fractioned metanephrines. All levels are significantly elevated. At this time the patient is diagnosed with a pheochromocytoma and plans are made for right adrenalectomy.

Prior to surgery, the patient is started on a nonselective α-blocker (phenoxybenzamine). Once α-blockade has been established, β-blockade with atenolol is begun. The day prior to surgery the patient is admitted to the hospital for intravenous hydration, endocrinology consult, and anesthesiology consult. The next day the patient undergoes laparoscopic right adrenalectomy. Postoperatively, the patient was admitted to the ICU where there was persistent hypotension for 24 hours. On postoperative day 3, the patient was hemodynamically stable and was discharged home in good condition with a blood pressure of 130/70. The surgical aspects of this case highlight several important points. First, preoperatively patients should receive α-blockade followed by β-blockade (especially if symptomatic). It is prudent to admit these patients for aggressive hydration prior to surgery. Furthermore, these cases are best approached via a multidisciplinary team consisting of a surgeon, an endocrinologist, and an anesthesiologist. Postoperatively patients need admission to the ICU to be monitored for hemodynamic instability secondary to removal of pheochromocytoma and residual effects of the α-blockade.

CASE STUDY 3

A 37-year-old male presents to the ED with a chief complaint of back pain for several months. He has been unable to get relief with over-the-counter medications, and seeks more potent pain medications. He does report recent malaise and 15 pound unintentional weight loss. He has no past medical or surgical history. Physical examination is normal except for a sense of fullness on the right side of the abdomen. Given his abnormal abdominal examination he undergoes a CT scan which demonstrates a 15 cm heterogeneous, enhancing mass superior to and involving the right kidney. Additionally, there are several large retroperitoneal nodes up to 2 cm and several enhancing lesions within the liver. Given these findings the patient was admitted to the hospital. He underwent needle biopsy of the mass which was consistent with adrenal cortical carcinoma (ACC). Given his metastatic disease the patient was not deemed a surgical candidate. He was started on mitotane for his systemic disease. Unfortunately, the patient expired from this disease 18 months later.

This case of ACC highlights several important points. First patients are either asymptomatic or have vague symptoms. These lesions are usually picked up incidentally on cross-sectional imaging. Second, these lesions tend to be large (>5 cm). Third, over 50% present with locally advanced or metastatic disease. Finally, the prognosis of patients with locally advanced or metastatic ACC is uniformly poor with 5-year survival rates reported at <5%.

Introduction

The adrenal glands are small retroperitoneal organs which secrete a variety of hormones that serve a pivotal role in a multitude of physiologic processes throughout the human body. Alterations in adrenal steroid synthesis result in a number of well-described syndromes. However, the diagnosis and treatment of these syndromes is challenging. This chapter serves to discuss the presentation, diagnosis, and treatment of the most common adrenal disorders encountered by urologists.

Anatomy and normal physiology

Normal anatomy and histology

The adrenal glands are paired retroperitoneal organs that lie superior to the kidneys within Gerota's fascia. The inferior phrenic artery, aorta, and renal artery provide the arterial blood supply to the adrenal gland. Venous drainage occurs via a solitary adrenal vein which drains into the inferior vena cava and renal vein on the right and left, respectively. Notably, the short right adrenal vein is a common site for troublesome bleeding during right adrenalectomy [1].

Microscopically, the adrenal is composed of an outer adrenal cortex and inner medulla. Embryologically, these layers are derived from the intermediate mesoderm and neuroectoderm, respectively. The adrenal cortex is further subdivided into the *zona glomerulosa* most superficially, *zona fasciculata*, and *zona reticularis* adjacent to the medulla. The normal function of these zones is to secrete aldosterone, cortisol, and sex steroids (dehydroepiandrosterone (DHEA), sulfated DHEA, and androstenedione), respectively. These steroids are all derived from cholesterol metabolism. The production of pregnenolone from cholesterol via mitochondrial side chain cleavage is the rate limiting step in the production of all adrenal cortex hormones. The adrenal medulla is composed of chromaffin cells. These cells function as an integral part of the sympathetic nervous system by secreting catecholamines (epinephrine, norepinephrine, and dopamine) [1].

Normal physiology

Aldosterone, secreted by the *zona glomerulosa*, is the primary mineralocorticoid in humans. Secretion is regulated primarily by angiotensin II and serum potassium levels with ACTH providing a less potent stimulus. Angiotensin II is formed under the influence of the renin–angiotensin system which is primarily regulated by effective circulating blood volume and sodium balance. Specifically, decreased renal perfusion pressure, decreased sodium delivery to the distal nephron, and serum hyperkalemia lead to increased secretion of aldosterone. The main function of aldosterone is to promote sodium reabsorption and potassium secretion in the distal nephron [1, 2].

Cortisol, the main glucocorticoid in humans, is secreted by the *zona fasciculata* under the influence of adrenocorticotropic hormone (ACTH) secreted by the anterior pituitary gland [2]. Secretion of cortisol occurs in a distinct circadian rhythm with highest levels occurring in the early morning. Cortisol has a key role in modulating numerous physiologic pathways including metabolism, immunity, and cardiovascular and nervous system function [1, 3].

Adrenal sex steroids secreted by the *zona reticularis* include **DHEA, DHEA-S, and androstenedione.** Production of these hormones is under the influence of ACTH. In the normal state, these hormones do not play a major role in adult physiology [1, 2].

Epinephrine is the major secretory product of the adrenal medulla (80%) [4]. Interestingly, the adrenal medulla is the primary source of epinephrine as the enzyme responsible for converting norepinephrine to epinephrine (phenylethanolamine N-methyltransferase) is located primarily in the adrenal gland [4]. Secretion of epinephrine and other catecholamines is regulated by preganglionic sympathetic fibers which innervate the adrenal medulla. The effect of catecholamines is variable throughout the body and depends on the target organ and the type of adrenergic receptor. Of note, the main metabolites of catecholamine degradation are **metanephrine, normetanephrine, and vanillylmandelic acid.** Quantitative analysis of serum and urine levels of these metabolites is important in the diagnosis of pheochromocytomas as will be discussed later in this chapter [1].

Cushing's syndrome

Overview and presentation

Cushing's syndrome describes the symptom complex associated with excess circulating glucocorticoids from the adrenal cortex. The incidence of Cushing's syndrome is 2–5 per million people per year [5, 6]. Causes of Cushing's syndrome can be subdivided into three main categories: **(1) ACTH dependent, (2) ACTH independent, and (3) exogenous.** Overall, exogenous Cushing's syndrome, secondary to the iatrogenic administration of synthetic glucocorticoids, is the most common etiology [7]. Considering only endogenous cases, ACTH-dependent Cushing's syndrome accounts for 80–85% of cases [7]. Importantly, other conditions (alcoholism, major depressive disorder, obesity, etc.) can cause dysregulation of the hypothalamus–pituitary–adrenal axis causing elevated cortisol levels in the absence of Cushing's syndrome (*pseudo-Cushing's syndrome*) [1]. These must be ruled out before establishing a diagnosis of Cushing's syndrome.

ACTH-dependent Cushing's syndrome results from pathology extrinsic to the adrenal gland. The majority of cases (80%) are due to hypersecretion of ACTH by a pituitary adenoma. This condition is known as **Cushing's disease.** The other major cause of ACTH-dependent Cushing's syndrome is **ectopic ACTH production** most commonly from a lung or pancreatic source [7].

ACTH-independent Cushing's syndrome is due to unregulated secretion of glucocorticoids from the adrenal cortex. Functional **adrenal adenomas and adrenal cortical carcinomas (ACC)** represent the majority of these cases and account for ~10% and 8% of cases of Cushing's syndrome, respectively. Rare entities including macronodular adrenal hyperplasia and primary pigmented nodular adrenocortical disease comprise the remainder of cases with each accounting for <1% of cases of Cushing's syndrome [1, 7].

Presentation

The clinical presentation of Cushing's syndrome is variable among patients and often nonspecific. Typically, patients have a classic appearance characterized by **central obesity with peripheral muscle wasting, moon faces, buffalo hump, and abdominal striae** [6]. In addition, patients often present with systemic symptoms including **hypertension and metabolic syndrome** [8]. Table 26.1 lists various signs and symptoms of Cushing's syndrome with their estimated prevalence. Other urology-specific complications of Cushing's syndrome include hypogonadal hypogonadism and urolithiasis [1].

Table 26.1 Signs and symptoms of Cushing's syndrome [8]

Signs and symptoms	Prevalence (%)
Central obesity	90–100
Rounded face (moon faces)	
Facial plethora	
Decreased libido	
Purple striae	70–90
Menstrual disturbances	
Hirsutism	
Erectile dysfunction	
Hypertension	
Muscle weakness	50–70
Posterior neck fat deposit (buffalo hump)	
Body bruising	
Glucose intolerance/diabetes	
Osteopenia/osteoporosis	
Emotional lability/depression	
Headache	20–50
Backache	
Limb edema	
Recurrent infections	
Hypokalemic alkalosis	
Nephrolithiasis	
Acne	0–20
Alopecia	

Diagnosis

Diagnosis begins with having a low threshold for working-up a patient for Cushing's syndrome as many signs and symptoms are nonspecific. Furthermore, exogenous administration of synthetic glucocorticoids and comorbidities causing pseudo-Cushing's syndrome must be excluded. The diagnostic work-up should then proceed in a systematic fashion as follows:

1 *Diagnosis of Cushing's syndrome:* Diagnosis of Cushing's syndrome was historically based on the **low-dose dexamethasone suppression test.** In patients with Cushing's syndrome, administration of dexamethasone fails to suppress cortisol levels the following morning. More commonly used tests now include a **24-hour urinary free cortisol measurement and late-night salivary cortisol test.**

2 *Determine dependence on ACTH:* The most direct way to determine ACTH dependence is by measuring **serum ACTH.** Obviously, a high-serum ACTH indicates an ACTH-dependent pathology.

3 *Identifying the etiology of ACTH-independent Cushing's syndrome:* **Abdominal cross-sectional imaging** to evaluate adrenal glands.

4 *Identifying the etiology of ACTH-dependent Cushing's syndrome:* Cross-sectional imaging of the head, chest, and abdomen is typically performed to diagnose a pituitary adenoma or ACTH-secreting tumor. However, the high prevalence of pituitary microadenomas and incidental findings within the lungs and pancreas limit the utility of imaging in establishing a diagnosis.

The **high-dose dexamethasone suppression test** was historically used to differentiate Cushing's disease

Table 26.2 General treatment strategies for Cushing's syndrome stratified by etiology

Etiology	Treatment
Exogenous Cushing's syndrome	1 Cessation of exogenous glucocorticoids
Cushing's disease	2 Transsphenoidal surgical resection--25% relapse rate 3 Consider radiotherapy or bilateral adrenalectomy[a] if surgical resection fails
Ectopic ACTH production	4 Resection of ACTH-secreting tumor if feasible 5 Bilateral adrenalectomy[a] if tumor is unresectable or unidentifiable
Adrenal adenoma	6 Unilateral adrenalectomy vs. partial adrenalectomy
Adrenal cortical carcinoma	7 Unilateral adrenalectomy
Macronodular hyperplasia	8 Bilateral adrenalectomy[a]

[a]Nelson's syndrome defined as the developing of an ACTH-secreting pituitary adenoma can result in 8–29% of patients after bilateral adrenalectomy. Patients typically present with visual changes and rarely with symptoms due to increased intracranial pressure [34].

(pituitary adenoma) from ectopic ACTH production. In this test, cortisol levels are suppressed in patients with Cushing's disease after a high dose of dexamethasone. However, the value of this test is now limited and **direct measurement of ACTH from the inferior petrosal sinus** following corticotrophin stimulation is now the gold standard [1, 6].

Treatment

Treatment of Cushing's syndrome depends on the etiology of the syndrome. Table 26.2 provides general treatment recommendations for the various etiologies of Cushing's syndrome. At times, definitive treatment of Cushing's syndrome is not possible and medical therapy must be employed to control the symptoms. These medications include **metyrapone, aminoglutethimide, mitotane, and ketoconazole** work by blocking enzymes involved in steroid synthesis [1].

Primary hyperaldosteronism (Conn's syndrome)

Overview

Primary aldosteronism, first described by Dr. Jerome Conn in 1955, is defined by aldosterone secretion occurring independent of the renin–angiotensin–aldosterone system [9]. The disease has a reported prevalence of 5–13% among hypertensive patients, and is most commonly diagnosed in the third to the sixth decade of life [10–12]. The etiology is most commonly an adrenal adenoma (35%) or idiopathic bilateral hyperplasia (60%). Other rare causes of primary aldosteronism include unilateral idiopathic hyperplasia (2%), ACC (<1%), ectopic aldosterone-secreting tumor (<1%), and familial hyperaldosteronism (<1%) [12].

Presentation

Classic characteristics of primary aldosteronism include **hypertension and hypokalemia**. Patients typically have moderate to severe hypertension that is more severe than patients without primary hyperaldosteronism [1]. Mean blood pressures in contemporary series have ranged from 154/98 to 184/112 [11, 12]. Although hypokalemia has classically been described in association with primary aldosteronism, between 63% and 91% of newly diagnosed patients will have normal serum potassium levels [10]. Other less common symptoms include muscle weakness, urinary frequency, headaches, nocturia, and polydipsia. Notably, hypernatremia does not occur due to mineralocorticoid escape.

Diagnosis

Diagnosis of primary aldosteronism includes screening, confirmation, and subtype differentiation.

1 *Screening:* Table 26.3 lists indications for screening for primary aldosteronism. Before initiating diagnostic tests, hypokalemia must be corrected and

Table 26.3 Indications for screening for primary aldosteronism [1]

Hypertension with hypokalemia
Resistant hypertension (poor control with >3 agents)
Adrenal incidentaloma with hypertension
Early onset of hypertension (<20) or stroke (<50)
Severe hypertension (>160/>110)
When considering causes of secondary hypertension
Unexplained hypokalemia
Target end organ damage disproportionate to degree of hypertension

aldosterone-antagonist medications must be stopped for at least 6 weeks. Primary aldosteronism is established by obtaining a morning **plasma aldosterone concentration (PAC) and plasma renin activity (PRA)**. The following values represent a positive screening test and are indicative of primary aldosteronism:

- PAC > 15 ng/dL
- PRA < 0.2 nd/dL
- PAC:PRA < 20:1

2 *Confirmation:* 50–70% of patients with a positive screening test will ultimately be diagnosed with primary aldosteronism. Four tests (fludrocortisone suppression test, oral sodium loading test, intravenous saline infusion test, and captopril suppression test) have been described to confirm the diagnosis of primary aldosteronism. Currently, the **oral sodium loading test** and **intravenous saline infusion test** are the most commonly used.

3 *Subtype differentiation:* Once a primary aldosteronism diagnosis has been established the next step is identifying patients who are surgical candidates (unilateral pathology). The initial test of choice is an adrenal CT scan. However, given that 20% of aldosterone-secreting adenomas are <1 cm and the potential presence of nonfunctional adenomas it is recommended that **adrenal vein sampling** be performed to lateralize the location of excess aldosterone secretion [1].

Treatment

Treatment of primary aldosteronism depends on disease subtype and a patient's suitability for surgical therapy. **Unilateral adrenalectomy** is reserved for patients with a confirmed unilateral source of excess aldosterone (adenoma, unilateral hyperplasia, and ACC). Surgical success, defined as requiring no antihypertensives postoperatively, occurs in 33–73% of patients [13–15]. Patients with nonsurgical disease (bilateral hyperplasia) and those who are not surgical candidates should be managed with **aldosterone receptor antagonists** (spironolactone or eplerenone) [1].

Pheochromocytoma

Overview

Pheochromocytomas are catecholamine-secreting tumors of the adrenal medulla. Approximately 1–25% of catecholamine-secreting tumors occur outside the adrenal in sympathetic ganglia and are referred to as paragangliomas [16]. The incidence of pheochromocytomas has been reported as 1–2 per 100,000 people per year [17]. Approximately 33% of pheochromocytomas occur in association with several familial syndromes including von Hippel–Lindau disease, von Recklinghausen's disease (neurofibromatosis type 1), and multiple endocrine neoplasia type 2A and 2B [18]. Familial cases typically occur at a younger age than sporadic cases which are most common in the fourth and fifth decades of life. The majority of pheochromocytomas are pathologically benign, but ~5% of patients will have malignant disease defined by the presence of metastases [1].

Presentation

Symptoms depend on the type and amount of catecholamines secreted. The classic triad of symptoms for a pheochromocytoma is **headache, episodic hypertension, and tachycardia** [1]. Of these, headache is the most common symptom occurring in up to 90% of patients [19]. Notably, more patients have sustained hypertension as compared to the classically described episodic hypertension. Table 26.4 lists symptoms associated with pheochromocytoma and their relative prevalence. Approximately 20% of patients with a pheochromocytoma are asymptomatic. Additionally, cases of familial pheochromocytoma will present at a younger age with a phenotype consistent with the familial syndrome.

Diagnosis

Diagnosis of pheochromocytoma includes both a biochemical and an imaging evaluation. Biochemical

Table 26.4 Signs and symptoms of pheochromocytoma [19]

Sign or symptom	Frequency (%)
Headache	60–90
Palpitations	50–70
Sweating	55–75
Pallor	40–45
Nausea	20–40
Flushing	10–20
Weight loss	20–40
Tiredness	25–40
Psychological symptoms	20–40
Sustained hypertension	50–60
Paroxysmal hypertension	30
Orthostatic hypotension	10–50
Hyperglycemia	40

evaluation documents an excess of catecholamines. Currently, **plasma-free metanephrines** is the best test with a sensitivity of 97–99% and specificity of 82–96% [20]. Typically, the initial diagnostic work-up includes plasma-free metanephrines, 24-hour urinary catecholamines, and 24-hour urine-fractioned metanephrines.

Imaging evaluation begins with either CT or MRI. Typical CT appearance is an attenuation of >10 HU on noncontrast-enhanced scans with slow washout after the administration of contrast [21]. Typical MRI characteristics include bright signal intensity on T2-weighted images and absence of signal drop out out-of-phase sequences [22]. In cases where the lesion cannot be localized with CT or MRI, metaiodobenzylguanidine (MIBG) scintigraphy can be used.

Treatment

The standard of care for pheochromocytomas is **unilateral adrenalectomy.** Perioperatively, patients should be treated first with α-blockade (phenoxybenzamine) followed by β-blockade (selective β_1-blockers). Additionally, the patient should be aggressively hydrated going into the operating room. Postoperatively, patients should be monitored in the intensive care unit as hypotension is common especially in the setting of a preoperative α-blockade [1]. Lifelong follow-up is mandatory for these patients as up to 16% of patients will recur and up to 50% of recurrences are malignant [23].

Adrenal insufficiency (Addison's disease)

Overview

Adrenal insufficiency is a deficiency of mineralocorticoids and glucocorticoids. It may occur in a chronic or acute (Addisonian crisis) fashion with the latter representing a life-threatening condition [24]. There are numerous etiologies of adrenal insufficiency with autoimmune diseases and infection (tuberculosis) representing the most common etiologies in developed and undeveloped countries, respectively. The etiologies most commonly seen by urologists include bilateral adrenalectomy, abrupt cessation of exogenous steroids, and interruption of normal adrenal steroid synthesis with medications (ketoconazole or abiraterone). Other etiologies include infiltrative diseases (amyloidosis), hemorrhage, and abnormalities of the pituitary or hypothalamus [1].

Presentation

Acute adrenal insufficiency is a life-threatening condition characterized by hypotension refractory to fluid resuscitation, abdominal pain, nausea, vomiting, and fever. These patients often represent a diagnostic dilemma and providers must keep a high index of suspicion for an Addisonian crisis.

Initial presentation of **chronic adrenal insufficiency** is characterized by nonspecific signs and symptoms including fatigue, anorexia, and vague aches and pains. Hyperpigmentation of the skin is a classic sign due to excess serum melanocortin, a by-product of ACTH production. Abnormal laboratory values including hyponatremia, hyperkalemia, and azotemia may be present in some patients [1].

Diagnosis

Diagnosis of acute adrenal insufficiency is made on clinical grounds. Appropriate therapy should be administered at the time of suspected diagnosis.

Diagnosis of chronic adrenal insufficiency is accomplished by the measurement of an early morning **cortisol and ACTH.** If abnormalities in these tests are discovered, a **corticotropin test** is performed to assess the adrenal's response to ACTH stimulation [1].

Treatment

Treatment of adrenal insufficiency involves the replacement of mineralocorticoids and glucocorticoids. Hydrocortisone and fludrocortisones are typically used in the chronic setting. 4 mg of dexamethasone or 100 mg of hydrocortisone is typically administered to patients with acute adrenal insufficiency.

Adrenal cortical carcinoma

Overview

ACC is a rare malignant tumor with an estimated incidence of 0.2–2 per million per year. These lesions occur more commonly in females and have a bimodal distribution with peaks both in childhood and during the fourth and fifth decades of life. The majority of lesions are unilateral occurring sporadically although a minority may be bilateral in association with various tumor syndromes such as Li–Fraumeni and Beckwith–Wiedemann syndromes [1, 25].

Presentation

Due to increased utilization of cross-sectional imaging, a significant number of ACCs are detected incidentally. However, up to 79% of tumors are biochemically active (most commonly cortisol), and patients may present with signs and symptoms associated with the tumor's secretory product [25]. All tumors can also present with constitutional symptoms including pain, nausea, vomiting, fever, and weight loss.

Diagnosis and staging

The diagnosis of ACC is based on radiographic characteristics. However, the functional status of all lesions should be evaluated for the purposes of pre- and postoperative planning. Radiographically, most lesions are large with an average size of 10–12 cm, and >90% being larger than 5 cm [26, 27]. Given the strong correlation between malignancy and adrenal tumor size, it is currently recommended that incidental adrenal tumors >4–6 cm undergo surgical excision [1]. Patients suspected of ACC should also be assessed for the presence of metastases which occur most commonly in the lung and liver.

On CT, lesions are typically irregular with heterogeneous enhancement and areas of hemorrhage and necrosis. Additionally, lesions demonstrate increased enhancement and delayed washout compared to adenomas [25, 28]. On MRI, lesions typically have a bright signal intensity on T2-enhanced images, and demonstrate avid enhancement on gadolinium-enhanced images [29].

Staging is typically via the TNM system. T1 and T2 tumors are confined to the adrenal gland and are differentiated by a size cutoff of 5 cm. T3 tumors exhibit local invasion into the periadrenal adipose tissue, and T4 lesions invade adjacent organs [1].

Treatment and prognosis

Adrenalectomy is the mainstay of treatment for ACC. Unfortunately, up to 49% of patients will present with locally advanced or metastatic disease for which surgery may not be curative [1]. Table 26.5 lists 5-year survival estimates by tumor stage. Metastatic disease is typically treated with **mitotane** which also has efficacy in the adjuvant setting after adrenalectomy for localized ACC.

Table 26.5 Prognosis of ACC by stage [1]

Stage	2004 UICC/WHO	At diagnosis (%)	5-year survival(%)
1	T1N0M0	3–4	33–66
2	T2N0M0	29–46	20–58
3	T1-T2N1M0 T3N0M0	11–19	18–24
4	T1-4N0-1M1 T3N1M0 T4N0-1M0	39–49	<5

Adenoma and other benign lesions

Adrenal adenoma

Adrenal adenomas are the most common adrenal lesion occurring in up to 7% of patients over 70 years [30]. Most lesions are detected incidentally and the overwhelming majority is biochemically inactive (>90%) [1, 30]. Contrast-enhanced CT scan is the gold standard in the diagnosis of adrenal adenomas. These lesions are homogeneous, smooth-bordered lesions which demonstrate hypoattenuation on unenhanced images due to high levels of intracellular lipid. Additionally, adenomas exhibit rapid washout on contrast-enhanced images [31]. The vast majority of these lesions are <4cm in size. Treatment is adrenalectomy for metabolically active lesions and lesions >4–6 cm due to the increased risk of malignancy. Lesions not meeting these criteria may be managed conservatively [1].

Other benign lesions

Other benign lesions include **oncocytoma and myelolipoma.** Myelolipomas are benign lesions diagnosed via the detection of macroscopic fat on cross-sectional imaging. These lesions are managed conservatively. Oncocytomas are indistinguishable from other adrenal lesions and are typically excised when larger than 4–6 cm. Some of these lesions can exhibit malignant potential [1].

Adrenal metastases

The adrenal is a common site of metastases. Primary tumors which frequently metastasize to the adrenals include melanoma, lung cancer, and renal cell carcinoma. In fact, in patients with a known primary tumor, up to 50% of incidentally detected adrenal lesions will represent a metastatic deposit

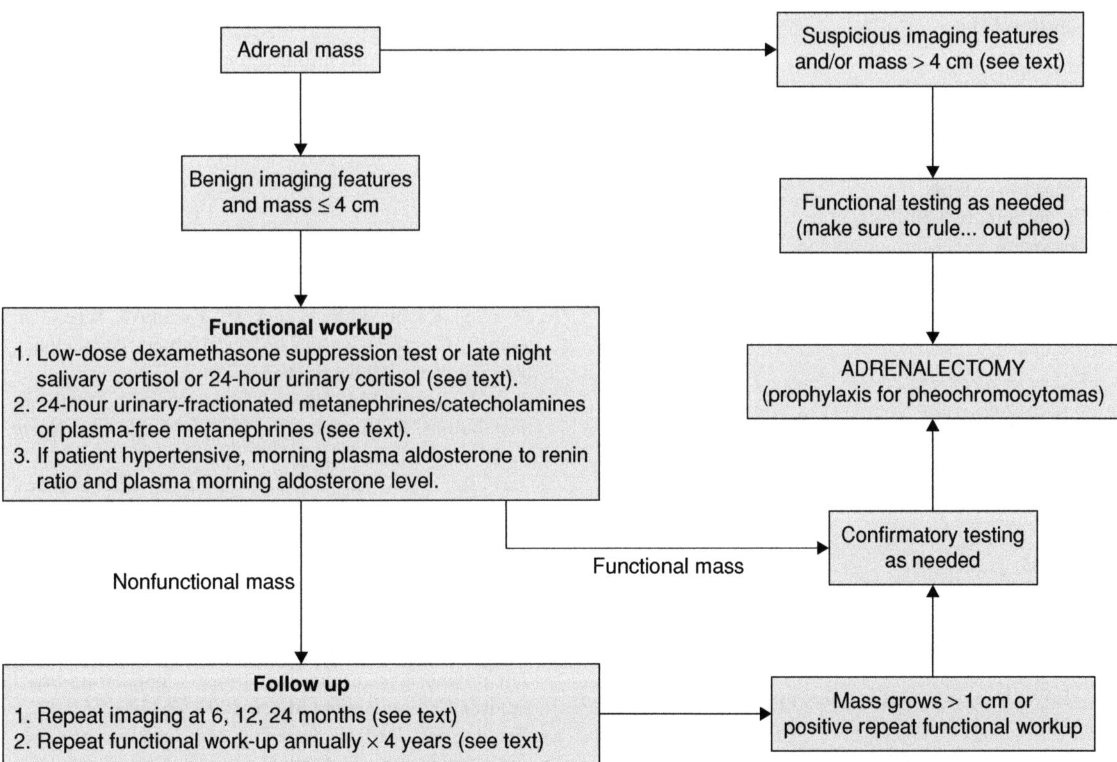

Figure 26.1 Algorithm for the work-up of incidentally detected adrenal lesions [1].

[32, 33]. Therefore, when evaluating an adrenal lesion, it is imperative to inquire about a patient's history of previous malignancies. Radiographically, these lesions appear similar to ACC as irregular, heterogeneous lesions. When metastatic disease is suspected, needle biopsy should be considered. Treatment depends on the primary tumor and ranges from systemic chemotherapy, surgical excision, or palliative care.

Summary: the incidentaloma

A common dilemma faced by urologists is the work-up of the incidentaloma, defined as an adrenal lesion >1 cm detected incidentally on radiographic studies. These lesions require complete radiographic and functional assessment as detailed in Table 26.5. Typically, functional lesions and lesions >4 cm should undergo surgical excision. Those managed conservatively should be followed with serial imaging to assess for interval growth. Tumor growth >1 cm in 6–12 months has been suggested as a relative indication for surgical intervention [1].

WHAT TO AVOID

- Do not operate on an adrenal lesion without a full biochemical work-up.
- Do not initiate β-blockade prior to α-blockade in patients with a pheochromocytoma.
- Do not wait for diagnostic testing when a patient has suspected acute adrenal insufficiency. These patients should be emergently treated with steroids.

KEY WEB LINK

http://www.nejm.org/doi/full/10.1056/NEJMcp065470

Multiple choice questions

1 What is the diagnostic test of choice for Cushing's syndrome?
  a Low-dose dexamethasone suppression test
  b High-dose dexamethasone suppression test
  c CT scan of abdomen/pelvis
  d Late-night salivary cortisol

2 The initial treatment of acute adrenal insufficiency includes:
  a Aggressive hydration
  b Dexamethasone 4 mg IV
  c Cortisol stimulation test
  d All of the above
  e a and b only

3 All of the following are forms of hereditary pheochromocytoma except:
  a Von Hippel–Lindau syndrome
  b Tuberous sclerosis
  c Neurofibromatosis I
  d MEN 2A

4 What medication has proven beneficial in the adjuvant setting after adrenalectomy for adrenal cortical carcinoma?
  a Mitotane
  b Ketoconazole
  c Aminoglutethimide
  d Steroids

5 What CT scan feature is most consistent with an adrenal adenoma?
  a Size >6 cm
  b Heterogeneous enhancement
  c Rapid wash-out of contrast on delayed images
  d Macroscopic fat

References

1 Kutikov A, Crispen PL, Uzzo RG. Pathophysiology, evaluation, and medical management of adrenal disorders. In: Wein AJ, Kavoussi LR, Novick AC, Partin AW, Peters CA, editors. *Campbell-Walsh Urology*. 10th ed. Philadelphia, PA: Saunders; 2011. pp. 1685–1736.
2 Arlt W, Stewart PM. Adrenal corticosteroid biosynthesis, metabolism, and action. *Endocrinol Metab Clin North Am* 2005;34:293–313, viii
3 Jacobson L. Hypothalamic-pituitary-adrenocortical axis regulation. *Endocrinol Metab Clin North Am* 2005;34:271–292, vii
4 Robertson D. The adrenal medulla and adrenomedullary hormones. In: Scott WH, editor. *Surgery of the Adrenal Glands*. Philadelphia, PA: JB Lippincott; 1990. pp. 55–68
5 Lindholm J, Juul S, Jorgensen JO, et al. Incidence and late prognosis of cushing's syndrome: a population-based study. *J Clin Endocrinol Metab* 2001;86:117–123
6 Findling JW, Raff H. Screening and diagnosis of Cushing's syndrome. *Endocrinol Metab Clin North Am* 2005;34:385–402, ix–x

7 Newell-Price J, Bertagna X, Grossman AB, Nieman LK. Cushing's syndrome. *Lancet* 2006;367:1605–1617
8 Pivonello R, De Martino MC, De Leo M, Lombardi G, Colao A. Cushing's syndrome. *Endocrinol Metab Clin North Am* 2008;37:135–149, ix
9 Conn JW. Presidential address. I. Painting background. II. Primary aldosteronism, a new clinical syndrome. *J Lab Clin Med* 1955;45:3–17
10 Mulatero P, Stowasser M, Loh KC, et al. Increased diagnosis of primary aldosteronism, including surgically correctable forms, in centers from five continents. *J Clin Endocrinol Metab* 2004;89:1045–1050
11 Rossi GP, Bernini G, Caliumi C, et al. A prospective study of the prevalence of primary aldosteronism in 1,125 hypertensive patients. *J Am Coll Cardiol* 2006;48: 2293–2300
12 Young WF. Primary aldosteronism: renaissance of a syndrome. *Clin Endocrinol (Oxf)* 2007;66:607–618
13 Sawka AM, Young WF, Thompson GB, et al. Primary aldosteronism: factors associated with normalization of blood pressure after surgery. *Ann Intern Med* 2001;135:258–261
14 Meyer A, Brabant G, Behrend M. Long-term follow-up after adrenalectomy for primary aldosteronism. *World J Surg* 2005;29:155–159
15 Schirpenbach C, Reincke M. Primary aldosteronism: current knowledge and controversies in Conn's syndrome. *Nat Clin Pract Endocrinol Metab* 2007;3:220–227
16 Ilias I, Pacak K. Current approaches and recommended algorithm for the diagnostic localization of pheochromocytoma. *J Clin Endocrinol Metab* 2004;89:479–491
17 Bravo EL, Tagle R. Pheochromocytoma: state-of-the-art and future prospects. *Endocr Rev* 2003;24:539–553
18 Benn DE, Robinson BG. Genetic basis of phaeochromocytoma and paraganglioma. *Best Pract Res Clin Endocrinol Metab* 2006;20:435–450
19 Lenders JW, Eisenhofer G, Mannelli M, Pacak K. Phaeochromocytoma. *Lancet* 2005;366:665–675
20 Lenders JW, Pacak K, Walther MM, et al. Biochemical diagnosis of pheochromocytoma: which test is best? *JAMA* 2002;287:1427–1434
21 Motta-Ramirez GA, Remer EM, Herts BR, Gill IS, Hamrahian AH. Comparison of CT findings in symptomatic and incidentally discovered pheochromocytomas. *AJR Am J Roentgenol* 2005;185:684–688
22 Namimoto T, Yamashita Y, Mitsuzaki K, et al. Adrenal masses: quantification of fat content with double-echo chemical shift in-phase and opposed-phase FLASH MR images for differentiation of adrenal adenomas. *Radiology* 2001;218:642–646
23 Amar L, Servais A, Gimenez-Roqueplo AP, Zinzindohoue F, Chatellier G, Plouin PF. Year of diagnosis, features at presentation, and risk of recurrence in patients with pheochromocytoma or secreting paraganglioma. *J Clin Endocrinol Metab* 2005;90:2110–2116
24 Asari R, Scheuba C, Kaczirek K, Niederle B. Estimated risk of pheochromocytoma recurrence after adrenal-sparing surgery in patients with multiple endocrine neoplasia type 2A. *Arch Surg* 2006;141:1199–1205; discussion 205
25 Roman S. Adrenocortical carcinoma. *Curr Opin Oncol* 2006;18:36–42
26 Ng L, Libertino JM. Adrenocortical carcinoma: diagnosis, evaluation and treatment. *J Urol* 2003;169:5–11
27 Fassnacht M, Allolio B. Clinical management of adrenocortical carcinoma. *Best Pract Res Clin Endocrinol Metab* 2009;23:273–289
28 Szolar DH, Korobkin M, Reittner P, et al. Adrenocortical carcinomas and adrenal pheochromocytomas: mass and enhancement loss evaluation at delayed contrast-enhanced CT. *Radiology* 2005;234:479–485
29 Ilias I, Sahdev A, Reznek RH, Grossman AB, Pacak K. The optimal imaging of adrenal tumours: a comparison of different methods. *Endocr Relat Cancer* 2007;14: 587–599
30 Young WF, Jr. Management approaches to adrenal incidentalomas. A view from Rochester, Minnesota. *Endocrinol Metab Clin North Am* 2000;29:159–185, x
31 Grumbach MM, Biller BM, Braunstein GD, et al. Management of the clinically inapparent adrenal mass ("incidentaloma"). *Ann Intern Med* 2003;138:424–429
32 Lenert JT, Barnett CC, Jr., Kudelka AP, et al. Evaluation and surgical resection of adrenal masses in patients with a history of extra-adrenal malignancy. *Surgery* 2001;130:1060–1067
33 Frilling A, Tecklenborg K, Weber F, et al. Importance of adrenal incidentaloma in patients with a history of malignancy. *Surgery* 2004;136:1289–1296
34 Assie G, Bahurel H, Coste J, et al. Corticotroph tumor progression after adrenalectomy in Cushing's disease: A reappraisal of Nelson's syndrome. *J Clin Endocrinol Metab* 2007;92:172–179

Answers to multiple choice questions

1 d
2 e
3 b
4 a
5 c

27 Testicular tumors

Varun Sharma[1] *and Markus Margreiter*[2]

[1]Department of Urology, IKDRC-ITS, Civil Hospital Campus, Ahmedabad, Gujarat, India
[2]Department of Urology, Medical University Vienna, Vienna General Hospital, Vienna, Austria

KEY POINTS

- Most common cancer in men—15–35 years old.
- Majority arises from the germ cells—seminoma or NSGCT.
- Undescended testicle, personal or family (first-degree relatives) history of testicular cancer, Klinefelter syndrome, and infertility are risk factors.
- Most common presentation is a painless lump or swelling in either testicle.
- Initial investigations—US, tumor markers, inguinal exploration, CXR, CT.
- Prognostic factors—stage, type, tumor markers, size and number of retroperitoneal lymph nodes.
- Treatment is based on prognostic factors above, and includes surveillance, RT, RPLND, and chemotherapy.
- Treatment for testicular cancer can cause infertility. Sperm banking should be discussed.

CASE STUDY 1

A 27-year-old man presents with a feeling of heaviness in his left testis for the past 6 months. Physical examination reveals enlargement of the left testis, while the right testis appears normal. There is a palpable left inguinal lymph node. An ultrasound reveals a 4 cm solid mass within the left testis. Laboratory tests revealed a serum β-hCG of 5 IU/L and α-fetoprotein of 2 ng/mL. The left testis is removed with an inguinal incision and with gross examination on sectioning reveals a firm, lobulated light tan mass without hemorrhage or necrosis. He receives radiation therapy.

The most common pure form of testicular cancer is seminoma, which is radiosensitive. The tumor markers are not markedly elevated. This form of testicular carcinoma has the best prognosis overall, when not mixed with other elements

CASE STUDY 2

A 35-year-old man goes to his physician for a routine examination. On physical examination there is a left inguinal mass. The right testis is palpated in the scrotum and is of normal size, but a left testis cannot be palpated in the scrotum. An ultrasound scan shows that there is an inguinal mass.

An undescended testis that is not treated in early childhood no longer functions and presents a risk for subsequent development of seminoma.

Handbook of Urology, First edition. J. Kellogg Parsons, John B. Eifler and Misop Han.
Published 2014 by John Wiley & Sons, Ltd.

Epidemiology

Testicular cancer accounts for 1–2% of all solid tumors in men with an incidence of 3–10/100,000 men per year [1]. Worldwide, the incidence has doubled in the last 40 years, with Scandinavian countries having the highest incidence [2]. In the United States, rates are fivefold greater among whites than blacks [3]. Bilateral tumors occur in 2–5%, synchronous (1–2%) or metachronous [4]. Right-sided tumors are more common. Testicular cancer is associated with cryptorchidism, which can be found in 7–10% of cases. Orchidopexy prior to puberty decreases relative risk from 4–5 to 2–3 [5]. Personal or family (among first-degree relatives) history of testicular tumors, Klinefelter syndrome, ITGCN (risk of GCT 50% and 70% at 5 and 7 years, respectively), infertility, testicular trauma, testicular microlithiasis, exogenous estrogens, and mumps orchitis are risk factors [6].

Biology and pathological classification

Testicular tumors are divided according to the tissue of origin:

- **Germ cell tumors** (Table 27.1)
- **Sex cord/gonadal stromal tumors**
- **Miscellaneous nonspecific stromal tumors**

Table 27.1 Key features of germ cell tumors

1 **Seminoma**	
a Classic	• Most common testicular cancer (60% of all testicular tumors) • Peak incidence: 35–39 years • Arise from ITGCN—considered as a common precursor for NSGCT subtypes (5)
b Spermatocytic seminoma	• <1% of GCTs • Benign • Does not arise from ITGCN and/or as part of mixed GCTs • No association with cryptorchidism • Does not express PLAP or i(12p) • Almost always cured with orchiectomy
2 **NSGCT**	
a Embryonal cell (EC) carcinoma	• Aggressive • High rates of metastasis • Most undifferentiated type • Can differentiate into other NSGCT • Presence and proportion of EC—independent risk factor for occult metastasis and relapse
b Yolk-sac tumor	• Pure form (endodermal sinus tumors) rare in adults • Most common testicular tumor in children and infants • Schiller–Duval body seen • Produce AFP (no hCG)
c Choriocarcinoma	• Composed of syncytiotrophoblasts (produce hCG) and cytotrophoblasts • Aggressive/hematogenous spread • Disseminated disease at presentation with elevated serum hCG levels • Prone to hemorrhage
d Teratoma	• Well (mature teratoma) to incompletely differentiated (immature teratoma) elements of at least two of the three germ cell layers • Normal tumor markers • Pure teratoma rare in adults but common in children • Resistant to chemotherapy
e Tumors with more than one histological type	

Relative risk of germ cell cancer for the sons of affected fathers is 4, and for brothers 8–10 [7]. Isochromosome 12p (i(12p)) is present in 70% of GCT and 66% have p53 abnormalities.

ITGCN consists of undifferentiated germ cells. It is a precursor lesion for GCT (except spermatocytic seminoma) and has 50% risk of developing an invasive GCT within 5 years [8]. Treatment options are radical orchiectomy and low-dose (20 Gy) radiation therapy.

Testicular tumors metastasize mostly to retroperitoneal lymph nodes (RPLN), lungs, mediastinum, and abdominal viscera. The landing zones (initial metastasis) differ between right and left. For the right, it is the interaortocaval, precaval, and preaortic nodes; for the left, they are the para-aortic, preaortic, and interaortocaval nodes. Tumor cells disseminate from the right to the left side. This serves as the basis of the templates for retroperitoneal lymph node dissection (RPLND).

Due to the impact of therapy for testicular cancer on fertility, men planning future paternity should undergo sperm cryopreservation before treatment is initiated.

Diagnosis and staging

The most common presentation is a palpable testicular mass (50–60%). Pain is the first symptom in about 20% of patients (10% present as epididymo-orchitis). Other presentations are dull ache at the affected testicle (30–40%), acute testicular pain (10–20%), symptoms of metastases: neck mass, cough, abdominal pain, diarrhea, back pain (10%), or gynecomastia (5%) [9].

Initial evaluation consists of scrotal ultrasound with a sensitivity around 100% (mandatory in initial workup) [10]. **Serum tumor makers** play an important role in diagnosis and follow-up as 70% of all patients with testicular cancer and 90% of all patients with nonseminoma have at least one of these markers elevated [11]. Post-orchiectomy, the levels normalize commensurate with serum half-life ($t_{1/2}$). If consistently elevated, metastatic or residual disease has to be suspected [12]. **Human chorionic gonadotropin (β-hCG)** is produced by syncytiotrophoblast cells with a half-life of 24–36 hours. It is elevated in 40–60% of patients with NSGCT and up to 30% seminomas. **α-fetoprotein (AFP)** is produced by yolk sac cells and is raised in 50–70% NSGCT [13]. Its half-life is 5–7 days. It is never produced by pure seminoma or choriocarcinoma and can be elevated in children <1 year of age. **Lactate dehydrogenase (LDH)** is a nonspecific marker with levels proportional to tumor volume. It is elevated in up to 60% of patients with advanced testicular cancer. **Placental alkaline phosphatase (PLAP)** correlates with tumor burden and is elevated in pure seminoma [14].

Inguinal exploration and radical orchiectomy is the initial step in the management of testicular tumors [15]. Transscrotal orchiectomy or biopsy is contraindicated because it leaves the inguinal spermatic cord intact and alters the lymphatic drainage of the testis, increasing the risk of local recurrence and pelvic or inguinal lymph node metastasis. Radical orchiectomy must be performed for local tumor control, histological confirmation of the diagnosis, and determination of the local extension for staging purposes. The basic principle is high ligation of the spermatic cord at the level of the internal ring as the first step. Biopsy of the contralateral testis should be considered if intratesticular abnormalities are seen on ultrasound, in the presence of an undescended testis, or in patients with marked testicular atrophy [16]. For solitary testicle or bilateral tumors, partial orchiectomy can be performed if tumor volume is <30% of the testis. Close follow-up is mandatory [17]. In patients with rapidly increasing β-hCG and symptoms of disseminated disease with a testicular mass, chemotherapy can be initiated immediately without waiting for a biopsy diagnosis. For clinical staging, mandatory workup includes abdominopelvic computed tomography (CT), liver function tests, and chest radiographs as initial staging studies (chest CT if elevated post-orchiectomy serum tumor markers, metastatic disease by physical examination or abdominopelvic CT, abnormal chest X-ray, lymphovascular invasion) [18].

Staging: TNM staging system (Table 27.2) and **Stage grouping for testicular tumors** [19] (Table 27.3)

For metastatic germ cell cancer the International Germ Cell Consensus Classification (IGCCCG) has been proposed as a prognostic-based staging system [20].

Table 27.2 TNM staging system

pT Primary tumor

pTX Primary tumor cannot be assessed

pT0 No evidence of primary tumor (e.g., histological scar in testis)

pTis Intratubular germ cell neoplasia (testicular intraepithelial neoplasia)

pT1 Tumor limited to testis and epididymis without vascular/lymphatic invasion: tumor may invade tunica albuginea but not tunica vaginalis

pT2 Tumor limited to testis and epididymis with vascular/lymphatic invasion, or tumor extending through tunica albuginea with involvement of tunica vaginalis

pT3 Tumor invades spermatic cord with or without vascular/lymphatic invasion

pT4 Tumor invades scrotum with or without vascular/lymphatic invasion

N Regional lymph nodes clinical

NX Regional lymph nodes cannot be assessed

N0 No regional lymph node metastasis

N1 Metastasis with a lymph node mass 2 cm or less in greatest dimension or multiple lymph nodes, none >2 cm in greatest dimension

N2 Metastasis with a lymph node mass >2 cm but not more than 5 cm in greatest dimension, or multiple lymph nodes, any one mass >2 cm but not >5 cm in greatest dimension

N3 Metastasis with a lymph node mass >5 cm in greatest dimension

N Pathological

pNX Regional lymph nodes cannot be assessed

pN0 No regional lymph node metastasis

pN1 Metastasis with a lymph node mass 2 cm or less in greatest dimension and five or fewer positive nodes, none >2 cm in greatest dimension

pN2 Metastasis with a lymph node mass >2 cm but not >5 cm in greatest dimension; or more than five nodes positive, none >5 cm; or evidence or extranodal extension of tumor

pN3 Metastasis with a lymph node mass >5 cm in greatest dimension

M Distant metastasis

MX Distant metastasis cannot be assessed

M0 No distant metastasis

M1 Distant metastasis

M1a Nonregional lymph node(s) or lung

M1b Other sites

S Serum tumor markers

Sx Serum marker studies not available or not performed

S0 Serum marker study levels within normal limits

LDH (U/l) hCG (mIU/mL) AFP (ng/mL)

S1 <1.5 × N <5000 <1000

S2 1.5–10 × N 5000–50,000 1000–10,000

S3 >10 × N >50,000 >10,000

N indicates upper limit of normal for LDH assay.

Table 27.3 Stage grouping for testicular tumors

Stage	Description
Stage I	Confined to the testicle, spermatic cord, or scrotum, with or without vascular invasion.
Stage IIA	Lymph node mass ≤2 cm, or multiple lymph node masses all ≤2 cm.
Stage IIB	Lymph node mass >2 cm and ≤5 cm, or multiple lymph node masses with any one mass >2 cm and ≤5 cm.
Stage IIC	Lymph node mass >5 cm.
Stage III	Nonregional nodal, pulmonary, or visceral metastases.

Treatment and prognosis of germ cell testicular tumors

Radical orchiectomy is the initial diagnostic and therapeutic step. Treatment after orchiectomy depends upon: (1) tumor stage and (2) histology.

Treatment for seminoma

Clinical stage (CS) I: Disease-specific survival for stage I disease is 99% irrespective of the management strategy [21]. Options are primary radiotherapy (RT), surveillance, or single-agent chemotherapy.

Primary radiotherapy (25–35 Gy in 15–20 daily fractions) to retroperitoneum ± ipsilateral pelvis (dog-leg configuration) with in-field recurrence <1%. There is no need for surveillance abdominopelvic CT but it has a risk for secondary malignancy.

Surveillance has the risk of limited utility of serum tumor markers to detect relapse. There is a need for long-term surveillance CT. Tumor >4 cm, invasion of the rete testis, and proliferation rate >70% are significant predictors of relapse. Long-term follow-up is mandatory (higher incidence of relapse after 5 years compared with NSGCT).

Primary chemotherapy with single agent (1–2 cycles of carboplatin) has a response rate of approximately 90%.

Surveillance is the preferred approach (low overall risk of relapse, no validated markers, and late toxicity with radiotherapy and carboplatin). In noncompliant patients or those unwilling to accept surveillance, RT is recommended (long-term efficacy and simplified follow-up).

Strict follow-up is needed (risk of recurrence is highest in the first 2 years) [22].

CS IIa/IIb: Treatment options include RT to para-aortic and ipsilateral iliac lymph nodes (30–36 Gy). Advantages are that routine surveillance CT is not necessary. Relapse rates are moderate (5–6% for stage IIA) and overall survival is almost 100% [23]. Induction chemotherapy (BEP×3 or EP×4) is given if bulky RPLN (>3 cm) and/or multiple retroperitoneal masses are present [24] (BEP = Bleomycin/etoposide/cisplatin; EP = Etoposide/cisplatin).

CS IIc/III: Treatment options include induction chemotherapy with low-risk patients receiving BEP×3 or EP×4 and intermediate-risk patients receiving BEP×4.

Residual masses after chemotherapy are seen in 58–80%. Spontaneous resolution occurs in 50–60% (at 13–18 months). If resected, histology is necrosis (90%) or viable malignancy (10%). Surgery is difficult due to the desmoplastic reaction after chemotherapy. FDG-PET scan has a high positive and negative predictive value for active disease in residual masses after chemotherapy, and should be done at 6 weeks after completion of chemotherapy to decrease false-positive results [25]. While residual masses <3 cm, normal markers and PET-negative masses >3 cm qualify for observation, residual mass >3 cm and PET-positive masses should undergo surgical resection [26]. If tumor markers are elevated, the patient should be treated as harboring NSGCT.

Patients who have a relapsing seminoma need further treatment. Chemo-naïve relapses need first-line chemotherapy. While patients having early relapse (within 2 years) after chemotherapy are given second-line chemotherapy, late relapse (after 2 years) are treated with cisplatin-based chemotherapy.

Treatment for NSGCT

Treatment after orchiectomy includes surveillance, RPLND, or chemotherapy depending upon the clinical stage

CS I: The cure rate of surveillance, RPLND, or chemotherapy exceeds 95%. Predominant risk factors for occult metastasis in this group of patients are lymphovascular invasion and predominant embryonal carcinoma component [27].

Advantage of surveillance is that orchiectomy alone cures 70–80% patients and relapsing patients can be salvaged thus avoiding the morbidity of RPLND or chemotherapy. Disadvantages are high risk of relapse, long-term (>5 yrs) surveillance, secondary malignant neoplasms due to intensive surveillance CT, and intensive therapy to treat relapse. If relapse occurs and it is >3 cm RP mass with raised markers and distant metastasis, chemotherapy should be given. If it is <3 cm with normal markers and no distant metastasis, RPLND is the treatment of choice.

Proponents of RPLND say that the retroperitoneum is the most common site of occult metastasis with 15–25% incidence of retroperitoneal teratoma (resistant to chemotherapy). There is a low risk of abdominopelvic recurrence following RPLND. As a monotherapy, it has lower long- and short-term morbidity with high salvage rates by chemotherapy in patients having relapse. If lymph nodes are positive, two cycles of BEP should be given.

Chemotherapy (BEP×2) offers the greatest chance of being relapse free with any single modality and can be delivered at community-based hospital. It does not treat teratoma and requires long-term surveillance with CT. Toxicity of these agents needs special care. It can be concluded that in patients with low-risk disease, surveillance should be offered and in high-risk disease, surveillance, RPLND, or primary chemotherapy are options and treatment should be individualized.

CS IS: These patients have elevated post-orchiectomy serum tumor markers without clinical or radiographic evidence of metastatic disease and are treated with induction chemotherapy (BEP×3/EP×4) [28].

CS IIa/IIb: Treatment options for these patients are RPLND and chemotherapy [29]. With RPLND, chemotherapy is avoided in patients with negative lymph nodes. Around 30% of these patients have retroperitoneal teratoma, which are resistant to chemotherapy and RPLND provides them a cure. Long-term cancer-specific survival is 98–100% with RPLND ± adjuvant chemotherapy. Additional chemotherapy is required in >50% patients and 13–15% have persistence of disease and need full induction chemotherapy. If lymph nodes are positive on resection, two cycles of BEP should be given.

With chemotherapy (BEP×3/EP×4), 60–78% have a complete response and it is easily available. But it has its own toxicity. These patients if relapse, have chemorefractory GCT.

For patients at risk for retroperitoneal teratoma and low risk for systemic disease (normal serum tumor markers, lymphadenopathy <3 cm), RPLND is a better option. In patients with elevated AFP or hCG or bulky lymph nodes (>3 cm), chemotherapy (BEP×3/EP×4) should be given [30].

CS IIc/III: These patients need induction chemotherapy according to the risk (good risk—BEP×3/EP×4; intermediate and poor risk—BEP×4).

Post-chemotherapy residual masses have necrosis, teratoma, and viable malignancy (± teratoma) in 40%, 45%, and 15% of cases, respectively. FDG-PET has no role in NSGCT post-chemotherapy residual masses. Residual mass >1 cm need surgical resection [31]. If residual masses are present at multiple sites, they need to be resected after RPLND. If viable malignancy is revealed on histopathology, chemotherapy with 2 cycles of EP or TIP or VIP/VeIP is given (TIP—paclitaxel/ifosfamide/cisplatin, VeIP—vinblastine/ifosfamide/cisplatin, VIP—etoposide/ifosfamide/cisplatin).

Relapsing NSGCT: If chemotherapy naïve, treatment is induction chemotherapy (BEP×3/EP×4). If it is an early (within 2 years) post-chemotherapy relapse, second-line chemotherapy (TIP4, VIP4, VeIP4) or high-dose chemotherapy is given and if it is a late relapse (after 2 years) salvage surgical resection is needed.

RPLND is the standard approach to the surgical management of NSGCT in both the primary and the post-chemotherapy setting. A template dissection or a nerve-sparing approach to minimize the risk of ejaculatory disorders should be performed. The "split and roll" technique minimizes the risk of an in-field recurrence. A full bilateral template RPLND should be performed in all patients undergoing RPLND in the post-chemotherapy setting. Nerve dissection techniques spare the paravertebral sympathetic chains, post-ganglionic efferent sympathetic nerves, and hypogastric plexus, thereby preserving ejaculatory function in >95% of cases [32].

Non-germ-cell testicular tumors

A **Sex cord/gonadal stromal tumors:** ***Leydig cell tumors*** are most common and present as painless testicular mass with precocious puberty in prepubertal boys (increased testosterone). Almost 90% are benign and cured with radical orchiectomy alone [13]. However, 10% are malignant, metastasize to the retroperitoneum, and need further RPLND. ***Sertoli cell tumors*** account for 1% of all testicular tumors [33]. These tumors are malignant and metastasize (usually in the retroperitoneal nodes thus needing RPLND) in 10%. ***Granulosa cell tumors*** are extremely rare, biologically similar to those in ovaries. They are predominantly benign and only rarely malignant.

B ***Gonadoblastoma*** constitute 0.5% of all testicular tumors. Usually seen in patients with gonadal dysgenesis [13]. Phenotypic females with primary amenorrhea comprise 80% patients. It is mostly benign and treated with orchiectomy alone. Nearly half of these tumors are bilateral. Hence, removal of the contralateral gonad is recommended. Around 50% develop invasive GCT (usually seminoma).

C ***Carcinoid of the testis*** is very rare, identical to gastrointestinal carcinoid. They usually present as a painless testicular mass without the typical carcinoid prodrome. Radical orchiectomy alone is usually curative. Metastasis is seen in 10% [34].

D ***Epidermoid cyst*** occur in the second decade and are uniformly benign [13]. Ultrasonography shows a well-circumscribed lesion with a hyperechoic central core. Surgical resection alone is curative.

E ***Adenocarcinoma of the rete testis*** is rare and highly malignant with 54% of patients having metastases at the time of diagnosis, and cancer-specific survival at 1 year <50%. Radical orchiectomy is indicated. The efficacy of adjuvant therapy (chemotherapy or radiation) is unproven [35].

F ***Testicular lymphoma*** present as a painless, diffuse testicular enlargement with constitutional symptoms seen in 25% of patients. Non-Hodgkin lymphoma is the most frequent testicular tumor in men >50 years old [13]. Initial treatment is with radical orchiectomy to obtain a tissue diagnosis. Subsequent treatment is with combination chemotherapy ± radiation [36].

G ***Metastasis*** in the testis are rare, primarily from prostate, lung, gastrointestinal tract, melanoma, and kidney [13].

Extratesticular tumors

They are tumors originating from the epididymis, spermatic cord, or testicular tunicae and usually present as a painless scrotal mass. ***Adenomatoid tumor*** is the most common type of paratesticular tumor with peak incidence in the fourth decade of life [37]. They are usually benign and surgical excision is curative [37]. ***Rhabdomyosarcoma*** are primarily seen in children and adolescents (80% occurring in patients <21 years old) [37]. Initial treatment is radical orchiectomy, followed by systemic chemotherapy. Overall 5-year disease-specific survival is 58–80% [37]. ***Mesothelioma*** present as a painless, firm scrotal mass with a hydrocele with peak incidence at 55–75 years. It is associated with asbestos exposure. Treatment is radical orchiectomy. These are aggressive with nearly 50% of patients developing metastatic disease or local recurrence. Disease-specific survival is 60% [37]. ***Cystadenoma*** originates from the epididymis and are usually benign. They are strongly **associated with von Hippel–Lindau disease** [37]. Surgical excision is curative.

WHAT TO AVOID (COMMON ERRORS IN DIAGNOSIS AND TREATMENT)

- Delay in diagnosis due to hesitation of the patient to tell about an abnormality in testis.
- Strict follow-up as per guidelines in patients opting for surveillance.
- Treatment-related secondary infertility.

KEY WEB LINKS

http://www.nccn.org/
http://www.campbellsurology.com/
http://urology.jhu.edu/

Multiple choice questions

1 Which of the following statements is true regarding testicular tumors?
  a Are embryonal cell carcinomas in 95% of cases.
  b Bilateral in 2% cases.
  c Teratomas are more common than seminomas.
  d Usually present after 50 years of age.

2 All of the following are true about GCTs of testis except:
  a GCTs are divided into seminomatous and nonseminomatous subtypes.
  b Nonseminomatous subtypes are most common in the third decade of life.
  c Seminomatous subtypes are most common in the fourth decade of life.
  d Seminomas represent about 20% of all GCTs.

3 All of the following are true about seminomatous type of GCTs except:
  a They are more common in the fourth decade.
  b Constitute about 50% of all GCTs and 70% of patients present with stage I disease.
  c Seminomas have an indolent course.
  d Chemotherapy is the treatment of choice in patients with stage I disease and stage II disease where the nodes are <5 cm in maximum diameter.

4 What is the major long-term effect of standard (modified bilateral) RPLND operation?
  a Retrograde ejaculation and infertility
  b Urinary incontinence
  c Fecal incontinence
  d Lymphedema of leg

References

1 Siegel R, Naishadham D, Jemal A. Cancer statistics, 2012. *CA Cancer J Clin* 2012; 62(1):10–29.

2 Carlsen E, Giwercman A, Keiding N, Skakkebaek NE. Evidence for decreasing quality of semen during past 50 years. *BMJ* 1992;305(6854):609–613.

3 McGlynn KA, Devesa SS, Sigurdson AJ, Brown LM, Tsao L, Tarone RE. Trends in the incidence of testicular germ cell tumors in the United States. *Cancer* 2003;97(1): 63–70.

4 Dieckmann KP, Broeckmann W, Brosig W, Jonas D, Bauer HW. Bilateral testicular germ cell tumors. Report of nine cases and review of the literature. *Cancer* 1986;57(6):1254.

5 Wood HM, Elder JS. Cryptorchidism and testicular cancer: separating fact from fiction. *J Urol* 2009;181(2):452–461.

6 Oliver RTD. Epidemiology of testis cancer: A clinical perspective. In: Vogelzang NJ, Scardino PT, Shipley WU, Coffey DS, editors. *Genitourinary Oncology*. Philadelphia, PA: Lippincott Williams and Wilkins; 2000. pp. 880–890.

7 Forman D, Chilvers C, Oliver R, Pike M. The aetiology of testicular cancer: Association with congenital abnormalities, age at puberty, infertility and exercise. United Kingdom Testicular Cancer Study Group. *BMJ* 1994;308(6941):1393–1399.

8 von der Maase H, Rorth M, Walbom-Jorgensen S, et al. Carcinoma in situ of contralateral testis in patients with testicular germ cell cancer: Study of 27 cases in 500 patients. *BMJ* 1986;293(6559):1398–1401.

9 Kennedy BJ. Testis cancer: Clinical signs and symptoms. In: Vogelzang NJ, Scardino PT, Shipley WU, Coffey DS, editors. *Genitourinary Oncology*. Philadelphia, PA: Lippincott Williams and Wilkins; 2000. pp. 877–879.

10 Garcia Vega E, Fernandez Rodriguez C, Sanchez Lombrana JL. [Behavioral profile of the patient with Crohn's disease]. *Rev Esp Enferm Dig* 1994;86(5):791–795.

11 Barzell WE, Whitmore WF. Clinical significance of biologic markers: Memorial Hospital experience. *Semin Oncol* 1979;6:48–52.

12 Klein EA. Tumor markers in testis cancer. *Urol Clin North Am* 1993;20(1):67–73.

13 Richie JP, Steele GG. Neoplasms of the testis. In: Walsh PC, Retik AB, Vaughan ED, Wein AJ, editors. *Campbell's Urology*. 8th ed. Philadelphia, PA: Saunders; 2002. pp. 2876–2919.

14 Bower M, Rustin GJS. Serum tumor markers and their role in monitoring germ cell cancers of the testis. In: Vogelzang NJ, Scardino PT, Shipley WU, Coffey DS, editors. *Genitourinary Oncology*. Philadelphia, PA: Lippincott Williams and Wilkins; 2000.

15 Jones RH, Vasey PA. Part I: testicular cancer–management of early disease. *Lancet Oncol* 2003;4(12):730–737.

16 Fossa SD, Chen J, Schonfeld SJ, et al. Risk of contralateral testicular cancer: a population-based study of 29,515 U.S. men. *J Natl Cancer Inst* 2005;97(14):1056–1066.

17 Maneschg C, Rogatsch H, Neururer R, Bartsch G, Hobisch A. Follow-up of organ preserving tumor enucleation in testicular tumors. *J Urol* 2000;163(4 Suppl):144.

18 See WA, Hoxie L. Chest staging in testis cancer patients: imaging modality selection based upon risk assessment as determined by abdominal computerized tomography scan results. *J Urol* 1993;150(3):874–878.

19 Steele GS, Kantoff PW, Richie JP. Staging and imaging of testis cancer. In: Vogelzang NJ, Scardino PT, Shipley WU, Coffey DS, editors. *Genitourinary Oncology*. Philadelphia, PA: Lippincott Williams and Wilkins; 2000. pp. 939–949.

20 International Germ Cell Consensus Classification: A prognostic factor-based staging system for metastatic germ cell cancers. International Germ Cell Cancer Collaborative Group. *J Clin Oncol* 1997;15(2):594–603.

21 Mead GM, Fossa SD, Oliver RT, et al. Randomized trials in 2466 patients with stage I seminoma: patterns of relapse and follow-up. *J Natl Cancer Inst* 2011;103(3):241–249.

22 Martin JM, Panzarella T, Zwahlen DR, Chung P, Warde P. Evidence-based guidelines for following stage 1 seminoma. *Cancer* 2007;109(11):2248–2256.

23 Classen J, Schmidberger H, Meisner C, et al. Radiotherapy for stages IIA/B testicular seminoma: final report of a prospective multicenter clinical trial. *J Clin Oncol* 2003;21(6):1101–1106.

24 Detti B, Livi L, Scoccianti S, et al. Management of Stage II testicular seminoma over a period of 40 years. *Urol Oncol* 2009;27(5):534–538.

25 De Santis M, Pont J. The role of positron emission tomography in germ cell cancer. *World J Urol* 2004;22(1):41–46.

26 Kollmannsberger C, Daneshmand S, So A, et al. Management of disseminated nonseminomatous germ cell tumors with risk-based chemotherapy followed by response-guided postchemotherapy surgery. *J Clin Oncol* 2010;28(4):537–542.

27 Groll RJ, Warde P, Jewett MA. A comprehensive systematic review of testicular germ cell tumor surveillance. *Crit Rev Oncol Hematol* 2007;64(3):182–197.

28 Culine S, Theodore C, Terrier-Lacombe MJ, Droz JP. Primary chemotherapy in patients with nonseminomatous germ cell tumors of the testis and biological disease only after orchiectomy. *J Urol* 1996;155(4):1296–1298.

29 Stephenson AJ, Bosl GJ, Motzer RJ, Bajorin DF, Stasi JP, Sheinfeld J. Nonrandomized comparison of primary chemotherapy and retroperitoneal lymph node dissection for clinical stage IIA and IIB nonseminomatous germ cell testicular cancer. *J Clin Oncol* 2007;25(35):5597–5602.

30 Stephenson AJ, Bosl GJ, Bajorin DF, Stasi J, Motzer RJ, Sheinfeld J. Retroperitoneal lymph node dissection in patients with low stage testicular cancer with embryonal carcinoma predominance and/or lymphovascular invasion. *J Urol* 2005;174(2):557–560; discussion 560.

31 Kuczyk M, Machtens S, Stief C, Jonas U. Management of the post-chemotherapy residual mass in patients with advanced stage non-seminomatous germ cell tumors (NSGCT). *Int J Cancer* 1999;83(6):852–855.

32 Sheinfeld J, Herr HW. Role of surgery in management of germ cell tumor. *Semin Oncol* 1998;25(2):203–209.

33 Mostofi FK, Sesterhenn IA, Davis CJ. Anatomy and pathology of testis cancer. In: Vogelzang NJ, Scardino PT, Shipley WU, Coffey DS, editors. *Genitourinary Oncology*. Philadelphia, PA: Lippincott Williams and Wilkins; 2000.

34 Singer AJ, Anders KH. Primary carcinoid of the testis 25 years after contralateral testicular seminoma. *Urology* 2001;57(3):554–555.

35 Spataro V, Caldiera S, Rusca T, Sessa C, Cavalli F. Adenocarcinoma of the rete testis. *J Urol* 2000;164(4):1307–1308.

36 Colevas AD, Kantoff PW, DeWolf WC, Canellos GP. Malignant lymphoma of the genitourinary tract. In: Vogelzang NJ, Scardino PT, Shipley WU, Coffey DS, editors. *Genitourinary Oncology*. Philadelphia, PA: Lippincott Williams and Wilkins; 2000. pp. 1120–1126.

37 Khoubehi B, Mishra V, Ali M, Motiwala H, Karim O. Adult paratesticular tumours. *BJU Int* 2002;90(7):707–715.

Answers to multiple choice questions

1 b
2 d
3 d
4 a

Section 7 Congenital and acquired disease

28 Obstructing congenital anomalies of the urinary tract

Kristina D. Suson

Pediatric Urology, Children's Hospital of Michigan, Detroit, MI, USA

KEY POINTS

- Obstructing anomalies often present with prenatal hydronephrosis, pain, urinary tract infections (UTIs), nausea/vomiting, hematuria, or nephrolithiasis.
- Lower tract anomalies may present with voiding complaints.
- Ultrasound, voiding cystourethrogram (VCUG), and diuretic renography are commonly employed diagnostic tests.
- Cystoscopy is used to characterize ureteroceles and to diagnose and treat posterior urethral valves (PUVs).
- PUVs require immediate intervention. In the absence of infection or negative impact on renal function, other pathologies may be observed.

CASE STUDY

A 5-year-old boy presents to the emergency room with flank pain and microscopic hematuria after a fall from a chair. CT scan (Figure 28.1) revealed marked right hydronephrosis with parenchymal thinning, consistent with ureteropelvic junction obstruction and adjacent fluid, likely representing a small urine leak. His mother remembered he had prenatal hydronephrosis, but this had resolved on postnatal ultrasound the day of delivery. Recently, he had started experiencing intermittent nausea, vomiting, and flank pain. After admission to the hospital, his posttraumatic pain persisted and a nephrostomy tube was placed. The patient underwent uncomplicated open pyeloplasty 2 weeks after nephrostomy tube placement.

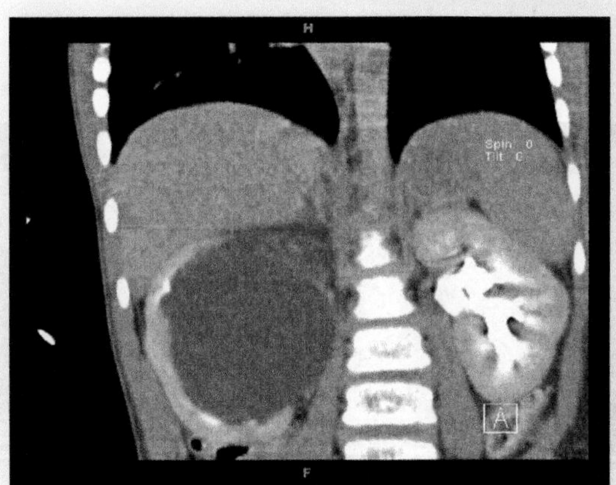

Figure 28.1 Incidentally noted right hydronephrosis on CT scan for abdominal pain and microscopic hematuria following minor trauma.

Handbook of Urology, First edition. J. Kellogg Parsons, John B. Eifler and Misop Han.
Published 2014 by John Wiley & Sons, Ltd.

Ureteropelvic junction obstruction

Epidemiology

Ureteropelvic junction (UPJ) obstruction is the most common cause of prenatal upper tract dilatation. It is more common in boys than girls. It occurs more frequently in the left kidney and may be bilateral in 10–40% of patients [1].

Etiology

UPJ obstruction is caused by intrinsic obstruction or extrinsic compression. With intrinsic obstruction, there is typically no stricture, but rather widely separated muscle fibers that do not contract well enough to enable renal drainage. Valvular mucosal folds, polyps, and fetal convolutions have also been described [1].

Extrinsic compression, more common in older patients, is typically caused by a crossing vessel. Inflammation from the vessel may lead to kinking and stenosis, exacerbating the obstruction [1].

Severe vesicoureteral reflux (VUR) with torturous ureters may lead to secondary obstruction [1].

Presentation

UPJ obstruction may present as prenatal hydronephrosis, abdominal mass, vomiting, pain, urinary tract infection (UTI), or hematuria (Figure 28.2) [1, 2].

Presence of associated anomalies may also warrant UPJ evaluation, including contralateral UPJ obstruction, renal dysplasia, multicystic kidney, renal agenesis, duplicated collecting systems, fused kidneys, ectopic kidneys, VUR, and VATER syndrome [1].

Diagnosis

Ultrasound is used to confirm prenatally diagnosed hydronephrosis and follow patients managed conservatively [3].

Voiding cystourethrogram (VCUG) rules out other causes of hydronephrosis or concomitant anomalies, such as VUR, ureteroceles, or posterior urethral valves (PUVs) [4].

Diuretic renography diagnoses obstruction and evaluates differential renal function. It may be repeated for worsening or unchanged hydronephrosis on interval ultrasounds [3].

The invasive Whitaker test measures the pressure gradient between the renal pelvis and the bladder and may help diagnose obstruction if diuretic renography is inconclusive [4].

In the future, urinary biomarkers may predict obstruction that requires intervention. Transforming growth factor β1, *N*-acetyl-β-D-glucosaminidase, monocyte chemotactic peptide-1, and endothelin-1 are increased, and epidermal growth factor is decreased [5].

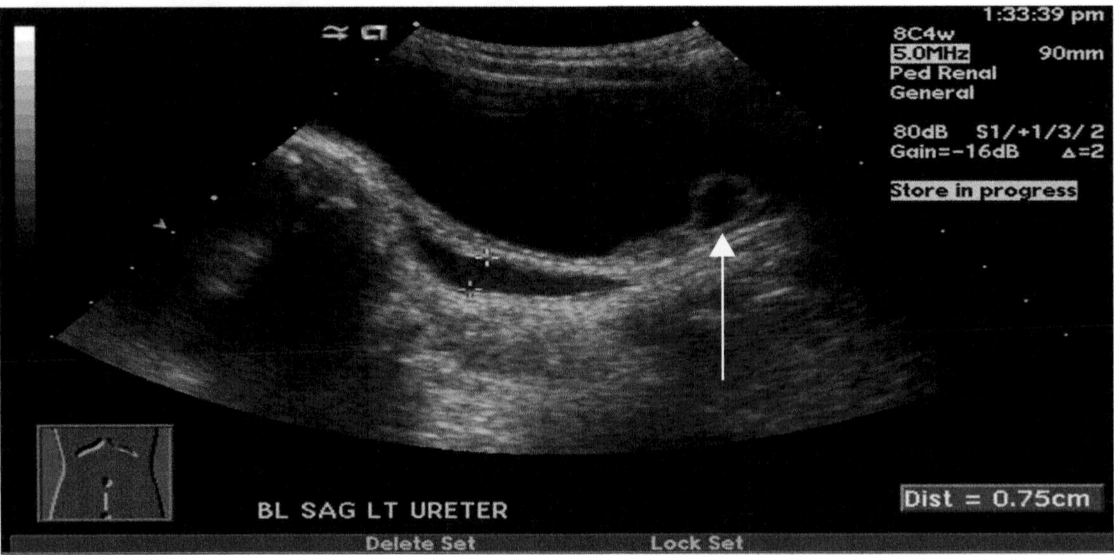

Figure 28.2 Ultrasound of ureterocele.

Prognosis

Hydronephrosis usually stabilizes or spontaneously improves [3, 6], with early intervention required for 15–20% of patients [5]. Patients with severe hydronephrosis (SFU grade 4) [6] or a prenatal renal pelvis diameter >20 mm are more likely to require pyeloplasty [7].

Management

Options include observation, pyeloplasty, ureterocalicostomy, and endopyelotomy.

Conservative management with interval renal ultrasounds and diuretic renography is safe [6], but relies upon standardized grading of hydronephrosis and parental compliance [3].

Early pyeloplasty is recommended for no drainage or reduced differential renal function on diuretic renography [6]. Other indications include reduction in function by greater than 5%, differential function less than 40%, pain, recurrent pyelonephritis, massive hydronephrosis, and poorly compliant family [5].

Dismembered pyeloplasties may be performed via flank, dorsal lumbotomy, or laparoscopic approaches with no difference in outcome [8]. Advocates of the open technique claim shorter operating time [8] and the option of reducing the renal pelvis [1]. The same complication and success rates have been reported in children at all ages treated laparoscopically [9]. The length of stay and narcotic requirements may be decreased in children aged 10 years and older [10]. Shorter length of stay [8, 11] may translate to decreased expense of parental lost wages and hospitalization [11].

Nondismembered pyeloplasty is safe and effective, both via open and laparoscopic approaches [12]. Options include Foley Y-V plasty, intubated ureterotomy, and spiral and vertical flaps [1].

Ureterocalicostomy can be performed via open or robot-assisted laparoscopic approach safely. It may be indicated if there is significant intraparenchymal dilatation with little redundancy in the renal pelvis or after failed pyeloplasty [13].

Endopyelotomy is safe after failed pyeloplasty, but is less effective than reoperative pyeloplasty [14].

Judicious use of internalized or externalized stents or nephrostomy tubes is recommended after UPJ correction [1, 15, 16].

Ureterocele

Terminology

Intravesical ureteroceles are within the bladder with an orifice above the bladder neck. The orifice of an extravesical ureterocele is below the bladder neck. A cecoureterocele has an orifice above the bladder neck, but prolapses out of the bladder [17].

Etiology

Theories of ureterocele development include rostral ureteral budding [18], ureteral maturation defect [18], or failure of Chwalle's membrane to rupture at the ureteral orifice [17]. In duplex systems, they are associated with the upper pole [17].

Presentation

Ureteroceles are detected on prenatal ultrasound. After birth, they may present with infection, incontinence, pain, prolapse [17], or urinary retention [19].

Diagnosis

On physical examination, ureteroceles may be visibly prolapsed. A palpable kidney may also suggest its presence [17].

On ultrasound (Figure 28.2), ureteroceles appear as thin-walled cystic structures within the bladder [17]. The bladder thickness, trabeculations, capacity, and residual help assess bladder function [17]. There may be hydroureteronephrosis, a duplicated collecting system with upper pole dilatation and parenchymal thinning [17]

VCUG delineates anatomy of the ureter and bladder and assesses for concomitant reflux [17].

MRI is useful for cases with subtle findings or distorted anatomy [17].

Diuretic renography assesses function and obstruction [17].

Intravenous pyelogram (IVP) may help delineate anatomy if little upper pole dilatation [17].

At cystoscopy, note the ureterocele position relative to urethra, bladder neck, and other orifices [17].

Management

The goals of therapy are to preserve renal function, prevent and remedy infection, obstruction and reflux, and to preserve continence [17]. Options include observation, endoscopic therapy, heminephrectomy/nephrectomy, ureteroureterostomy, and bladder reconstruction.

Observation is limited to patients without infections, with either no obstruction or minimal function, and limited or no VUR [17].

Two techniques have been described for endoscopic ablation. With incision, a single incision is made through the intravesical ureterocele with a Collins knife, electrocautery hook, Bugbee, or laser. Success rates of ureterocele and hydronephrosis decompression approach 90%, but 75% of patients develop VUR [20]. With the watering can puncture technique, a laser is used to poke 10–20 holes in the ureterocele. It successfully decompresses over 90% of ureteroceles and 82% of hydronephrosis, while only creating VUR in 36% [20]. When postincisional reflux does occur, it may be in the ipsilateral upper or lower pole, or contralateral kidney. As it will resolve spontaneously in most patients, initial therapy should be close surveillance rather than surgical correction [21].

If there is no function of the kidney or upper pole, nephrectomy or heminephrectomy may be considered. Endoscopic incision or bladder reconstruction is typically also required to prevent recurrent infections [22]. Open, laparoscopic, or robot-assisted approaches are described. The goal is preservation of the lower unit, regression of ureterocele/reflux, and reduction in incidence of infections [23].

To avoid upper tract surgery in a duplex system with a nonrefluxing lower pole, ureteroureterostomy is an option. This can be performed through flank, Gibson, Pfannenstiel, or inguinal herniorrhaphy-type incisions [24]. One caution is the potential "yo-yo" effect of urine refluxing up to the upper pole and creating urinary stasis [17].

Bladder reconstruction may be performed as a primary therapy or after endoscopic ablation. Most patients are continent and free of lower urinary tract symptoms [25]. Surgical options include excision or marsupialization of the ureterocele, recreation of the bladder floor, and reimplantation [17, 26].

Megaureter

Definition

The normal ureteral diameter is <5 mm, with diameter >7 mm considered a megaureter [1]. There are four classifications: nonobstructed/nonrefluxing, obstructed, refluxing, and obstructed and refluxing [27].

Epidemiology

Nonrefluxing megaureters are responsible for roughly 25% of prenatal upper tract dilatation, with nonobstructed/nonrefluxing the most common variant. They are more common in males, and the left ureter is affected more often than the right [27].

Presentation

Many patients are referred with prenatal hydroureteronephrosis. After birth, common presentations are febrile UTI and urolithiasis [27]. Associated findings include renal agenesis/dysplasia [27] and megacalyces [28].

Etiology

An obstructed megaureter is caused by an aperistaltic segment between 0.5 and 4 cm long that cannot adequately transport urine [27]. The cause is not completely understood, but it is likely a distal ureter maturation defect [18]. Molecular factors may include transforming growth factor $\beta 1$ [27] or leukocyte antigen-related family protein tyrosine phosphatases [29]. It likely involves inappropriate collagen deposition or arrangement of smooth muscle cells [27].

Diagnosis

Ultrasound reveals hydroureteronephrosis and is useful in follow-up [27].

VCUG distinguishes between refluxing and nonrefluxing megaureters [27].

Diuretic renography delineates differential function and can diagnose obstruction. The drainage curve should include the ureter to avoid false negatives. It should also account for the degree of dilation, as massive dilation may give false positives [27].

The invasive Whitaker test compares pressure in renal pelvis to that of bladder, with pressure >22 cm H_2O considered diagnostic of obstruction [27].

Management

Management options include observation, temporizing procedures, and reimplantation. Most patients can be managed conservatively with prophylactic antibiotics and interval imaging, and will remain stable or improve spontaneous [27, 30, 31]. Surgical indications include recurrent febrile UTIs, hematuria, pain, or worsening function

[27, 32]. Children with more severe hydroureteronephrosis, longer time to resolution, or unequal differential function are more likely to undergo surgery [31, 32]. Gender and laterality do not influence spontaneous resolution [32]. Some patients may require temporizing measures that enable drainage while allowing ureteral maturation to complete [27]. Such options include cutaneous ureterostomy [27] and endoscopic or open stent placement [27, 30, 33]. Balloon dilation with postprocedural stent for 6–8 weeks has also been described [34]. Reimplantation is the definitive treatment. The narrow, aperistaltic segment of ureter is excised, and the ureter is reimplanted in a nonrefluxing fashion with a tunnel to ureteral diameter ratio of at least 5:1. If the diameter is >10 mm, the ureter may be tapered with excision or folding of the excess ureter. A psoas hitch can help create sufficient floor length for an adequate tunnel [27].

Prognosis

Renal function is preserved in most patients; those with decreased renal function typically have dysplasia present at birth [31, 32].

Posterior urethral valves

Epidemiology

PUV only affects males and occurs in 1 in 8000 to 25,000 live births. Its incidence is decreasing secondary to prenatal diagnosis and subsequent termination of pregnancy [35].

Classification

The traditional classification scheme describes three types of valves. Type 1 valves, representing 95% of valves, are two sails that connect in the area of the verumontanum, and extend and expand distally in the region of the bulbomembranous urethra. Type 2 valves are probably not true valves but rather a nonobstructive fold between the verumontanum and the bladder neck that represents muscle hypertrophy. Type 3 valves comprise the remaining 5% and are a circumferential membrane lying distal to the verumontanum [35].

Pathophysiology

PUVs are potentially caused by inappropriate incorporation of mesonephric ducts into the cloaca [35]. The bladder struggles against obstruction and becomes hypertrophied secondary to increased storage and voiding pressures. This leads to severe ureteral dilatation with poor coaptation and contraction, obstructive uropathy, and renal dysplasia. If unilateral VUR develops, it may protect the opposite kidney from dysplasia [35].

Presentation

Neonates present with prenatal hydroureteronephrosis and bladder thickening, pulmonary hypoplasia, renal insufficiency, and ascites [35]. Older children present with febrile UTI or voiding complaints [36].

Diagnosis

Ultrasound classically demonstrates hydroureteronephrosis, a distended bladder with wall thickening, and a dilated posterior urethra [35].

VCUG may reveal VUR, a trabeculated bladder, diverticulae, a high bladder neck, and a dilated posterior urethra. Often the valves are visualized [35].

Diuretic renography is used to evaluate differential renal function and secondary obstruction [35].

Serum BUN and creatinine should be followed, remembering that initial values represent maternal levels [35].

Management

Immediately place a catheter to ensure bladder drainage [35]. If the infant is too small for cystoscopic instruments, consider vesicostomy. This may improve renal function relative to primary ablation [37]. If bladder-level drainage does not prevent infections or allow kidney drainage, upper tract diversion is warranted [35]. Definitive treatment is valve ablation. VCUG and cystourethroscopy are both used for follow-up to verify treatment success, although VCUG may miss residual valve leaflets [38]. Additionally, consider circumcision, as this reduces risk of UTI by over 80% [39]. If pyelonephritis cannot be prevented and the bladder is adequately rehabilitated, some patients require ureteral reimplantation [35]. In patients who require renal transplantation, urologic complications, including urethral strictures, stones, and retention, are more common. Urodynamic evaluation is vital to determine who must perform clean intermittent catheterization or under augmentation cystoplasty [35].

Antenatal interventions do not appear to improve renal outcomes [40]. Indicated if oligohydramnios is identified between 20 and 32 weeks gestation [35], options include vesicoamniotic shunts and fetal cystoscopy [41]. Some studies suggest that prenatal bladder drainage may improve survival [42].

Prognosis

Up to 50% of patients will develop end-stage renal disease (ESRD) [35] in childhood or adulthood [43]. By the mid-30s, the risk of ESRD from valves starts to decrease [43]. Early diagnosis, *in utero* lung pathology, bilateral VUR, and recurrent childhood UTI increase the risk of ESRD [43]. For children without prenatal hydronephrosis, severe preoperative or increasing hydronephrosis and bilateral VUR increase the ESRD risk [36]. Urinomas may be protective; boys with urinomas have lower nadir creatinine levels and are less likely to require renal replacement therapy [44].

Bladder dysfunction, with retention, weak stream, or double voiding, is seen in 40–60% of patients [45, 46]. Postnatal diagnosis and severe VUR increase the risk for bladder dysfunction [45]. Early valve ablation helps protect bladder function [47]. Bladder dysfunction increases the risk for renal dysfunction [45]. Prepubertal incontinence was traditionally assumed to result from weak sphincter/bladder neck, but may be secondary to detrusor instability, as most patients do achieve continence [46]. Bladder dysfunction may require intensive therapy, including urodynamics, anticholinergics, α-blockers, clean intermittent catheterization, timed voiding, and/or continuous nocturnal bladder drainage [35].

WHAT TO AVOID

- Obtaining a postnatal ultrasound within 48 hours of birth, as transitory neonatal dehydration may minimize degree of hydronephrosis [4].
- Rough handling of the ureter during surgical interventions.
- Overfilling the bladder during cystoscopic evaluation of ureteroceles, as it can compress the ureterocele, making it difficult to identify [17].
- Inadequately draining endoscopically treated ureteroceles.
- Failing to account for degree of hydroureteronephrosis when interpreting diuretic renography.
- Missing the diagnosis of PUV in older boys with persistent lower urinary tract symptoms.

KEY WEB LINKS

SFU Grading of Hydronephrosis
http://www.uab.edu/images/peduro/SFU/sfu_grading_on_web/sfu_grading_on_web.htm

Ureteropelvic Junction Obstruction AUA Foundation Information Page
http://www.urologyhealth.org/urology/index.cfm?article=43

Ureterocele AUA Foundation Information Page
http://www.urologyhealth.org/urology/index.cfm?article=42

Megaureters AUA Foundation Information Page
http://www.urologyhealth.org/urology/index.cfm?article=3

Posterior Urethral Valves
http://www.puvs.org/

Multiple choice questions

1 A 29-year-old P1G0000 female is referred to your clinic. On her 20-week prenatal ultrasound, her male fetus was found to have severe bilateral hydronephrosis. You tell her that which of the following conditions is most likely to result in long-term sequelae and will require treatment?

a UPJ
b Ureterocele
c VUR
d PUVs
e Primary obstructing megaureter

2 You are following a 6-month-old baby boy with SFU grade 3 left hydronephrosis. Which of the following findings would make you consider pyeloplasty?

a Ultrasound finding of stable hydronephrosis with preservation of cortical tissue
b VCUG with no evidence of VUR
c MAG-3 with equivocal T½ of 15 minutes
d MAG-3 with prolonged $T_{1/2}$ and differential function of left kidney 37% and right kidney 63%
e IVP showing an enlarged left collecting system with prompt nephrogram and delayed drainage

3 You are referred a 3-month-old baby boy with bilateral hydroureteronephrosis to the level of the bladder, negative VCUG, and equivocal MAG-3. What is your initial treatment plan?

a Bilateral cutaneous ureterostomies
b Bilateral tapered ureteral reimplants

c Interval imaging and prophylactic antibiotics
d Interval imaging and no prophylactic antibiotics
e Vesicostomy

References

1 Carr MC, Casale P. Chapter 120: anomalies and surgery of the ureter in children. In: Wein A, Kavoussi LR, Novick AC, Partin AW, Peters CA, editors. *Campbell-Walsh Urology.* 10th ed. Philadelphia, PA: Elsevier; 2011.

2 Kajbafzadeh AM, Tourchi A, Nezami BG, Khakpour M, Mousavian AA, Talab SS. Miniature pyeloplasty as a minimally invasive surgery with less than 1 day admission in infants. *J Pediatr Urol* 2011;7(3):283–288.

3 Karnak I, Woo LL, Shah SN, Sirajuddin A, Ross JH. Results of a practical protocol for management of prenatally detected hydronephrosis due to ureteropelvic junction obstruction. *Pediatr Surg Int* 2009;25(1):61–67.

4 Churchill BM, Feng WC. Chapter 20: ureteropelvic junction anomalies: congenital ureteropelvic junction problems in children. In: Gearhart JP, Rink RC, Mouriquand PDE, editors. *Pediatric Urology*. Philadelphia, PA: Saunders Elsevier; 2010. pp. 248–271.

5 Madsen MG, Nørregaard R, Frøkiær J, Jørgensen TM. Urinary biomarkers in prenatally diagnosed unilateral hydronephrosis. *J Pediatr Urol* 2011;7(2):105–112.

6 Ross SS, Kardos S, Krill A, et al. Observation of infants with SFU grades 3-4 hydronephrosis: worsening drainage with serial diuresis renography indicates surgical intervention and helps prevent loss of renal function. *J Pediatr Urol* 2011;7(3):266–271.

7 Uluocak N, Ander H, Acar O, Amasyali AS, Erkorkmaz U, Ziylan O. Clinical and radiological characteristics of patients operated in the first year of life due to ureteropelvic junction obstruction: significance of renal pelvis diameter. *Urology* 2009;74(4):898–902.

8 Braga LH, Lorenzo AJ, Bägli DJ, et al. Comparison of flank, dorsal lumbotomy and laparoscopic approaches for dismembered pyeloplasty in children older than 3 years with ureteropelvic junction obstruction. *J Urol* 2010;183(1):306–311.

9 Subotic U, Rohard I, Weber DM, Gobet R, Moehrlen U, Gonzalez R. A minimal invasive surgical approach for children of all ages with ureteropelvic junction obstruction. *J Pediatr Urol* 2011;8(4):354–358.

10 Tanaka ST, Grantham JA, Thomas JC, Adams MC, Brock JW, 3rd, Pope JC, 4th. A comparison of open vs laparoscopic pediatric pyeloplasty using the pediatric health information system database—do benefits of laparoscopic approach recede at younger ages? *J Urol* 2008;180(4):1479–1485.

11 Behan JW, Kim SS, Dorey F, et al. Human capital gains associated with robotic assisted laparoscopic pyeloplasty in children compared to open pyeloplasty. *J Urol* 2011;186(4 Suppl):1663–1667.

12 Polok M, Chrzan R, Veenboer P, et al. Nondismembered pyeloplasty in a pediatric population: results of 34 open and laparoscopic procedures. *Urology* 2011;78(4):891–894.

13 Casale P, Mucksavage P, Resnick M, Kim SS. Robotic ureterocalicostomy in the pediatric population. *J Urol* 2008;180(6):2643–2648.

14 Veenboer PW, Chrzan R, Dik P, Klijn AJ, de Jong TP. Secondary endoscopic pyelotomy in children with failed pyeloplasty. *Urology* 2011;77(6):1450–1454.

15 Braga LH, Lorenzo AJ, Farhat WA, Bägli DJ, Khoury AE, Pippi Salle JL. Outcome analysis and cost comparison between externalized pyeloureteral and standard stents in 470 consecutive open pyeloplasties. *J Urol* 2008;180(4 Suppl):1693–1698; discussion 1698–1699.

16 Chacko JK, Piaggio LA, Neheman A, González R. Pediatric laparoscopic pyeloplasty: lessons learned from the first 52 cases. *J Endourol* 2009;23(8):1307–1311.

17 Peters C, Schlussel R, Mendelsohn C. Chapter 121: ectopic ureter, ureterocele, and ureteral anomalies. In: Wein AJ, Kavoussi LR, Novick AC, Partin AW, Peters CA, editors. *Campbell-Walsh Urology.* 10th ed. Philadelphia, PA: Elsevier; 2011.

18 Uetani N, Bouchard M. Plumbing in the embryo: developmental defects of the urinary tracts. *Clin Genet* 2009;75(4):307–317.

19 Asgari SA, Mansour Ghanaie M, Simforoosh N, Kajbafzadeh A, Zare' A. Acute urinary retention in children. *Urol J* 2005;2(1):23–27.

20 Palmer BW, Greger H, Mannas DB, Kropp BP, Frimberger D. Comparison of endoscopic ureterocele decompression techniques. Preliminary experience—is the watering can puncture superior? *J Urol* 2011;186(4 Suppl):1700–1703.

21 Jesus LE, Farhat WA, Amarante AC, et al. Clinical evolution of vesicoureteral reflux following endoscopic puncture in children with duplex system ureteroceles. *J Urol* 2011;186(4):1455–1458.

22 Pearce R, Subramaniam R. Partial nephroureterectomy in a duplex system in children: the need for additional bladder procedures. *Pediatr Surg Int* 2011;27(12):1323–1326.

23 Denes FT, Danilovic A, Srougi M. Outcome of laparoscopic upper-pole nephrectomy in children with duplex systems. *J Endourol* 2007;21(2):162–168.

24 Prieto J, Ziada A, Baker L, Snodgrass W. Ureteroureterostomy via inguinal incision for ectopic ureters and ureteroceles without ipsilateral lower pole reflux. *J Urol* 2009;181(4):1844–1848; discussion 1848–1850.

25 Beganovic A, Klijn AJ, Dik P, De Jong TP. Ectopic ureterocele: long-term results of open surgical therapy in 54 patients. *J Urol* 2007;178(1):251–254.
26 Lewis JM, Cheng EY, Campbell JB, et al. Complete excision or marsupialization of ureteroceles: does choice of surgical approach affect outcome? *J Urol* 2008;180(4 Suppl):1819–1822; discussion 1822–1823.
27 Merlini E, Spina P. Primary non-refluxing megaureters. *J Pediatr Urol* 2005;1(6):409–417.
28 Vargas B, Lebowitz RL. The coexistence of congenital megacalyces and primary megaureter. *AJR Am J Roentgenol* 1986;147(2):313–316.
29 Uetani N, Bertozzi K, Chagnon MJ, Hendriks W, Tremblay ML, Bouchard M. Maturation of ureter-bladder connection in mice is controlled by LAR family receptor protein tyrosine phosphatases. *J Clin Invest* 2009;119(4):924–935.
30 Arena F, Baldari S, Proietto F, Centorrino A, Scalfari G, Romeo G Conservative treatment in primary neonatal megaureter. *Eur J Pediatr Surg* 1998;8(6):347–351.
31 Gimpel C, Masioniene L, Djakovic N, et al. Complications and long-term outcome of primary obstructive megaureter in childhood. *Pediatr Nephrol* 2010;25(9):1679–1686.
32 Calisti A, Oriolo L, Perrotta ML, Spagnol L, Fabbri R. The fate of prenatally diagnosed primary nonrefluxing megaureter: do we have reliable predictors for spontaneous resolution? *Urology* 2008;72(2):309–312.
33 Farrugia MK, Steinbrecher HA, Malone PS. The utilization of stents in the management of primary obstructive megaureters requiring intervention before 1 year of age. *J Pediatr Urol* 2011;7(2):198–202.
34 Torino G, Collura G, Mele E, Garganese MC, Capozza N. Severe primary obstructive megaureter in the first year of life: preliminary experience with endoscopic balloon dilation. *J Endourol* 2011;26(4):325–329.
35 Casale A. Chapter 126: posterior urethral valves. In: Wein AJ, Kavoussi LR, Novick AC, Partin AW, Peters CA, editors. *Campbell-Walsh Urology*. Philadelphia, PA: Elsevier; 2011.
36 Engel DL, Pope JC, 4th, Adams MC, Brock JW, 3rd, Thomas JC, Tanaka ST. Risk factors associated with chronic kidney disease in patients with posterior urethral valves without prenatal hydronephrosis. *J Urol* 2011;185(6 Suppl):2502–2506.
37 Godbole P, Wade A, Mushtaq I, Wilcox DT. Vesicostomy vs primary ablation for posterior urethral valves: always a difference in outcome? *J Pediatr Urol* 2007;3(4): 273–275.
38 Smeulders N, Makin E, Desai D, et al. The predictive value of a repeat micturating cystourethrogram for remnant leaflets after primary endoscopic ablation of posterior urethral valves. *J Pediatr Urol* 2011;7(2): 203–208.
39 Mukherjee S, Joshi A, Carroll D, Chandran H, Parashar K, McCarthy L. What is the effect of circumcision on risk of urinary tract infection in boys with posterior urethral valves? *J Pediatr Surg* 2009;44(2):417–421.
40 Salam MA. Posterior urethral valve: outcome of antenatal intervention. *Int J Urol* 2006;13(10):1317–1322.
41 Morris RK, Ruano R, Kilby MD. Effectiveness of fetal cystoscopy as a diagnostic and therapeutic intervention for lower urinary tract obstruction: a systematic review. *Ultrasound Obstet Gynecol* 2011;37(6):629–637.
42 Clark TJ, Martin WL, Divakaran TG, Whittle MJ, Kilby MD, Khan KS. Prenatal bladder drainage in the management of fetal lower urinary tract obstruction: a systematic review and meta-analysis. *Obstet Gynecol* 2003;102(2):367–382.
43 Heikkila J, Holmberg C, Kyllönen L, Rintala R, Taskinen S. Long-term risk of end stage renal disease in patients with posterior urethral valves. *J Urol* 2011;186(6): 2392–2396.
44 Wells JM, Mukerji S, Chandran H, Parashar K, McCarthy L. Urinomas protect renal function in posterior urethral valves—a population based study. *J Pediatr Surg* 2010;45(2):407–410.
45 Otukesh H, Sharifiaghdas F, Hoseini R, et al. Long-term upper and lower urinary tract functions in children with posterior urethral valves. *J Pediatr Urol*, 2009;6(2): 143–147.
46 Holmdahl G, Sillen U. Boys with posterior urethral valves: outcome concerning renal function, bladder function and paternity at ages 31 to 44 years. *J Urol* 2005;174(3):1031–1034; discussion 1034.
47 Youssif M, Dawood W, Shabaan S, Mokhless I, Hanno A. Early valve ablation can decrease the incidence of bladder dysfunction in boys with posterior urethral valves. *J Urol* 2009;182(4 Suppl):1765–1768.

Answers to multiple choice questions

1 d Requires ablation of the valves at a minimum and may result in ESRD and bladder dysfunction.
2 d A differential function <40% is an indication for surgery.
3 c Children with congenital megaureters may be safely followed with prophylactic antibiotics and interval imaging.

29 Developmental abnormalities of the genitalia: disorders of sexual differentiation, hypospadias, and cryptorchidism

Eric Z. Massanyi

The James Buchanan Brady Urological Institute and Department of Urology, The Johns Hopkins School of Medicine, Baltimore, MD, USA

KEY POINTS

- Sex-determining region of the Y chromosome (SRY) initiates a cascade of events that leads to the development of testicular tissue in the bipotential gonad *in utero*.
- The urogenital tract is identical in both sexes during the first 8 weeks of development.
- Congenital adrenal hyperplasia (CAH) accounts for the majority (60%) of disorders of sexual differentiation (DSD).
- Streaks and dysgenetic gonads associated with Y chromosome material are at increased risk of developing gonadoblastoma and should be prophylactically removed.
- An individual diagnosed with hypospadias and cryptorchidism should be evaluated for possible disorders of sexual differentiation.
- Infants suspected of having hypospadias should not be circumcised at birth.
- Individuals with undescended testes are at increased risk of infertility and germ cell tumors.

Disorders of sexual differentiation

Normal sexual development

The developing fetus has bipotential gonads during the first 6 weeks of human development. Masculinization requires the presence of testis determining factor (TDF) located on the sex-determining region of the Y chromosome (SRY). SRY subsequently initiates a process that leads to testicular development from the primordial gonads. The testes then differentiate into Leydig cells, which produce testosterone, and Sertoli cells, which produce Müllerian inhibition substance (MIS). MIS is responsible for the regression of the female ductal system. Testosterone acts in a paracrine fashion to develop the vas deferens, epididymis, and seminal vesicle. External genitalia begin to change in males during the eighth week of gestation from androgen activity. Testosterone is converted by 5α-reductase II to produce dihydrotestosterone (DHT). DHT leads to elongation of the genital tubercle, fusion of the urethral and labioscrotal folds, and development of the prostate from the urogenital sinus. In the absence of androgen activity, the internal ducts and external genitalia feminize (Figure 29.1) [1].

Presentation

Disorders of sexual differentiation (DSD) often present with ambiguous genitalia during neonatal examination. This can be considered undermasculinization of a male, virilization of a female, or abnormal development due to dysgenetic gonads. Common findings include clitoromegaly, phallus with nonpalpable gonads, female with palpable gonads, and hypospadias with cryptorchidism [2].

Handbook of Urology, First edition. J. Kellogg Parsons, John B. Eifler and Misop Han. © 2014 by John Wiley & Sons, Ltd.
Published 2014 by John Wiley & Sons, Ltd.

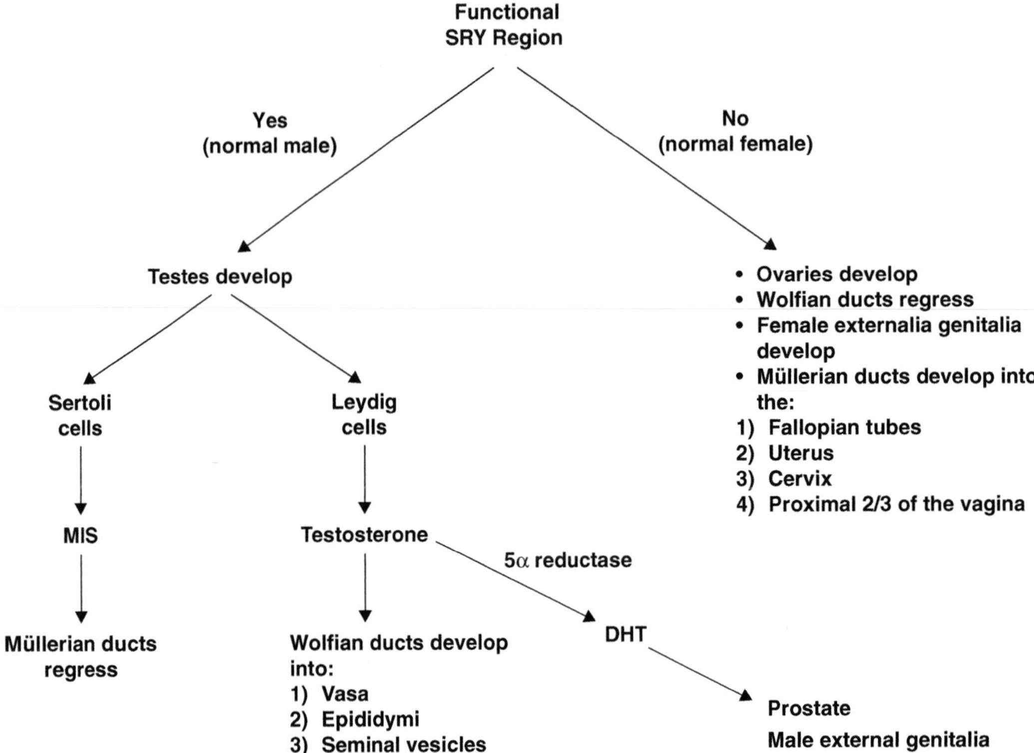

Figure 29.1 Normal sexual development.

Evaluation and workup

Careful history of the neonate's family is important in suspecting and diagnosing DSD. Investigation of maternal exposures to androgens, family history of DSD, history of infertility, and prior infant deaths are important. Physical examination should include inspection of the phallus for hypospadias and urethral position; visualization of the labia/scrotum for rugae, palpable gonads, and fusion; and inspection assessment for hyperpigmentation. After the neonate is determined to be stable, serum electrolytes, hormone assays, and a karyotype should be obtained. Further evaluation should include a pelvic sonogram to identify Müllerian structures and a urogenitogram. If further workup is required, anesthesia can be utilized for examination, endoscopy, and laparoscopy [3].

Female DSD

Rarely, 46,XX DSD can arise from maternal exposure to androgens or virilizing tumors. The most common cause of DSD is congenital adrenal hyperplasia (CAH). CAH is caused by an autosomal recessive defect in one of the three enzymes responsible for cortisol synthesis. This leads to increased androgen production (Figure 29.2). Increased ACTH by way of feedback from decreased cortisol production can lead to hyperpigmentation.

The most common type of CAH is 21-hydroxylase deficiency. A defect in this enzyme accounts for 90–95% of CAH. The incidence is 1 in 50,000 live births. Most (50–70%) are so-called "salt wasters" due to impaired aldosterone production. Genital ambiguity varies in females. The neonate may present with vomiting, dehydration, failure to thrive, and adrenal crisis. Diagnosis is made by detection of elevated levels of 17-hydroxyprogesterone and progesterone levels. Elevation of 17-hydroxyprogesterone can be detected prenatally.

11β-Hydroxylase deficiency accounts for <5% of all CAH. Diagnosis is made by elevated levels of deoxycortisol and deoxycorticosterone (DOC). DOC leads

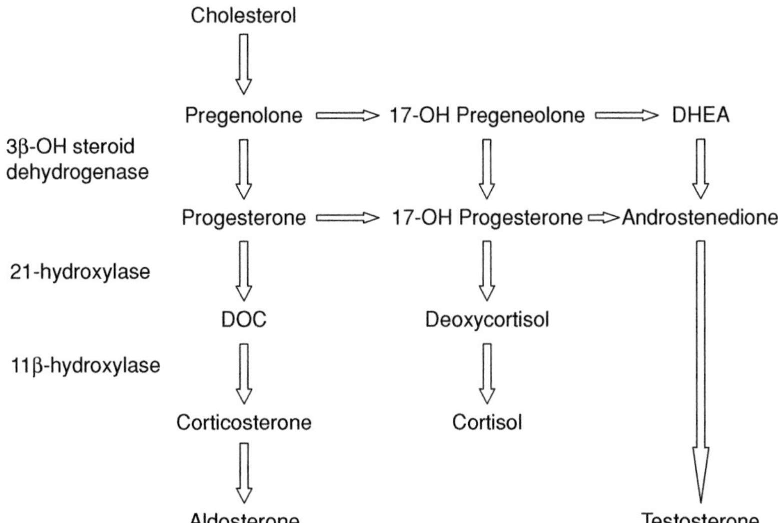

Figure 29.2 Cortisol synthesis.

to salt retention. Presentation may include hypertension, hyperpigmentation, virilization of females, and precocious puberty in males.

3β-Hydroxysteroid dehydrogenase deficiency accounts for only 1% of all cases of CAH. Diagnosis is made by elevated levels of 17-hydroxyprenolone and dehydroepiandrosterone (DHEA). Typically, patients present with severe salt wasting. Genital ambiguity may be seen in both females and males due to impaired androstenedione production.

Treatment of CAH is individualized for each patient. The mainstay of treatment is cortisol and mineralocorticoid replacement when indicated. This is typically accomplished with hydrocortisone and flucortisone (in salt wasters). Ambiguous genitalia may require clitoroplasty and/or vaginoplasty in severe cases [4].

Male DSD

Generally, 46,XY DSD arises from defective testosterone synthesis, or more commonly, from a defect in the androgen receptor. External genitalia are variable, usually accompanied by palpable gonads. Müllerian structures are suppressed by MIS. These individuals are often treated with exogenous testosterone.

Cholesterol is converted to testosterone through five enzymatic steps. A defect in any one of these enzymes can impair testosterone synthesis. Defects are associated with incomplete virilization. Affected individuals may have concomitant mineralocorticoid and glucocorticoid production. Sterility is common among these individuals.

5α-Reductase II deficiency is an autosomal condition most commonly seen among inbred populations. Normal virilization of the external genitalia requires DHT. Often, these children are raised female until masculinization of varying degrees occurs at puberty. Micropenis and penoscrotal hypospadias may be noted among those who present earlier. Affected individuals will have an elevated testosterone:DHT ratio. Treatment is individualized; most individuals undergo genitoplasty and are raised as males.

Complete androgen insensitivity is caused by a defect in the androgen receptor and affects 1 in 20,000–40,000 individuals. Patients are phenotypic females and commonly present with amenorrhea at puberty. Some individuals are diagnosed earlier due to palpable gonads, often presenting as hernias. MIS still suppresses Müllerian ducts. However, a rudimentary uterus is found in one-third of cases. Prophylactic gonadectomy is recommended due to increased risk of gandoblastoma or seminoma. Reifenstein syndrome is an X-linked disorder which leads to incomplete androgen insensitivity. It is caused by either a decreased number of androgen receptors or decreased affinity of the receptors to androgens. Presentation varies, and treatment is individualized [5].

MIS deficiency is a sex-linked autosomal recessive condition that arises from mutations that affect the production of MIS by Sertoli cells or its receptors. It is also known as *hernia uteri inguinalis*. Individuals have normal external genitalia with retained internal Müllerian structures. Cryptorchidism is common; oftentimes, the Müllerian structures are recognized during orchidopexy. Retained Müllerian structures are usually removed with careful preservation of the vas deferens [6].

Ovotesticular DSD

The diagnosis of true hermaphroditism is given to individuals who have both ovarian and testicular tissues. This can occur as two separate distinct gonads or as ovotestes. Karyotype is most commonly 46,XX, but may also be mosaics of 46,XX/46,XY or 47,XXX/56,XY. A small number are 46,XY. Ambiguous genitalia are usually found on presentation. Diagnosis requires gonadal biopsy and identification of both ovarian and testicular tissues. Internal ducts vary according to ipsilateral gonadal histology. Management is individualized, but usually involves removal of discordant structures. Females may be fertile. Males are usually sterile and prophylactic gonadectomy is recommended [7].

Gonadal dysgenesis

Mixed gonadal dysgenesis (MGD) is defined by the presence of patients with one testis and one streak gonad. Karyotype is most commonly mosaic 45,XO/46,XY. It is the second leading cause of ambiguous genitalia. The streak gonad has impaired testosterone and MIS production. The contralateral testis also has diminished testosterone production. Patients are at increased risk of Denys–Drash syndrome and Wilms' tumor. External genitalia vary from normal to predominantly feminized. Affected individuals are infertile and may have retained Müllerian structures secondary to decreased MIS production by the streak gonad. Prophylactic gonadectomy is recommended [8].

Pure gonadal dysgenesis

Patients with pure gonadal dysgenesis have bilateral streak gonads. Karyotype is either 46,XX or 46,XY. Phenotype is typically female. They are sexually infantile, but lack the other stigmata associated with Turner syndrome (see section Turner syndrome). Patients are treated with cyclic estrogen and progesterone replacement. If Y chromosomal material is present, prophylactic gonadectomy is required [9].

Turner syndrome

Turner syndrome usually is caused by the karyotype 45,XO. It leads to a female phenotype, bilateral streak gonads, short stature, broad chest, webbed neck, and sexual infantilism. Turner syndrome is associated with coarctation of the aorta and renal abnormalities, including horseshoe kidney, duplication, malrotation, and agenesis. A small minority of patients may contain Y chromosomal material. These patients require prophylactic gonadectomy [10].

Klinefelter syndrome

Klinefelter syndrome is defined by a karyotype that contains both a Y chromosome and more than one X chromosome (i.e., XXY, XXXY, etc.). Affected individuals are phenotypically male with poorly developed secondary sex characteristics. Patients may present with gynecomastia. Patients are infertile due to azoospermia. Testicular histology demonstrates hyaline replacement of seminiferous tubules. Patients will exhibit low testosterone levels and increased levels of follicle-stimulating hormone (FSH) and luteinizing hormone (LH). Treatment involves androgen supplementation and reduction mammoplasties [11].

Hypospadias

Introduction

Hypospadias is a developmental anomaly characterized by arrested penile development. It is characterized by proximal opening of the urethral meatus, dorsal hooding of the foreskin, and ventral penile curvature (chordee). Phallic development is dependent upon androgenic stimulation between the ninth and twelfth weeks of gestation. Androgen stimulation leads to elongation of the genital tubercle and fusion of the urethral folds. Lack of androgenic stimulation during this critical time period can lead to hypospadias and its associated findings.

The incidence of hypospadias is 1 in 250 live births. Hypospadias is noted to also occur in 6–8%

of affected individuals' fathers and 14% of male siblings. Severe hypospadias is associated with DSD and karyotype is warranted, especially if diagnosed with concomitant cryptorchidism. Hypospadias can cause difficulty with both sexual intercourse and urinating from a standing position [12].

Treatment

The need for further urinary tract evaluation is unnecessary in those diagnosed with isolated hypospadias. Any child with suspected hypospadias should not be circumcised; the foreskin can be used for surgical repair should it be necessary. If surgical repair is elected, timing of surgery should be between 6 and 18 months of age. Preoperative hormones in the form of β-hCG, testosterone, or DHT have been administered to increase penile size and vascularity. Surgery should be individualized to the patient. Correction may require more than one operation (i.e., staged approach).

General principles of surgical repair include orthoplasty, urethroplasty, glansplasty, and skin closure. Curvature less than 30° is most often corrected by midline dorsal placation (Nesbit repair). Curvature exceeding 30° may require ventral lengthening by corporotomy with dermal grafting. Most urethroplasties are accomplished by tubularization of the urethral plate, often with a dorsal midline relaxing incision to widen the plate. Tissue flaps and grafts can be utilized, if necessary.

Complications may include bleeding, infection, fistula, meatal stenosis, urethral stricture, diverticulum, and dehiscence. Most complications require a second surgery for a successful outcome. In these cases, surgery should be delayed for at least 6 months to allow tissues to heal from prior surgeries [13].

Cryptorchidism

Introduction

Cryptorchidism is defined by failure of one or both testes to properly descend into the scrotum. The incidence is 3% among full-term infant boys and 0.8% among 1-year-old boys. Normal descent of the testes occurs around the 28th week of gestation. A testosterone surge that occurs 6–12 weeks after birth may stimulate postnatal descent in some boys. It is therefore important to wait 4 months after birth before surgical correction is performed. Cryptorchidism is associated with Prader–Willi syndrome and other defects of the hypothalamic–pituitary–testis axis. DSD should be suspected if diagnosed with concomitant hypospadias. Most cases, however, are sporadic.

Rationale for treatment

Seven percent of normal men are subfertile. Approximately 10% of men with a unilateral undescended testis are subfertile, and 33% of men with bilateral undescended testes are subfertile. Orchidopexy performed at an early age has been shown to improve long-term infertility. Normal germ cell counts have been shown to diminish after 1 year of age.

Tumors are estimated to develop in 0.5–1% of undescended testes. Orchidopexy performed before the age of puberty decreases the risk of cancer. The contralateral, descended testis is not at increased risk for developing malignancy [14].

Evaluation

A careful history, including maternal exposures and family history of cryptorchidism, infertility, and testicular malignancy, is paramount. It is also important to evaluate whether or not the testis has ever been seen or palpated by the parents or caregivers.

A cryptorchid or undescended testis should not be confused with a retractile testis. A retractile testis can be pulled into the scrotum from a position near the external inguinal ring and will remain in place until cremasteric muscle contraction causes it to ascend. Patients with retractile testes are not at increased risk for infertility or cancer. A nonpalpable testis can indicate either the testis is in a location that cannot be palpated (i.e., intra-abdominal) or a vanishing testis, also known as a *nubbin*. Further evaluation is necessary in any patient with a nonpalpable testis [15].

No imaging test is accurate enough to detect intra-abdominal testes. Laboratory tests are usually unnecessary. A boy born with bilateral undescended testes may benefit from a serum testosterone, FSH, and LH to evaluate for testicular viability. Increased FSH and LH are suggestive of anorchia. If FSH and LH levels are normal or minimally elevated (<3Xs normal), an hCG stimulation test may be utilized to detect a rise in testosterone from a viable testis. MIS can also be measured to evaluate for testicular viability.

Treatment

β-hCG or gonadotropin-releasing hormone (GnRH) has been used to stimulate descent by some clinicians. Hormonal stimulation is more often used to distinguish a retractile testis from an undescended testis.

Surgical correction by the way of orchidopexy is the preferred treatment of cryptorchidism. This can be accomplished by laparoscopy or through a scrotal incision, but it is most commonly approached by way of an inguinal incision. After the gubernaculum is divided and the hernia sac is dissected from the cord, the testis is evaluated to ensure that enough length is present to place the testis into a subdartos pouch into the ipsilateral scrotum. If more length is needed, the peritoneum can be dissected free of the spermatic cord in the abdomen or the transversalis fascia can be opened to move the cord medial to the epigastric vessels (Prentiss maneuver). Rarely, the testicular arteries are transected (Fowler–Stevens) and the testis is preserved by collateral blood supply. This has been described as both one- and two-stage procedures [16].

Laparoscopy may be employed for suspected intra-abdominal testes. Management is dependent upon intraoperative findings. If blind-ending internal spermatic vessels are identified, no further treatment is necessary. If a spermatic cord entering an inguinal ring is identified, inguinal exploration is carried out. Finally, if an intra-abdominal testis is identified, the testis should be brought down to the scrotum using the open surgical principles outlined above.

WHAT TO AVOID/KEY PITFALLS

- Patients with undiagnosed CAH may be in extremis secondary to glucocorticoid deficiency; electrolytes should be obtained before any further workup.
- Individuals born with 5α-reductase deficiency raised as females may be virilized at puberty if prophylactic gonadectomy is not performed.
- Adequate time must be given before performing a second surgery on a patient with hypospadias to allow for adequate tissue healing and neovascularization.
- A neonate with an undescended testis should be given at least 4 months before intervention to allow for a postnatal testosterone surge to stimulate descent.
- A testis that can be manipulated down to the scrotum and remains in place before cremasteric contraction is a retractile testis and does not warrant further treatment.

KEY WEB LINKS

Guidelines on DSD from the Consortium on the Management of Disorders of Sex Development
http://www.accordalliance.org/dsdguidelines/htdocs/clinical/index.html

European Association of Urology's Guidelines on Paediatric Urology
http://www.uroweb.org/fileadmin/user_upload/Guidelines/Paediatric%20Urology.pdf

Clinical Guidelines on the Management of 21-hydroxylase Deficiency from the Endocrine Society
http://www.endo-society.org/guidelines/upload/FINAL-Standalone-CAH-Guideline.pdf

CASE STUDY

A 6-month-old male born full term via uncomplicated vaginal delivery presents to the office with a diagnosis of left undescended testis. The patient was diagnosed at birth, but the parents are seeking medical attention now. Up until now, the baby has been feeding well, gaining weight, and is otherwise healthy.

Upon examination, the baby is noted to have an uncircumcised phallus with penoscrotal hypospadias and moderate chordee. On the right, there is a mild hydrocele, but no definite testicle. Something is palpable near the right internal ring. No testicle is palpable on the left.

Urinalysis, serum electrolytes, 17-hydroxyprogesterone, 11-deoxycortisol, testosterone, and urine 17-ketosteroids are all within normal limits. A pelvic ultrasound reveals a structure posterior to the bladder resembling a uterus. Urogenitogram reveals a collection of dye in the posterior urethra with a possible cervical impression. Karyotype is 46,XX.

Multiple choice questions

1 The next best step in the treatment of this child is
   a Gonadal biopsy
   b Gonadectomy
   c Bilateral orchidopexy
   d Hypospadias repair
   e Abdominal MRI

2 The most likely diagnosis in this patient is:
   a Mixed gonadal dysgenesis
   b Congenital adrenal hyperplasia
   c True hermaphroditism
   d Pure gonadal dysgenesis
   e Androgen insensitivity syndrome

References

1 Wiener JS, Marcelli M, Lamb DJ. Molecular determinants of sexual differentiation. *J Urol* 1996;14:278–294.
2 Lee PA, Houk CP, Ahmed SF, et al. Consensus statement on management of intersex disorders. International Consensus Conference on Intersex. *Pediatrics* 2006;118:488–500.
3 Ahmed SF, Rodie M. Investigation and initial management of ambiguous genitalia. *Best Pract Res Clin Endocrinol Metab* 2010;24:197–218
4 Daimond D. Sexual differentiation: normal and abnormal. In: Wein AJ, editor. *Campbell-Walsh Urology*. 9th ed. Philadelphia, PA: Saunders; 2007. pp. 3799–3829.
5 Werner R, Grötsch H, Hiort O. 46,XY disorders of sex development--the undermasculinised male with disorders of androgen action. *Best Pract Res Clin Endocrinol Metab* 2010;24:263–277.
6 Rey R, Mebarki F, Forest MG, et al. Anti-müllerian hormone in children with androgen insensitivity. *J Clin Endocrinol Metab* 1994;79:960–964.
7 Kousta E, Papathanasiou A, Skordis N. Sex determination and disorders of sex development according to the revised nomenclature and classification in 46,XX individuals. *Hormones* 2010;9:218–231.
8 Arcari AJ, Bergadá I, Rey RA, Gottlieb S. Predictive value of anatomical findings and karyotype analysis in the diagnosis of patients with disorders of sexual development. *Sex Dev* 2007;1:222–229.
9 Val P, Swain A. Mechanisms of disease: normal and abnormal gonadal development and sex determination in mammals. *Nat Clin Pract Urol* 2005;2:616–627.
10 Morgan T. Turner syndrome: diagnosis and management. *Am Fam Physician* 2007;76:405–410.
11 Wikström AM, Dunkel L. Klinefelter syndrome. *Best Pract Res Clin Endocrinol Metab* 2011;25:239–250.
12 Roberts J. Hypospadias surgery past, present and future. *Curr Opin Urol* 2010;20:483–489.
13 Snodgrass W, Bush N. Tubularized incised plate proximal hypospadias repair: continued evolution and extended applications. *J Pediatr Urol* 2011;7:2–9.
14 Wood HM, Elder JS. Cryptorchidism and testicular cancer: separating fact from fiction. *J Urol* 2009;181:452–461.
15 Belman AB, Rushton HG. Is the vanished testis always a scrotal event? *BJU Int* 2001;87:480–483.
16 Elyas R, Guerra LA, Pike J, et al. Is staging beneficial for Fowlers-Stephens orchiopexy? A systematic review. *J Urol* 2010;183:2012–2018.

Answers to multiple choice questions

1 a
2 c

30 Pediatric urinary infections, vesicoureteral reflux, and voiding dysfunction

Eric Z. Massanyi

The James Buchanan Brady Urological Institute and Department of Urology, The Johns Hopkins School of Medicine, Baltimore, MD, USA

KEY POINTS

- *Escherichia coli* is the most common pathogen among pediatric urinary tract infections.
- The incidence of urinary tract infection is higher among uncircumcised males only in the first year after birth.
- Voiding cystourethrogram (VCUG) is necessary to grade the severity of vesicoureteral reflux (VUR).
- Pyelonephritic scarring is the leading cause of pediatric hypertension.
- Ureteroneocystostomy is the most effective treatment for VUR.
- VUR may be secondary to dysfunctional elimination syndrome and treatment should focus on correction of voiding dysfunction prior to surgery.
- Dysfunctional voiding is commonly associated with bowel dysfunction and both should be treated together.

Pediatric urinary tract infections

Classification

Urinary tract infections (UTIs) have been classified in many ways. Generally, UTIs are described based on their location, whether symptoms are present, and whether or not the infection is new, persistent, or represents reinfection. Most infections are localized to the bladder and are referred to as cystitis. An infection that involves at least one kidney is called pyelonephritis. Bacterial colonization without symptoms is known as asymptomatic bacteriuria. Infections that are symptomatic resolve with treatment, and become symptomatic again, may represent recurrent UTI. However, it should be noted that the term "recurrent" is not adequately descriptive. Persistent UTI is diagnosed when the same organism is cultured after a period of noninfection. Reinfection describes a new infection by a different organism.

Epidemiology

The incidence of UTI in males is greater only during the first year after birth. The incidence in uncircumcised boys is 1%. The risk is increased 5–20 times among uncircumcised boys [1]. After the age of 1 year, the incidence of UTI among females is 10 times greater than males. Females have a 60–80% chance of reinfection within 5 years of initial UTI [2].

Etiology

Escherichia coli is the most common uropathogen [3]. Enterobacteriaceae of all types may be responsible for pediatric UTI, including *Klebsiella*, *Proteus*, *Enterobacter*, and *Pseudomonas* species. Other rarer pathogens include *Staphylococcus*, *Enterococcus*, and nonbacterial species. Most symptomatic infections will have colony counts greater than 100,000. However, colony counts of

Handbook of Urology, First edition. J. Kellogg Parsons, John B. Eifler and Misop Han.
Published 2014 by John Wiley & Sons, Ltd.

10,000 with symptoms should be considered infection among children [4].

Several virulence factors among certain strains of *E. coli* have been identified. Various surface structures, such as pili and fimbriae, allow for increased attachment of the bacteria to the urothelium. Some increase the risk of pyelonephritis [5].

Host factors also contribute to risk of infection and progression to pyelonephritis. Foreskin increases the risk of infection among males [1]. Vesicoureteral reflux (VUR) allows less virulent pathogens to cause pyelonephritis. Voiding dysfunction is often linked to UTI and may be secondary to incomplete emptying of the bladder, which increased the risk of UTI [6]. Other factors, such as sexual activity, anatomical anomalies, urinary calculi, and foreign bodies, also increase the risk of UTI.

Diagnosis

Common signs and symptoms of adult UTI, such as urinary frequency, urgency, incontinence, and dysuria, may not be present or are difficult to recognize among younger children [7]. Vague signs such as poor feeding, irritability, diarrhea, and so on may be more common. Fevers are suggestive of pyelonephritis.

Any child suspected of UTI should have urine obtained and cultured. Bag specimens are easily contaminated and thus are only useful when negative. Catheterized specimens may be traumatic, but are more reliable. The most reliable specimen among very young children can be obtained by suprapubic aspiration. Voided specimens should be reserved only for children who are toilet trained.

Any child younger than 5 years with a UTI or any child with a febrile UTI should be evaluated with renal ultrasonography and voiding cystourethrogram (VCUG) to rule out hydronephrosis and/or VUR. 99mTc dimercaptosuccinic acid (DMSA) renography can be used to evaluate a child for evidence of acute pyelonephritis or renal scarring. DMSA used to evaluate for scarring should be delayed at least 6 months after febrile UTI [8].

Treatment

Antimicrobial therapy is indicated for any child diagnosed with UTI. The choice of antimicrobial agent and duration of treatment depend on the patient and severity of the infection. Cystitis should be treated for 3–5 days. Pyelonephritis or febrile UTI should be treated for 10–14 days with broad-spectrum therapy until cultures are finalized. If a child appears septic or does not respond to oral therapy, hospitalization and parenteral antimicrobials are indicated. Asymptomatic bacteriuria does not warrant antimicrobial therapy [9].

It is appropriate to place patients on low-dose antimicrobial prophylaxis following first UTI until an evaluation for VUR and hydronephrosis has been completed and/or treated. Most commonly, amoxicillin is used in neonates. After 2 months of age, children can be placed on either nitrofurantoin or trimethoprim–sulfamethoxazole. Fluoroquinolones are currently not approved for use in children, as tendon rupture and abnormal bone development have been reported [10].

Vesicoureteral reflux

Classification and general information

VUR occurs when urine in the bladder flows retrograde into the upper urinary tracts toward the kidney(s). Infected urine can cause renal scarring and renal insufficiency. The incidence of scarring is related to the grade of reflux. Sterile reflux of urine does not cause renal scarring after birth. However, antenatal reflux of urine can lead to renal dysplasia [11]. The most common cause of pathologic antenatal hydronephrosis is VUR, and children with a diagnosis of persistent hydronephrosis after birth should undergo VCUG to determine if VUR is present [12].

VUR is diagnosed by the visualization of contrast in the upper urinary tracts on VCUG and is graded as follows:

Grade I: distal segment of the ureter is visualized

Grade II: reflux is visualized in the renal calices without evidence of dilation

Grade III: mild dilation or blunting of the renal calices

Grade IV: dilated ureter and marked distention of the renal pelves and calices

Grade V: severe tortuosity of the ureter and distention of the calices and pelves

Epidemiology

VUR affects 1–5% of all children [13]. The age of onset correlates to age of toilet training. VUR is present in 32% of affected individuals' siblings [14]. Among daughters of affected females, 50% will have VUR [15]. While males are more commonly found to have VUR secondary to antenatal hydronephrosis, the incidence of VUR is nearly four times higher in females among those diagnosed after a UTI [16]. VUR is found in 40% of children diagnosed with pyelonephritis and 70% of infants diagnosed with UTI [17]. VUR is more prevalent among Caucasians compared with African Americans.

Etiology

VUR is often secondary to a short intramural tunnel length as the ureter enters the bladder. Normal filling of the bladder causes mechanical compression of this tunnel, thus preventing reflux. If the tunnel length is too short or abnormally positioned, VUR may occur.

Secondary VUR occurs by increased intravesical pressure from obstruction or inability to empty the bladder. Treatment involves relief of the intravesical pressure.

Renal scarring may occur in as much as 60% of patients with UTI and VUR. Higher-grade reflux increases the likelihood of renal scarring. By-products of inflammation during infection result in local ischemic changes direct tissue injury. If scarring is not present by the age of 6 years, the risk of future scarring is significantly less. It is important to note that renal scarring is the most common cause of pediatric hypertension [18].

Diagnosis

Most commonly, VUR is diagnosed after the finding of antenatal hydronephrosis or UTI. However, careful history may also elicit other findings commonly associated with VUR, such as dysfunctional voiding, constipation, fevers without diagnosis, and flank pain.

Physical examination may reveal hypertension or below-average height and weight secondary to renal scarring. Other findings include abdominal mass and unrecognized neurological disease, such as sacral depression or abnormal perineal sensation and/or reflexes.

Urinalysis should be obtained in any patient suspected of having UTI, VUR, or voiding dysfunction. Pyuria and nitrites are indicators of infection and culture should be obtained. Proteinuria may be a sign of renal damage. Rarely, serum creatinine can be elevated in those children with profound renal damage.

All children with a history of antenatal hydronephrosis or UTI should undergo both renal ultrasonography and VCUG. However, VCUG may be traumatic for patients and requires radiation. The decision to obtain a VCUG should be individualized for each patient and his or her family. The diagnosis of VUR can only be made after a VCUG is obtained in suspected individuals. A nuclear cystogram can be used to make the diagnosis; however, grading is only possible with VCUG. Ultrasonography is useful only to diagnose hydronephrosis and conspicuous renal abnormalities. Suspicion of scarring can be diagnosed with a DMSA renogram.

Treatment

Goals in the treatment of VUR include prevention of UTI and renal scarring. Oftentimes, VUR will resolve spontaneously. Generally, higher grade and advanced age at diagnosis portend poorer resolution rates compared to those who are diagnosed at an earlier age or with lower grades of reflux. VUR in males is also more likely to resolve compared to females. VUR is closely related to bladder and bowel dysfunction. Those without bladder and bowel dysfunction or those who have been successfully treated also have a greater chance of spontaneous resolution.

All children diagnosed with VUR should be placed on antimicrobial prophylaxis until resolution of VUR, surgical treatment, or among children of advanced age who have no evidence of UTIs, renal scarring, or bladder and bowel dysfunction. Antimicrobial prophylaxis is effective in lowering the occurrence of febrile UTIs among children with VUR. Infants can be safely placed on amoxicillin until 2 months of age. At that time, either nitrofurantoin or trimethoprim–sulfamethoxazole can be used with equal effectiveness. The choice of antimicrobial may depend upon the patient's allergies, tolerance, side effects, resistance, and cost. While other antimicrobials have been used successfully as prophylaxis, it should be noted that nitrofurantoin is the only antimicrobial agent that does not lead to increased resistance among uropathogens.

Surgical management is another treatment option and represents definitive treatment. Indications include breakthrough infections while on antimicrobial prophylaxis, lack of compliance, failure of VUR to resolve spontaneously with time, high-grade reflux with renal scarring or renal insufficiency, and parental preference. The success rates of surgical correction are high. Traditionally, ureteroneocystostomy (UNC) or "ureteral reimplant" is performed either through an intravesical or extravesical approach. The principle of UNC is to ensure that the ureter passes through the bladder wall with a length-to-diameter ratio of at least 5:1. Success rates are roughly 98% with this method [13]. The procedure can also be accomplished with laparoscopy or robotic assistance in experienced hands. UNC usually requires hospitalization and urinary catheter following surgery. While the procedure is usually well tolerated, complications may occur along with prolonged hospitalization and patient discomfort.

A less-invasive form of surgical treatment has been used successfully in patients with VUR. Subureteric injection of a bulking agent can be accomplished endoscopically with minimal morbidity and can be performed as an outpatient. The principle of the procedure is to inject a bulking agent under the mucosa of the ureteral orifice to improve coaptation. Success rates range from 65% to 90% [19]. Generally, it is less effective with higher grades of reflux. Agents used for this procedure include dextranomer/hyaluronic acid, collagen, Teflon, and silicone microspheres.

Treatment of VUR should be individualized for each patient. Most young patients with low-grade reflux can be observed or maintained on antimicrobial prophylaxis until resolution of reflux. Children who are older with high-grade reflux usually will require definitive surgical correction of the reflux. Any child with breakthrough UTIs or new renal scarring should also undergo surgical correction.

Voiding dysfunction

Introduction

The physiology and dynamics of normal bladder behavior during development is very complex. Much of the micturition cycle depends upon intact neural pathways that develop antenatally. Coordination of the spinal reflexes, bladder, and urethral sphincter make normal bladder storage and emptying possible. While voiding dysfunction can be secondary to neurological abnormality, it may also be present without any identifiable neurologic abnormality. This chapter will focus on the nonneuropathic voiding dysfunction in children.

After birth, bladder development continues into childhood. Micturition frequency is often as much as 15–20 times per day among newborns. As the bladder grows, micturition frequency decreases until the child is toilet trained. The bladder capacity can be estimated by a child's age as follows: volume (in ounces) = age of the child (in years) + 2. By 5 years of age, 90–95% of children are dry during the day and 80–85% are dry at night [20].

Pediatric urinary incontinence

By 12 years of age, 99% of children are dry during the day and night. Urinary incontinence may be a sign of infection, stress in the home, abuse, or dysfunctional elimination syndrome (DES) [21]. It is important to evaluate patients who present with incontinence for both psychosocial and neurologic abnormalities. Patterns of incontinence (i.e., stress, urge, continuous, nocturnal, diurnal, etc.) should also be noted. It is important to assess each child for constipation and history of toilet training. Initial evaluation should include urinalysis and culture. Urodynamics should be considered. If an anatomical abnormality is suspected (i.e., urethral stricture, ectopic ureter, etc.), a VCUG or cystoscopy may be warranted.

Treatment should be aimed at reinforcing normal voiding habits. Treatment will be dictated by the type of incontinence and findings during evaluation. Continuous incontinence in a female suggests ectopic ureter and should be treated appropriately. Postmicturition incontinence may be a consequence of labial adhesions. Giggle incontinence occurs only during periods of heavy laughter, is more common in females, and usually resolves spontaneously [22]. Timed voiding, biofeedback, and anticholinergics are the options.

Dysfunctional elimination syndrome

Several different conditions that were previously treated as separate diseases are now felt to be all part of a spectrum of conditions involving both the urinary and gastrointestinal tracts. The etiology and mechanism for DES is largely unknown. Severe cases can lead to profound bladder dysfunction (i.e., Hinman syndrome, voluntary detrusor sphincter dyssynergia, etc.). Urodynamics may show overactive detrusor contractions with an obvious neurologic cause. A large "dumbbell-shaped" bladder or a "spinning top" urethra may be seen on radiographic evaluation. Hydronephrosis and secondary VUR may also occur. Typically, a history of constipation, poor fluid intake, and UTIs are common among patients with DES. Other variations of DES may exist [23].

Treatment may take months to years in some patients. The focus of treatment should be on timed voiding and relief of constipation. Discomfort experienced during elimination can negatively impact a child's ability to voluntarily empty his or her bladder and bowels. Biofeedback is also effective in teaching children how to relax their pelvic floor muscles. Anticholinergics and clean intermittent catheterization may be utilized in severe cases. It is also important to provide antimicrobial prophylaxis for any child with a diagnosis of VUR. However, surgery should not be considered until DES has been effectively or maximally treated. Children with DES and VUR are more prone to developing breakthrough UTIs compared to those without DES [24].

Nocturnal enuresis

Nocturnal enuresis (NE) affects 15–20% of 5-year-old children. The prevalence of NE decreases at a rate of 15% per year such that only 1% of 15-year-olds are affected. Among children with NE, 75% have primary NE (never were dry) [25]. The risk of developing NE is substantially increased among the offspring of parents with a history of NE. The pathogenesis of NE is poorly understood. Some have suggested that is associated with developmental delay, sleep disorders, and psychological stress. NE may also be associated with lower serum vasopressin levels compared to those without NE.

After a detailed history and physical examination, children are initially treated with behavioral modification. Motivational techniques and alarms have been used successfully, especially in older children [26]. Desmopression (DDAVP) may be given as a nasal spray or oral tablet to decrease urine output and increase urine osmolality at night. A potential dangerous side effect of the medication is hyponatremia; patients on therapy should be monitored with periodic serum sodium measurements. DDAVP is successful 60% of the time and is more effective when used in combination with behavioral therapy. It should be noted that DDAVP only treats the symptoms of DDAVP. Once the therapy is stopped, relapse is almost inevitable. Imipramine is another medication that has been used with varied levels of success.

WHAT TO AVOID/KEY PITFALLS

- Urinalysis and cultures from bag specimens are unreliable and should only be used to rule out UTI.
- VUR may or may not be seen with hydronephrosis. It is important to rule out VUR with a VCUG in any child with a febrile UTI or repeated UTIs.
- VUR may resolve spontaneously. It is appropriate to observe infants diagnosed with high-grade VUR who do not have evidence of renal scarring or breakthrough infections.
- Dysfunctional elimination may be present in those with VUR. Do not recommend surgical correction of VUR before attempting to treat constipation and dysfunctional elimination.
- When treating NE with DDAVP, it is important to monitor serum sodium. Hyponatremia is a potential dangerous side effect of the medication.

KEY WEB LINKS

Clinical Practice Guideline for the Diagnosis and Management of the Initial UTI in Febrile Infants and Children 2–24 Months
http://aappolicy.aappublications.org/cgi/reprint/pediatrics;128/3/595.pdf–

Guidelines on the Management of Vesicoureteral Reflux in Children from the American Urological Association
http://www.auanet.org/content/guidelines-and-quality-care/clinical-guidelines/main-reports/vesi_reflux.pdf

Clinical Practice Guideline on the Evaluation and Treatment of Constipation in Infants and Children from the North American Society for Pediatric Gastroenterology, Hepatology, and Nutrition
http://www.naspghan.org/user-assets/Documents/pdf/PositionPapers/constipation.guideline.2006.pdf

CASE STUDY

An 18-month-old female presents to the office after an episode of febrile UTI. The mother reports that her child had a decreased appetite and was fussy for a period of 36 hours when her temperature was recorded to be as high as 40.1°C. She took her child to the emergency department. Serum electrolytes and creatinine were normal. A bagged urine culture was positive for *E. coli*, and she was started on a course of cephalexin. The child became well within 24 hours of starting the medication.

The child's mother had no prenatal care. She does report a history of UTIs during her teenage years. The mother states that her daughter is not toilet trained, and often cries when her diaper is soiled. Examination reveals a healthy baby with a height and weight appropriate for her age. Some stool is felt in the left abdominal area. Office urinalysis is negative. An ultrasonogram performed in the office reveals grade II hydronephrosis on left and grade I hydronephrosis on the right.

A VCUG is performed a day later. Bilateral grade III VUR is visualized. A discussion regarding all treatment options ensues.

Multiple choice questions

1 The mother chooses to observe her child. The next step in the treatment of her child is

a DMSA renogram
b Repeat VCUG in 6 months
c Clean intermittent catheterization
d Antimicrobial prophylaxis
e Colonic enema

2 The likelihood that her 3-year-old brother also has VUR is

a 15%
b 32%
c 50%
d 70%
e 92%

3 Resolution or improvement in her VUR may be achieved by

a A high-fiber diet and stool softeners
b Increasing the frequency of her diaper changes
c Cranberry juice
d Anticholinergics
e Increasing the dose of her antimicrobial prophylaxis

References

1 Circumcision policy statement. American Academy of Pediatrics. Task Force on Circumcision. *Pediatrics* 1999;103:686–693.

2 Rushton HG. Urinary tract infections in children. Epidemiology, evaluation, and management. *Pediatr Clin North Am* 1997;44:1133–1169.

3 Hoban DJ, Nicolle LE, Hawser S, Bouchillon S, Badal R. Antimicrobial susceptibility of global inpatient urinary tract isolates of Escherichia coli: results from the Study for Monitoring Antimicrobial Resistance Trends (SMART) program: 2009-2010. *Diagn Microbiol Infect Dis* 2011;70:507–511.

4 Coulthard MG, Nelson A, Smith T, Perry JD. Point-of-care diagnostic tests for childhood urinary-tract infection: phase-contrast microscopy for bacteria, stick testing, and counting white blood cells. *J Clin Pathol* 2010;63:823–829.

5 Majd M, Rushton HG, Jantausch B, Wiedermann BL. Relationship among vesicoureteral reflux, P-fimbriated Escherichia coli, and acute pyelonephritis in children with febrile urinary tract infection. *J Pediatr* 1991;119:578–585.

6 Chen JJ, Mao W, Homayoon K, Steinhardt GF. A multivariate analysis of dysfunctional elimination syndrome, and its relationships with gender, urinary tract infection and vesicoureteral reflux in children. *J Urol* 2004;171:1907–1910.

7 Bhat RG, Katy TA, Place FC. Pediatric urinary tract infections. *Emerg Med Clin North Am* 2011;29: 637–653.

8 Ansari Gilani K, Modaresi Esfeh J, Gholamrezanezhad A, et al. Predictors of abnormal renal cortical scintigraphy in children with first urinary tract infection: the importance of time factor. *Int Urol Nephrol* 2010;42: 1041–1047.

9 Tullus K. Difficulties in diagnosing urinary tract infections in small children. *Pediatr Nephrol* 2011;26: 1923–1926.

10 Noel GJ, Bradley JS, Kauffman RE, et al. Comparative safety profile of levofloxacin in 2523 children with a focus on four specific musculoskeletal disorders. *Pediatr Infect Dis J* 2007;26:879–891.

11 Peters C, Rushton HG. Vesicoureteral reflux associated renal damage: congenital reflux nephropathy and acquired renal scarring. *J Urol* 2010;184:265–273.
12 Massanyi EZ, McMahon DR. Hydronephrosis, obstructive uropathy, and multicystic dysplastic kidney. In: Chand DH, editor. *Clinician's Manual of Pediatric Nephrology*. 1st ed. Hackensack, NJ: World Scientific Publishing; 2011. pp. 687–702.
13 Elder JS, Peters CA, Arant BS, Jr., et al. Pediatric Vesicoureteral Reflux Guidelines Panel summary report on the management of primary vesicoureteral reflux in children. *J Urol* 1997;157:1846–1851.
14 Hollowell JG, Greenfield SP. Screening siblings for vesicoureteral reflux. *J Urol* 2002;168:2138–2141.
15 Noe HN, Wyatt RJ, Peeden JN, Jr., Rivas ML. The transmission of vesicoureteral reflux from parent to child. *J Urol* 1992;148:1869–1871.
16 Farhat W, McLorie G, Geary D, et al. The natural history of neonatal vesicoureteral reflux associated with antenatal hydronephrosis. *J Urol* 2000;164:1057–1060.
17 Fanos V, Cataldi L. Antibiotics or surgery for vesicoureteric reflux in children. *Lancet* 2004;364:1720–1722.
18 Dillon MJ. Recent advances in evaluation and management of childhood hypertension. *Eur J Pediatr* 1979;132:133–139.
19 Kirsch AJ, Perez-Brayfield MR, Scherz HC. Minimally invasive treatment of vesicoureteral reflux with endoscopic injection of dextranomer/hyaluronic acid copolymer: The Children's Hospitals of Atlanta experience. *J Urol* 2003;170:211–215.
20 Fergusson DM, Horwood LJ, Shannon FT. Factors related to the age of attainment of nocturnal bladder control: an 8-year longitudinal study. *Pediatrics* 1986;78: 884–890.
21 von Gontard A, Baeyens D, Van Hoecke E, Warzak WJ, Bachmann C. Psychological and psychiatric issues in urinary and fecal incontinence. *J Urol* 2011;185: 1432–1436.
22 Chandra M, Saharia R, Shi Q, Hill V. Giggle incontinence in children: a manifestation of detrusor instability. *J Urol* 2002;168:2184–2187.
23 Nijman RJ. Role of antimuscarinics in the treatment of nonneurogenic daytime urinary incontinence in children. *Urology* 2004;63:45–50.
24 Koff SA, Wagner TT, Jayanthi VR. The relationship among dysfunctional elimination syndromes, primary vesicoureteral reflux and urinary tract infections in children. *J Urol* 1998;160:1019–1022.
25 Forsythe WI, Redmond A. Enuresis and spontaneous cure rate. Study of 1129 enuretis. *Arch Dis Child* 1974;49:259–263.
26 Blum NJ. Nocturnal enuresis: behavioral treatments. *Urol Clin North Am* 2004;31:499–507.

Answers to multiple choice questions

1 d
2 b
3 a

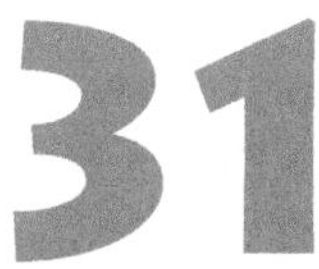

Pediatric genitourinary oncology

Eric Z. Massanyi

The James Buchanan Brady Urological Institute and Department of Urology, The Johns Hopkins School of Medicine, Baltimore, MD, USA

KEY POINTS

- Wilms' tumor (WT) is easily recognized histologically by its classic triphasic pattern of epithelial, stromal, and blastemal elements.
- WT is associated with allelic heterogeneity of 11p.
- WT rarely crosses the midline.
- Congenital mesoblastic nephroma is the most common renal tumor among infants and its course is usually benign.
- Any patient suspected of having neuroblastoma should undergo a bone marrow biopsy to evaluate for metastatic disease.
- Children with testicular masses that have normal levels of alpha-fetoprotein (AFP), no signs of metastasis, and pathology-proven teratoma may undergo testis-sparing excision of their tumors.
- Rhabdomyosarcomas are treated with surgery followed by adjuvant chemotherapy. Alveolar variants have a poor prognosis.

Wilms' tumor (Nephroblastoma)

Epidemiology

Representing 80% of genitourinary tumors of children younger than 5 years, Wilms' tumor (WT) is the most common genitourinary tumor of childhood [1]. The incidence is 8 per 1,000,000. Three hundred and fifty new cases are diagnosed each year in the United States. Males and females are affected equally. The tumor seems to have a higher incidence among African Americans compared with Caucasians and Asians. The majority of tumors are solitary; however, 5% are bilateral and 12% are multifocal. Twenty percent of affected children have a family history of other genitourinary malignancies [2].

Associated anomalies

WT is associated with aniridia. Aniridia has an overall incidence of 1 in 50,000. The incidence of aniridia among patients with a WT is 1 in 70. Approximately one-third of patients with aniridia will develop a WT.

WAGR syndrome represents a collection of conditions including WT, aniridia, genitourinary anomalies, and mental retardation. It is associated with deletions of 11p13. Other congenital anomalies may be seen, including ear deformities, hernias, hypospadias, cryptorchidism, and ambiguous genitalia [3].

WT is also associated with hemihypertrophy. Hemihypertrophy has an overall incidence of 1 in 14,000. Among patients with WT, the incidence is 1 in 32. Hemihypertrophy is also associated with embryonal carcinoma, pigmented nevi, and hemangiomas [4].

Beckwith–Wiedemann syndrome is characterized by patients with hemihypertrophy, macroglossia, and other congenital anomalies, including mental retardation, microcephaly, visceromegaly, and omphalocele. It is associated with 11p15 deletions. WT is seen in 4–10% of patients with Beckwith–Wiedemann syndrome [5].

Handbook of Urology, First edition. J. Kellogg Parsons, John B. Eifler and Misop Han.
Published 2014 by John Wiley & Sons, Ltd.

Denys–Drash syndrome is also associated with WT and 11p13 deletions. These patients may have ambiguous genitalia, renal mesangial sclerosis, and end-stage renal disease [6].

Histopathology

Gross specimens are usually surrounded by a pseudocapsule. The histology in 90% of WT reveals a triphasic pattern of three tissue types: epithelial, blastemal, and stromal. This is known as "favorable" type histology and carries a good prognosis. About 5–10% of patients are diagnosed with the anaplastic variant, which portends a very poor prognosis and accounts for 50% of deaths from WT. Clear cell or rhabdoid histologies can also be seen.

A nephrogenic rest is a focus of abnormally persistent nephrogenic blastemal cells that can develop into WT. In clusters, they are histologically identical to WT and are termed nephroblastomatosis. One percent of patients without WT are found to have nephroblastomatosis at autopsy. However, 45% of patients with unilateral and 100% of patients with bilateral WT are found to have these entities at autopsy [7].

Genetics

WT is associated with allelic heterogeneity of 11p. The following loci are felt to be important in the pathogenesis of WT. *WT1* is located on 11p13, and *WT2* is located on 11p15. 16q has also been implicated. Despite recent advances in our understanding of the genetics associated with WT, only 10% of sporadic cases have an identified genetic defect [8].

Presentation

The presentation of WT is usually that of a healthy-appearing child with a palpable abdominal mass. It rarely crosses the midline. Hematuria is rare and usually only microscopic. Other congenital anomalies may be seen in approximately 15% of patients at the time of diagnosis. Renin-mediated hypertension may also be present.

Evaluation

Diagnostic imaging is warranted in any child with a palpable abdominal mass. Ultrasonography is useful for imaging the kidneys and vena cava. Computerized tomography can aid in the evaluation of smaller tumors, liver lesions, or lymph nodes. Magnetic resonance imaging is also useful for evaluating vascular structures.

Staging

In the United States, staging is completed after surgical resection, if possible. The European staging is based on imaging studies [9]. Stage I tumors include those that are completely resected with no gross spillage or residual tumor. Stage II indicates a focus of regional spread either in the form of a positive surgical margin, gross spillage, or extrarenal vascular tumor thrombus. Stage III indicates incomplete resection or unresectable tumor, large tumor spill, or positive lymph nodes. Stage IV indicates distant metastases. Stage V indicates synchronous bilateral tumors. Prognosis is based on histology and stage [10, 11] (Table 31.1).

Treatment

Treatment in the United States is based on the National Wilms' Tumor Study Group (NWTSG) protocol. Patients younger than 2 years with Stage I tumors less than 550 g should undergo a nephrectomy followed by observation. Among children aged 2 years and older, those with Stage I and II tumors with favorable histology should undergo a nephrectomy followed by chemotherapy. Patients with anaplastic histology or Stages III and IV tumors should undergo nephrectomy, followed by radiation and chemotherapy. Patients with bilateral tumors (Stage V) should undergo

Table 31.1 Wilms' tumor prognosis by stage

Stage	Histology	Survival (%)
I	Favorable	98.7
	Unfavorable	82.6
II	Favorable	93.8
	Unfavorable	81.2
III	Favorable	93.0
	Unfavorable	72.0
IV	Favorable	89.5
	Unfavorable	55.9

biopsy, followed by chemotherapy. Reassessment of the child after chemotherapy is necessary to dictate further treatment [9].

Classically, patients undergo a chevron or midline incision so that the contralateral kidney can be evaluated. With modern imaging, exploration of the contralateral kidney may not be necessary. Partial nephrectomy should be considered in any child with renal insufficiency, bilateral tumors, or solitary kidney. Lymph node sampling is needed for proper staging [9].

In the United States, neoadjuvant chemotherapy is administered to patients with bilateral tumors, solitary kidney, tumors with major vascular involvement, or if the tumor is felt to be unresectable [1]. Neoadjuvant chemotherapy has been shown to decrease intraoperative morbidity but has no effect on long-term survival [12].

Other renal tumors

Congenital mesoblastic nephroma

Congenital mesoblastic nephroma is the most common renal tumor among infants. The mean age at diagnosis is 3.5 months. Histologically, it is characterized by a solitary hamartoma which infiltrates the renal stoma. These tumors are found more commonly in males and are almost always unilateral. Treatment is nephrectomy and course is almost universally benign [13].

Multilocular cystic nephroma

Multilocular cystic nephroma is an uncommon benign renal tumor. Fifty percent occur in young children, and fifty percent occur in young adult women. Among children, it is more common among males. Surgical resection is curative. Recurrence is possible with incomplete resection [13].

Clear cell sarcoma

Clear cell sarcoma is a highly malignant tumor that is diagnosed at a mean age of 3.5 years. Histology reveals polygonal cells with round oval nuclei [14]. Improved prognosis is seen with lower stage, earlier age at diagnosis, absence of tumor necrosis, and treatment with doxorubicin [15]. Long-term follow-up is needed as over 30% of relapses occur 3 years or more after treatment. Clear cell sarcomas are associated with brain and bone metastases. The mainstay of treatment is radiation and chemotherapy. Overall survival is poor [13].

Rhabdoid tumor

Rhabdoid tumors are the most aggressive and lethal renal tumors of childhood. The median age at diagnosis is 16 months. Rhabdoid tumors of the kidney may present as WTs. Metastases may occur anywhere in the abdomen, lungs, or brain [16]. Treatment consists of radiation and chemotherapy. Prognosis is extremely poor.

Neuroblastoma

Epidemiology

Neuroblastoma is the most common malignant tumor of infancy and second most common solid tumor of childhood. Most cases are diagnosed in children younger than 4 years. Children who are diagnosed at the age younger than 1 year tend to have a better outcome. The incidence is higher among those with Type I neurofibromatosis, Hirschsprung's disease, and Turner syndrome. There appears to be a slightly higher incidence among males. Most tumors are found in the abdomen. Among abdominal neuroblastomas, approximately two-thirds are adrenal in origin. Patients with adrenal neuroblastomas have a better prognosis than those with extra-adrenal tumors [17].

Genetics

Neuroblastoma may be hereditary or sporadic. Deletion in chromosome 1p with loss of heterozygosity is associated with a poor prognosis. N-myc oncogene amplification is associated with advanced stages of disease, rapid progression, and poor prognosis. Deletions in 11q or 14q may also be seen in 25–50% of cases [18].

Pathology

The tumor arises from neural crest cells. Masses are usually highly vascular and appear grossly purple. Small, round blue cells are seen microscopically. Prognosis is determined by the Shimada histological grading system.

Presentation

The typical presentation of a neuroblastoma is that of a child with a firm and irregular mass that may cross the midline. Seventy percent of patients present with synchronous metastases. Subcutaneous nodules, liver lesions, and bone lesions are common locations of metastases. Neuroblastomas may secrete catecholamines. Increased catecholamine release can cause hypertension, flushing, and palpitations.

Diagnosis

The first step in the diagnostic evaluation of a child with a suspected neuroblastoma is bone marrow aspirate, which proves to be positive 70% of the time. A 24-hour urine collection for vanillylmandelic acid (VMA) may aid in diagnosis as approximately 90% of patients with neuroblastoma have elevated levels of catecholamines. Additional imaging may be necessary. Computerized tomography usually reveals speckled calcifications in a suprarenal mass. Magnetic resonance imaging aids in the diagnosis of vascular and bone involvement. An MIBG scan can be used for equivocal cases and help with staging.

The International Neuroblastoma Staging System is used to stage tumors proven to be neuroblastoma. Stage 1 tumors are localized and with complete resection. Stage 2a tumors are localized tumors without complete gross resection and negative lymph nodes. Stage 2b implies ipsilateral positive lymph nodes and contralateral negative lymph nodes. Stage 3 tumors are unresectable or contain contralateral positive lymph nodes. Stage 4 is given to those with distant metastases. Stage 4S is reserved for children younger than 1 year with Stage 1 or 2 tumors with spread to skin, liver, or bone marrow. Patients with Stage 4S have a better prognosis and often undergo spontaneous regression [19].

Treatment

Surgery is the mainstay of treatment in most cases. Recently, organ-sparing surgery has been advocated. Adjuvant radiation and/or chemotherapy may be given if there is an evidence of residual tumor. Neoadjuvant chemotherapy may be given in cases of unresectable tumors or those with respiratory and bowel compromise. Radiation is not curative. It is primarily used for palliation of metastases or residual masses. Rarely, bone marrow transplant may be given to those after chemotherapy and total body irradiation [20].

Testicular tumors

Epidemiology

The incidence of testicular tumors in children is approximately 2 to 3 per 1,000,000 annually. Testicular tumors represent nearly 2% of all pediatric neoplasms. The majority of tumors present in patients younger than 2 years. Yolk sac tumors were thought to be the most common variant; however, many now believe that teratoma is the most common etiology of testicular tumors in children [21].

Teratoma

Teratomas are usually well-differentiated testicular tumors in children. The tumor can be considered benign in children younger than 2 years. Ultrasononographic appearance usually reveals a heterogeneous mass with internal echoes. As with other benign lesions of the testes, patients with pathology-proven teratoma can undergo testis-sparing surgical excision if adjacent testicular parenchyma is prepubertal [22].

Yolk sac tumor

Yolk sac tumors are the second most common testicular tumors. These occur primarily in infants. More than 90% of those diagnosed with yolk sac tumors will have elevated alpha-fetoprotein (AFP). The tumors appear pale gray, encapsulated, and well-circumscribed grossly. Microscopically, Schiller–Duval bodies may be seen. Presentation is usually that of a painless scrotal mass. More than 90% of lesions are localized to the testis upon presentation. However, the tumor can metastasize. The most common site of metastasis is the lung. Unlike adults, spread is usually hematogenous. Therefore, routine lymph node dissection is not necessary. Platinum-based chemotherapy is the treatment of choice for metastatic disease. An orchiectomy should be performed in any child suspected of having a testicular tumor with elevation in AFP, metastasis, or pathology-proven yolk sac tumor. Enucleation or testis-sparing excision is not indicated in these settings. Orchiectomy is curative in the large majority of children with testicular tumors [21].

Leydig cell tumor

Leydig cell tumors are the most common gonadal stromal cell tumor. Others include Sertoli cell tumors and juvenile granulosa cell tumors. The peak incidence is approximately 4–5 years of age and accounts for 10% of precocious puberty in males younger than 9 years. The tumors are typically benign and unilateral. Leydig cell tumors typically secrete testosterone; however, elevation of corticosteroids, estrogen, or progesterone may also be seen. Androgen-secreting tumors are differentiated from primary pituitary lesions by low levels of follicle-stimulating hormone (FSH) and luteinizing hormone (LH) from feedback inhibition. Inguinal orchiectomy is usually curative with Leydig cell tumors or other stromal tumors of the testes [23].

Rhabdomyosarcoma

Epidemiology

Rhabdomyosarcoma is the most common soft tissue sarcoma of childhood. Twenty percent of rhabdomyosarcomas are found in the genitourinary tract. A bimodal incidence with peaks between 2–6 years and 15–19 years of age has been noted. However, they are mostly present early in life. It is associated with Li–Fraumeni syndrome and neurofibromatosis. Abnormalities of the 2q37 locus are thought to be important. Rhabdomyosarcomas tend to spread by local invasion. Hematogenous and lymphatic spread are also possible, but less common [24].

There are three pathologic variants: embryonal, pleomorphic, and alveolar. Embryonal comprises the majority of cases and typically occurs in younger children. Sarcoma botryoides resembles a "bunch of grapes" and represents the pleomorphic variant. The alveolar variant represents an anaplastic and undifferentiated variant with a poor prognosis. Spindle-cell variants also exist [25].

Presentation

The clinical presentation depends largely on the size and origin of the tumor. Urologic manifestations may include dysuria, hematuria, hydronephrosis, or abdominal mass. It may involve the bladder, prostate, paratesticular tissue, vagina, vulva, or uterus [26].

Diagnosis

Magnetic resonance imaging is the best imaging modality to assess and stage pelvic tumors. Computerized tomography and ultrasonography can also be used with less accuracy.

Staging is based on the TNM system. T1 tumors are confined and T2 tumors extend into adjacent organs. Nodes are either negative (N0), positive (N1), or unknown (Nx). Distant metastases are either not present (M0) or present (M1).

Treatment

Treatment begins with biopsy of the lesion and assessment of local extension. This is usually followed by adjuvant VAC-based chemotherapy. Radiation may be used in addition. Reassessment by the way of MRI is usually completed after chemotherapy. Further surgical resection may be necessary for patients with recurrence or incomplete response [27].

WHAT TO AVOID/KEY PITFALLS

- Patients diagnosed with bilateral WTs may suffer from chronic renal insufficiency if surgical resection is undertaken. These patients should undergo neoadjuvant chemotherapy in order to shrink tumor burden prior to surgical resection.
- Proper staging of WT depends on the status of the adjacent lymph nodes. Do not forget to obtain lymph nodes during resection or patient will be upstaged to Stage III.
- Neuroblastomas in children younger than 1 year have a good prognosis even with metastasis to the skin, liver, or bone marrow. These tumors may undergo spontaneous regression.
- Elevated levels of AFP may be seen in normal children up to 1 year of age.
- Rhabdomyosarcoma may recur after initial treatment with surgery and chemotherapy. Do not forget to reassess patients radiographically after the initial treatment is over.

KEY WEB LINKS

Information on those with 11p deletion/WAGR Syndrome and Wilms' Tumor
http://www.wagr.org/home.html

Treatment recommendations for neuroblastoma by the National Cancer Institute
http://www.cancer.gov/cancertopics/pdq/treatment/neuroblastoma/HealthProfessional/page1

European Association of Urology's guidelines on testicular cancer
http://www.urosource.com/fileadmin/user_upload/Guidelines/22891_Testicular_Cancer.pdf

CASE STUDY

A 2-year-old male presents to your office with a left-sided palpable testicular mass that was discovered by his pediatrician during a well-child visit.

The child was born full term with bilateral descended testes. The child's medical history is otherwise unremarkable. Physical examination reveals a healthy, alert, and cooperative young boy with a soft abdomen and a visibly enlarged left hemiscrotum secondary to a palpable testicular mass.

An ultrasonogram revealed a 12-mm well-circumscribed intratesticular mass with internal echoes. A serum AFP was found obtained and found to be 6 ng/mL (normal).

Multiple choice questions

1 The most likely diagnosis in this patient is
- a Hydrocele
- b Teratoma
- c Yolk sac tumor
- d Leydig cell tumor
- e Orchitis

2 The most likely place for a testicular neoplasm to metastasize among children of this age is
- a Brain
- b Liver
- c Retroperitoneal Lymph Nodes
- d Lungs
- e Kidney

3 All of the following findings would preclude the patient from undergoing a testis-sparing excision of his testicular mass *except*:
- a An elevated AFP
- b Yolk sac tumor on frozen section
- c Adjacent postpubertal testicular parenchyma
- d A solitary lung metastasis
- e Testicular microlithiasis

References

1 Ko EY, Ritchey ML. Current management of Wilms' tumor in children. *J Urol* 2009;5:56–65.

2 Wu HY, Snyder HM, 3rd, D'Angio GJ. Wilms' tumor management. *Curr Opin Urol* 2005;15:273–276.

3 Fischbach BV, Trout KL, Lewis J, Luis CA, Sika M. WAGR syndrome: a clinical review of 54 cases. *Pediatrics* 2005;116:984–988.

4 Abraham P. What is the risk of cancer in a child with hemihypertrophy? *Arch Dis Child* 2005;90:1312–1313.

5 Green DM, Breslow NE, Beckwith JB, Norkool P. Screening of children with hemihypertrophy, aniridia, and Beckwith-Wiedemann syndrome in patients with Wilms tumor: a report from the National Wilms Tumor Study. *Med Pediatr Oncol* 1993;21:188–192.

6 Niaudet P, Gubler MC. WT1 and glomerular diseases. *Pediatr Nephrol* 2006;21:1653–1660.

7 Kirsch AJ, Snyder HM. What's new and important in pediatric urologic oncology. *AUA Update Series* 1998;17:11.

8 Coppes MJ, Egeler RM. Genetics of Wilms' tumor. *Semin Urol Oncol* 1999;17:2–10.

9 de Kraker J, Graf N, van Tinteren H, et al. Reduction of postoperative chemotherapy in children with stage I intermediate-risk and anaplastic Wilms' tumour (SIOP 93-01 trial): a randomised controlled trial. *Lancet* 2004;364:1229–1235.

10 Dome JS, Cotton CA, Perlman EJ, et al. Treatment of anaplastic histology Wilms' tumor: results from the Fifth National Wilms' Tumor Study. *J Clin Oncol* 2006;24:2352–2358.

11 Metzger ML, Dome JS. Current therapy for Wilms' tumor. *Oncologist* 2005;10:815–826.

12 Zugor V, Schott GE, Lausen B, Kühn R, Labanaris AP. Clinical and surgical experience with Wilms' tumor. Long-term results of a single institution. *Anticancer Res* 2010;30:1735–1739.

13 Rithcey ML, Shamberger RC. Pediatric urologic oncology. In: Wein AJ, editor. *Campbell-Walsh Urology*. 9th ed. Philadelphia, PA: Saunders; 2007. pp. 3870–3906.

14 Schmidt D, Beckwith JB. Histopathology of childhood renal tumors. *Hematol Oncol Clin North Am* 1995;9:1179–1200.

15 Argani P, Perlman EJ, Breslow NE, et al. Clear cell sarcoma of the kidney: a review of 351 cases from the National Wilms' Tumor Study Group Pathology Center. *Am J Surg Pathol* 2000;24:4–18.

16 D'Angio GJ, Rosenberg H, Sharples K, Kelalis P, Breslow N, Green DM. Position paper. Imaging methods for primary renal tumors of childhood: cost versus benefits. *Med Pediatr Oncol* 1993;21:205–212.
17 Heck JE, Ritz B, Hung RJ, Hashibe M, Boffetta P. The epidemiology of neuroblastoma: a review. *Paediatr Perinat Epidemiol* 2009;23:125–143.
18 Tonini GP. Neuroblastoma: the result of multistep transformation? *Stem Cells* 1993;11:276–282.
19 Brisse HJ, McCarville MB, Granata C, et al. Guidelines for imaging and staging of neuroblastic tumors: consensus report from the International Neuroblastoma Risk Group Project. *Radiology* 2011;261:243–257.
20 Niethammer D, Handgretinger R. Clinical strategies for the treatment of neuroblastoma. *Eur J Cancer* 1995;31:568–571.
21 Bahrami A, Ro JY, Ayala AG. An overview of testicular germ cell tumors. *Arch Pathol Lab Med* 2007;131: 1267–1280.
22 Shukla AR, Woodard C, Carr MC, et al. Experience with testis sparing surgery for testicular teratoma. *J Urol* 2004;171:161–163.
23 Al-Agha OM, Axiotis CA. An in-depth look at Leydig cell tumor of the testis. *Arch Pathol Lab Med* 2007;131:311–317.
24 Wu HY, Snyder HM, 3rd, Womer RB. Genitourinary rhabdomyosarcoma: which treatment, how much, and when? *J Pediatr Urol* 2009;5:501–506.
25 Parham DM. Pathologic classification of rhabdomyosarcomas and correlations with molecular studies. *Mod Pathol* 2001;14:506–514.
26 Stehr M. Pediatric urologic rhabdomyosarcoma. *Curr Opin Urol* 2009;19:402–406.
27 Driscoll K, Isakoff M, Ferrer F. Update on pediatric genitourinary oncology. *Curr Opin Urol* 2007;17:281–286.

Answers to multiple choice questions

1 b
2 d
3 e

32 The exstrophy–epispadias complex

Kristina D. Suson
Pediatric Urology, Children's Hospital of Michigan, Detroit, MI, USA

KEY POINTS

- The defect of classic bladder exstrophy (CBE) includes an exposed bladder, vesicoureteral reflux, externally rotated pelvis, and genital abnormalities.
- Epispadias can range from a misplaced or widened urethra to one that is splayed to the bladder neck.
- Goals of reconstruction for CBE, epispadias, and cloacal exstrophy are renal preservation, continence, and functional and cosmetic genitalia.
- While some children will become dry with closure or bladder neck reconstruction, others will require continent urinary diversion.
- Long-term concerns include bladder cancer, urolithiasis, or metabolic consequences from bladder augmentation.

CASE STUDY

A full-term infant with a prenatal diagnosis of bladder exstrophy is born via spontaneous vaginal delivery. On evaluation, there are no palpable gonads and a vaginal orifice is visualized. On initial evaluation, her bladder seems large but polypoid. The umbilical clamp is removed after tying it with two 0 silk sutures (Figure 32.1). An ultrasound of her spine reveals no abnormalities. A pelvic X-ray reveals a 3.5 cm pubic diastasis (Figure 32.2). She is taken to the operating room on the second day of life for examination under anesthesia, with hopes of closing her bladder without osteotomies. Her bladder is not pliable enough to close without tension, thus you remove the polyps and plan for examination under anesthesia in 4 months.

Classic bladder exstrophy

Epidemiology

Classic bladder exstrophy (CBE) has an incidence of around 1:40,000 live births, roughly equivalent male:female. Risk factors include family history, advanced maternal age, Caucasian race, and *in vitro* fertilization [1].

Embryology

Failure or incomplete movement of lateral body wall folds toward the midline results in lack of fusion and an abdominal wall defect with protrusion of the bladder [2].

Handbook of Urology, First edition. J. Kellogg Parsons, John B. Eifler and Misop Han.
Published 2014 by John Wiley & Sons, Ltd.

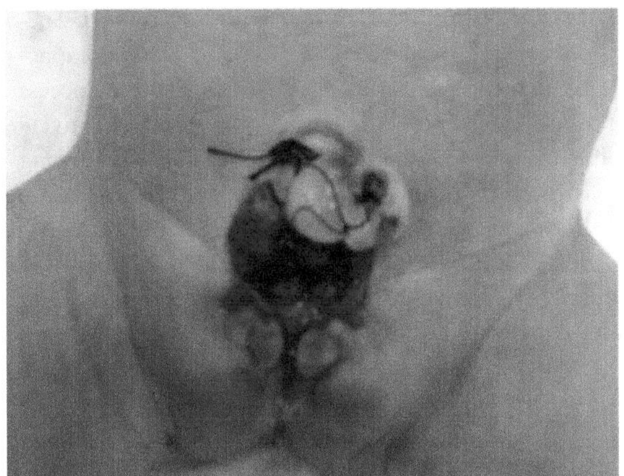

Plate 32.1 Exstrophy bladder

Anatomy

The defining feature of CBE is that the bladder opens to the abdominal wall (Figure 32.1). The size of the bladder template and potential presence of polyps impact surgical decision making. Lack of ureteral obliquity on entering the bladder leads to vesicoureteral reflux [1]. Concomitant renal anomalies are seen in 2.8% [3].

The genital structures are also affected. In males, the penis has shorter, wider corporal bodies with widely separated crural attachments secondary to pubic diastasis. There is prominent dorsal chordee and a shortened urethral groove [1, 4]. The testicles are frequently undescended. While of normal size, the prostate does not wrap around the urethra [1]. In females, the vagina is shorter [1], and uterine prolapse is common, especially without adequate pubic symphysis approximation [5].

Skeletal anomalies include an externally rotated pelvis with widened pubic diastasis (Figure 32.2). There is also an increased risk of spinal abnormalities and patellofemoral instability [6]. Concomitant colorectal anomalies, including imperforate anus, rectal stenosis, and rectal prolapse are seen in 1.8% [7]. In addition to the midline fascial defect [2], indirect inguinal hernias are common [1].

Prenatal diagnosis

The diagnosis of exstrophy can be made prenatally. Suggestive ultrasound findings include absence of the bladder, low umbilicus, widened pubic rami, small genitalia, and lower abdominal mass [1].

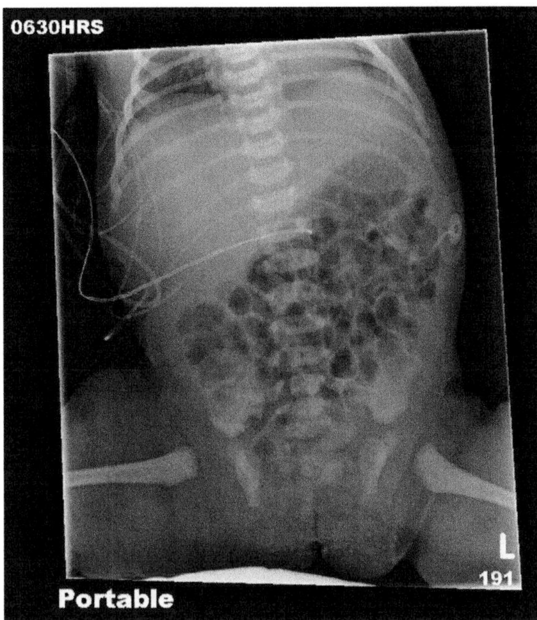

Figure 32.2 Plain film demonstrating widened pubic diastasis.

Management

After birth, a plain X-ray and renal ultrasound are obtained to assess the pubic diastasis and kidneys. The bladder is protected with saline irrigation and nonadherent plastic wrap until closure [1].

The goals of reconstruction are to secure abdominal closure, urinary continence, preservation of renal function, and functional and cosmetic external genitalia [1]. In the modern staged repair of exstrophy (MSRE), closure occurs at birth or when the bladder size permits. In males, the epispadias is repaired at 6–12 months of age. When the child desires continence and is willing to participate in a voiding/catheterizing program, bladder neck reconstruction (BNR) or diversion is performed [8]. Closure success rates of ≥95% [9, 10] and minimum 3-hour daytime dry periods in 72–96% of patients with BNR [11–14] are reported.

The complete primary repair of exstrophy (CPRE) includes BNR and epispadias repair at the time of closure [15]. Many patients will require additional procedures [16]. Closure success rates of 69–100% [17–19] and minimum 3-hour daytime dry periods in 19–78% of patients [16, 18] after closure and/or BNR are reported.

Radical soft tissue mobilization is an alternative three-stage procedure that avoids osteotomy. The ischial and pubic periosteum are elevated, mobilizing the attachments of the sphincter muscles and neurovascular structures, and wrapping them around the neourethra [20]. A closure success rate of 81% [20] and minimum 3-hour daytime dry periods in 35–37% of patients [20, 21] are reported.

Urologic complications of closure include failure (dehiscence, prolapse, vesicocutaneous fistula), posterior bladder outlet obstruction, urethrocutaneous fistula, premature tube/stent removal, and intrapubic stitch erosion [22].

Osteotomies may be used with MSRE or CPRE [6] and are recommended with closure after 72 hours or pubic diastasis >4 cm [23]. Types of osteotomies include posterior iliac, anterior iliac, combined anterior and posterior (horizontal and vertical), anterior pubic, posterior resection, and anterior diagonal. Nonabsorbable suture or internal hardware is typically used to reapproximate the symphysis. After surgery, modified Bryant's traction, external fixation with modified Buck's traction, spica casting, or mummy wraps may be used for immobilization [6].

Complications from osteotomy include urethral obstruction by suture/hardware, pelvic asymmetry, nerve palsies, osteotomy delayed or nonunion, gait abnormalities, leg length inequality, persistent pain, osteomyelitis, hardware migration, or skin erosions. Pin site infections, pressure ulcers, and compartment syndrome may result from immobilization [6, 22].

In the long term, osteotomies may not affect orthopedic outcomes positively or negatively. Pubic diastasis increases regardless of whether osteotomy was performed. Most children have normal activity/sports participation regardless of osteotomy, although osteotomy may decrease risk of later hip dysplasia and osteoarthritis [6].

Continence

Occasionally, continence may result from closure alone in MSRE or CPRE [14, 16]. Otherwise, BNR, sometimes with bladder augmentation (BA) and appendicovesicostomy, or continent urinary diversion with bladder neck transaction may be necessary [11]. Successful initial bladder closure [12] and bladder capacity of at least 100 mL [23] are critical to the success of BNR, while previous attempts at BNR negatively influence voided continence [14, 24]. Following BNR, there is an initial improvement over 1–2 years [13], although some authors suggest that continence is mostly achieved in adolescence [25]. Patients may experience bladder function deterioration and require later repeated reconstruction [14, 26].

Long-term complications

The relative risk of developing bladder cancer may be 700× and relative risk of death from cancer up to 65× that of general population. Some reconstructive approaches are linked to cancer risk. Procedures that store urine and stool concomitantly, like ureterosigmoidostomy, have long been associated with increased risk of malignancy [27]. BA is debated to increase risk, but other risk factors, including exstrophy, tobacco, or immunosuppression are probable confounders and augmentation is unlikely to further increase the risk [28].

Urolithiasis is another long-term complication. BA, BNR, cloacal exstrophy [29], and catheterizing through a continent stoma [30] increase the risk, as do risks present in the general population, such as urinary tract infection, foreign body, and urinary stasis [29]. Recurrence rates of nearly 40% have been reported, typically associated with urinary tract infection and struvite stones [29]. Reservoir stones may be prevented with irrigation protocols that include normal saline and/or antibiotic solutions [30].

There can be significant metabolic sequelae to BA. Metabolic acidosis can cause fatigue, anorexia, weight loss, polydipsia, and lethargy. Treatment options include sodium bicarbonate, sodium citrate, or citric acid solutions, ± for bone loss. There may be decreased linear growth. Bone demineralization and osteomalacia are treated with calcium and vitamin D. Patients with gastric segment reconstruction are at risk of dehydration and metabolic alkalosis. Those with an ileal augment could develop vitamin B12 deficiency, with megaloblastic anemia and neurologic damage, if there was excessive terminal ileal resection. This is treated or prevented with monthly intramuscular B12 injections [31]. Hypokalemia and hyperammonemia syndrome are also reported [31].

Penile loss of the corporal bodies and/or glans is a potentially devastating consequence. Most reported cases occur in patients undergoing radical soft tissue mobilization or CPRE [32–34]. It is caused by penile ischemia at the time of closure or epispadias repair with damage to the pudendal or accessory vessels, or vessel compression by pubic apposition [32].

Epispadias

Definition

In males, epispadias can range from dorsal malpositioning of the urethra on the glans with an intact sphincter to a penopubic defect with a splayed sphincter and incontinence [23]. Patients with distal glans epispadias may have an abnormal bladder neck and posterior urethra with incontinence despite a seemingly complete urethra [35]. The penile deformity includes dorsal chordee and penile shortening [23].

Epidemiology

Epispadias occurs at an incidence of 1:117,000; 70% of cases are complete epispadias with incontinence [23].

Associated anomalies

A widened pubic diastasis and vesicoureteral reflux are frequently identified [23].

Management

Continence with preservation of upper tracts and functional and cosmetic penile reconstruction are the reconstructive goals [23]. The staged approach includes early urethroplasty, followed by BNR for continence [23].

One reconstructive option is the modified Cantwell–Ransley epispadias repair. The urethral plate is dissected off of the corpora proximally but remains in continuity with the distal glans. The urethra is tubularized, and the corporal bodies are rotated medially over the urethra [1]. In complete penile disassembly, another option, the urethral plate is completely separated from each hemicorpus and hemiglans, and the corporeal glanular bodies are separated from each other. The urethral plate is tubularized and brought ventral to the corporal bodies. Following penile straightening, if the meatus does not reach the glans, it is matured to the ventral aspect of penis, creating a hypospadiac meatus. Finally, the glansplasty is completed [36]. For both options, surgical complications include urethral fistula, stenosis, residual penile curvature, and persistent incontinence [37].

With epispadias, adequate bladder capacity is the major predictor of voiding continence [23]. Urethroplasty before 12 months of age may enable higher bladder capacities, while urethroplasty after 29 months of age may negatively impact bladder growth [38].

Outcomes

Over 70% of patients achieve continence [23, 39]. Penile reconstruction enables most patients to achieve straight penis with normal erectile function, with ~80% of those patients reporting satisfactory intercourse [23].

Female epispadias

Female epispadias is rare, with an incidence of around 2:1,000,000 [23]. The urethra may be patulous, split dorsally along most of the urethra, or split along the entire urethra including a gap in the sphincter. There is a bifid clitoris, depressed mons with nonhair-bearing skin, and diminutive labia minora with little to no clitoral hood [23]. Vesicoureteral reflux is common, as is a widened pubic diastasis [23].

As in boys, goals of therapy include continence with preservation of renal function, and functional and cosmetic external genitalia [23]. In single-stage reconstruction, urethroplasty and bladder neck plication (with or without cystoscopic guidance) are performed simultaneously [40–42]. In staged reconstruction, urethroplasty and feminizing genitoplasty are performed early to help increase bladder capacity for later BNR and ureteral reimplantation. Continence rates >85% are reported [23].

Cloacal exstrophy

Epidemiology

Cloacal exstrophy occurs at an incidence of 1:200,000 to 1:400,000 live births [43] and a roughly equivalent male:female [23]. Historically, there was a very high mortality rate with only 22% survival reported in the

1960–1970s [43]. Currently over 90% survive, thus current goals include urinary continence, ambulation, and improved cosmesis [44].

Prenatal diagnosis

Prenatal diagnosis is important as some parents elect termination or seek centers of excellence [45, 46]. Ultrasound findings include nonvisualization of the bladder, omphalocele, myelomeningocele, lower limb deformities, renal anomalies, and hydrocephalus [1, 45].

Anatomy

There are typically two exstrophied hemibladders, with an intervening exstrophied intestinal segment [23]. 40–60% of patients have renal anomalies [23]. Males often have complete separation of the phallic halves, undescended testes, and inguinal hernias. Females have a widely separated bifid clitoris; there may also be Müllerian anomalies [23]. Two defining gastrointestinal findings are imperforate anus [23] and omphalocele [23, 44]; malrotation [23], a hindgut remnant [47], duplication anomalies [23], and short gut syndrome [47] may also be present. Bony anomalies are more severe than in CBE and may include extreme pubic diastasis and pelvic external rotation [48], vertebral malformation, scoliosis, club foot, limb length discrepancy, and limb deformities [46]. Spinal abnormalities, such as spina bifida, sacral agenesis, or tethered cord [46], are common. Less commonly, hydrocephalus, Chiari malformation, and craniosynostosis may occur [46].

Common surgeries

Urologically, MSRE and CPRE are both employed in the management of cloacal exstrophy [23]. The use of staged osteotomy with external fixation and gradual apposition of the pubic bones is recommended [49]. Most patients will require continent urinary diversion, as opposed to BNR, for continence [6]. Imperforate anus management options include end ileostomy, end colostomy from tubularized cecal plate, or hindgut pull-through procedures [47]. Additionally, gastric segments, small bowel, and hindgut are used for genitourinary reconstruction [23, 47]. Orthopedic procedures, such as spinal fusion, club foot procedure, or amputation [46], may be necessary. At birth, neurosurgery takes precedence, specifically closure of spinal defects or shunts. Laminectomy, excision of cord lipoma, cranial expansion, and cervicomedullary decompression may also be necessary [46].

Gender reassignment

Traditionally, pediatric urologists performed gender reassignment on 46XY cloacal exstrophy patients because of severe penile deformity. Currently, most prefer male gender assignment secondary to testosterone imprinting during development. Males may expect fertility if they avoid gonadectomy and utilize assisted reproductive technology. Despite female gender of rearing, genetic males may reassign their gender as they get older or have unclear sexual identity [50].

WHAT TO AVOID

- Closing the bladder and abdominal wall under tension.
- Compromising penile blood flow by damaging or compressing pudendal or accessory vessels.
- Losing patients to follow up and missing late complications such as neoplasm, urolithiasis, or metabolic derangements.
- Missing the diagnosis of female epispadias in a female with persistent continuous incontinence.
- Underevaluating patients with cloacal exstrophy; early involvement neurosurgery, orthopedics, and general surgery is recommended.
- Performing irreversible procedures, like gonadectomy, on 46XY cloacal exstrophy patients without adequately counseling the family.

KEY WEB LINKS

Association of Bladder Exstrophy Community
http://www.bladderexstrophy.com/

Bladder Exstrophy AUA Foundation Information Page
http://www.urologyhealth.org/urology/index.cfm?article=91

Epispadias AUA Foundation Information Page
http://www.urologyhealth.org/urology/index.cfm?article=126

Cloacal Exstrophy AUA Foundation Information Page
http://www.urologyhealth.org/urology/index.cfm?article=92

Multiple choice questions

1 A neonate with classic bladder exstrophy is transferred to your institution on the second day of life. After your examination of the infant and pertinent radiographic studies, you tell the team which of the following finding will preclude your ability to close the bladder immediately without osteotomies.

a Age
b Small bladder template
c Pubic diastasis of 3.5 cm
d Creatinine 0.8
e Minimal bladder polyps

2 A 4-year-old girl who is interested in being dry is brought to your clinic for consideration of BNR. She was closed successfully at 24 hours without osteotomies and was immobilized with spica casting. Her most recent bladder capacity was 70 mL. Which characteristic makes successful BNR least likely?

a No osteotomies at closure
b Spica casting immobilization
c Age
d Gender
e Bladder capacity

3 An 8-year-old incontinent boy whose CBE was closed at birth with osteotomies and underwent epispadias repair at 1 year is referred to your clinic to discuss the next step. His mother is unsure of his bladder capacity. Which of the following reconstruction options would not be an option for this patient?

a BNR
b BNR with appendicovesicostomy
c BNR with augmentation and appendicovesicostomy
d Bladder neck transection with augmentation and appendicovesicostomy
e Ileal conduit urinary diversion

References

1 Purves JT, Gearhart JP. Chapter 30: The bladder exstrophy-epispadias-cloacal exstrophy complex. In: Gearhart JP, Rink RC, Mouriquand PDE, editors. *Pediatric Urology*. Philadelphia, PA: Saunders Elsevier; 2010. pp. 386–415.
2 Sadler TW, Feldkamp ML. The embryology of body wall closure: relevance to gastroschisis and other ventral body wall defects. *Am J Med Genet C Semin Med Genet* 2008;148C(3):180–185.
3 Stec AA, Baradaran N, Gearhart JP. Congenital renal anomalies in patients with classic bladder exstrophy. *Urology* 2012;79(1):207–209.
4 McLorie GA, Bellemore MC, Salter RB. Penile deformity in bladder exstrophy: correlation with closure of pelvic defect. *J Pediatr Surg* 1991;26(2):201–203.
5 Ebert AK, Falkert A, Brandl R, Hirschfelder H, Koller M, Rösch WH. Pelvic-floor imaging using three-dimensional ultrasonography and magnetic resonance imaging in the long term follow-up of the bladder-exstrophy-epispadias complex. *BJU Int* 2010;105(2): 248–253.
6 Suson KD, Sponseller PD, Gearhart JP. Bony abnormalities in classic bladder exstrophy: The urologist's perspective. *J Pediatr Urol* 2013;9(2):112–122.
7 Stec AA, Baradaran N, Tran C, Gearhart JP. Colorectal anomalies in patients with classic bladder exstrophy. *J Pediatr Surg* 2011;46(9):1790–1793.
8 Mathews R, Gearhart JP. Modern staged reconstruction of bladder exstrophy–still the gold standard. *Urology* 2005;65(1):2–4.
9 Aadalen RJ, O'Phelan EH, Chisholm TC, McParland FA, Jr, Sweetser TH, Jr. Exstrophy of the bladder: long-term results of bilateral posterior iliac osteotomies and two-stage anatomic repair. *Clin Orthop Relat Res* 1980;(151):193–200.
10 Sponseller PD, Jani MM, Jeffs RD, Gearhart JP. Anterior innominate osteotomy in repair of bladder exstrophy. *J Bone Joint Surg Am* 2001;83-A(2):184–193.
11 Capolicchio G, McLorie GA, Farhat W, Merguerian PA, Bägli DJ, Khoury AE. A population based analysis of continence outcomes and bladder exstrophy. *J Urol* 2001;165(6 Pt 2):2418–2421.
12 Surer I, Baker LA, Jeffs RD, Gearhart JP. Modified Young-Dees-Leadbetter bladder neck reconstruction in patients with successful primary bladder closure elsewhere: a single institution experience. *J Urol* 2001;165(6 Pt 2):2438–2440.
13 Chan DY, Jeffs RD, Gearhart JP. Determinants of continence in the bladder exstrophy population: predictors of success? *Urology* 2001;57(4):774–777.
14 Shaw MB, Rink RC, Kaefer M, Cain MP, Casale AJ. Continence and classic bladder exstrophy treated with staged repair. *J Urol* 2004;172(4 Pt 1):1450–1453; discussion 1453.
15 Borer JG, Gargollo PC, Hendren WH, et al. Early outcome following complete primary repair of bladder exstrophy in the newborn. *J Urol* 2005;174(4 Pt 2): 1674–1678; discussion 1678–1679.
16 Gargollo PC, Borer JG, Diamond DA, et al. Prospective followup in patients after complete primary repair of bladder exstrophy. *J Urol* 2008;180(4 Suppl):1665–1670; discussion 1670.

17 Shoukry AI, Ziada AM, Morsi HA, et al. Outcome of complete primary bladder exstrophy repair: single-center experience. *J Pediatr Urol* 2009;5(6):496–499.
18 Kibar Y, Roth CC, Frimberger D, Kropp BP. Our initial experience with the technique of complete primary repair for bladder exstrophy. *J Pediatr Urol* 2009;5(3):186–189.
19 Shnorhavorian M, Grady RW, Andersen A, Joyner BD, Mitchell ME. Long-term followup of complete primary repair of exstrophy: The Seattle experience. *J Urol* 2008;180(4 Suppl):1615–1619; discussion 1619–1620.
20 Kelly JH. Vesical exstrophy-repair using radical mobilization of soft-tissues. *Pediatr Surg Int* 1995; 10(5–6):298–304.
21 Jarzebowski AC, McMullin ND, Grover SR, Southwell BR, Hutson JM. The Kelly technique of bladder exstrophy repair: Continence, cosmesis and pelvic organ prolapse outcomes. *J Urol* 2009;182(4 Suppl):1802–1806.
22 Schaeffer AJ, Purves JT, King JA, Sponseller PD, Jeffs RD, Gearhart JP. Complications of primary closure of classic bladder exstrophy. *J Urol* 2008;180(4 Suppl):1671–1674; discussion 1674.
23 Gearhart JP, Mathews RI. Chapter 124: Exstrophy-epispadias complex. In: McDougal WS, Wein AJ, Kavoussi LR, Novick AC, Partin AW, Peters CA, Ramchandani P, editors. *Campbell-Walsh Urology*, 10th ed. Philadelphia, PA: Saunders; 2011.
24 Mouriquand PD, Bubanj T, Feyaerts A, et al. Long-term results of bladder neck reconstruction for incontinence in children with classical bladder exstrophy or incontinent epispadias. *BJU Int* 2003;92(9):997–1001; discussion 1002.
25 Jochault-Ritz S, Mercier M, Aubert D. Short and long-term quality of life after reconstruction of bladder exstrophy in infancy: Preliminary results of the QUALEX (QUAlity of Life of bladder EXstrophy) study. *J Pediatr Surg* 2010;45(8):1693–1700.
26 Woodhouse CR, Redgrave NG. Late failure of the reconstructed exstrophy bladder. *Br J Urol* 1996;77(4):590–592.
27 Smeulders N, Woodhouse CR. Neoplasia in adult exstrophy patients. *BJU Int* 2001;87(7):623–628.
28 Husmann DA, Rathbun SR. Long-term follow up of enteric bladder augmentations: The risk for malignancy. *J Pediatr Urol* 2008;4(5):381–385; discussion 386.
29 Silver RI, Gros DA, Jeffs RD, Gearhart JP. Urolithiasis in the exstrophy-epispadias complex. *J Urol* 1997;158 (3 Pt 2):1322–1326.
30 Hensle TW, Bingham J, Lam J, Shabsigh A. Preventing reservoir calculi after augmentation cystoplasty and continent urinary diversion: The influence of an irrigation protocol. *BJU Int* 2004;93(4):585–587.
31 Gilbert SM, Hensle TW. Metabolic consequences and long-term complications of enterocystoplasty in children: A review. *J Urol* 2005;173(4):1080–1086.
32 Cervellione RM, Husmann DA, Bivalacqua TJ, Sponseller PD, Gearhart JP. Penile ischemic injury in the exstrophy/epispadias spectrum: New insights and possible mechanisms. *J Pediatr Urol* 2010;6(5):450–456.
33 Berrettini A, Castagnetti M, Rigamonti W. Radical soft tissue mobilization and reconstruction (Kelly procedure) for bladder exstrophy [correction of exstrophy] repair in males: initial experience with nine cases. *Pediatr Surg Int* 2009;25(5):427–431.
34 Purves JT, Gearhart JP. Complications of radical soft-tissue mobilization procedure as a primary closure of exstrophy. *J Pediatr Urol* 2008;4(1):65–69.
35 Canon S, Reagan R, Koff SA. Pathophysiology and management of urinary incontinence in case of distal penile epispadias. *J Urol* 2008;180(6):2636–2642; discussion 2642.
36 Kibar Y, Roth C, Frimberger D, Kropp BP. Long-term results of penile disassembly technique for correction of epispadias. *Urology* 2009;73(3):510–514.
37 Perovic SV, Djinovic RP. New insight into surgical anatomy of epispadiac penis and its impact on repair. *J Urol* 2008;179(2):689–695; discussion 695–696.
38 Kufner M, Gearhart JP, Mathews R. Impact of epispadias repair on bladder growth in boys with classic bladder exstrophy. *J Pediatr Urol* 2010;6(6):578–581.
39 Braga LH, Lorenzo AJ, Bägli DJ, Khoury AE, Pippi Salle JL. Outcome analysis of isolated male epispadias: Single center experience with 33 cases. *J Urol* 2008;179(3):1107–1112.
40 Cheikhelard A, Aigrain Y, Lottmann H, Lortat-Jacob S. Female epispadias management: perineal urethrocervicoplasty versus classical Young-Dees procedure. *J Urol* 2009;182(4 Suppl):1807–1811.
41 Kajbafzadeh AM, Talab SS, Elmi A, Tourchi A. Single-stage subsymphyseal cystoscopic-guided bladder neck plication and urethrogenitoplasty in female epispadias: presentation of long-term follow-up. *BJU Int* 2011; 108(7):1200–1207.
42 Lazarus J, van den Heever A, Kortekaas B, Alexander A. Female epispadias managed by bladder neck plication via a perineal approach. *J Pediatr Urol*, 2011;8(3): 244–248.
43 Hurwitz RS, Manzoni GA, Ransley PG, Stephens FD. Cloacal exstrophy: a report of 34 cases. *J Urol* 1987;138(4 Pt 2):1060–1064.
44 Mathews R, Jeffs RD, Reiner WG, Docimo SG, Gearhart JP. Cloacal exstrophy–improving the quality of life: The Johns Hopkins experience. *J Urol* 1998;160 (6 Pt 2):2452–2456.
45 Keppler-Noreuil K, Gorton S, Foo F, Yankowitz J, Keegan C. Prenatal ascertainment of OEIS complex/cloacal exstrophy – 15 new cases and literature review. *Am J Med Genet A* 2007;143A(18):2122–2128.

46 Suson KD, Novak TE, Gupta AD, Benson J, Sponseller P, Gearhart JP. Neuro-orthopedic manifestations of the omphalocele exstrophy imperforate anus spinal defects complex. *J Urol* 2010;184(4 Suppl):1651–1655.

47 Sawaya D, Goldstein S, Seetharamaiah R, et al. Gastrointestinal ramifications of the cloacal exstrophy complex: A 44-year experience. *J Pediatr Surg* 2010;45(1): 171–175; discussion 175–176.

48 Sponseller PD, Bisson LJ, Gearhart JP, Jeffs RD, Magid D, Fishman E. The anatomy of the pelvis in the exstrophy complex. *J Bone Joint Surg Am* 1995;77(2):177–189.

49 Mathews R, Gearhart JP, Bhatnagar R, Sponseller P. Staged pelvic closure of extreme pubic diastasis in the exstrophy-epispadias complex. *J Urol* 2006;176(5):2196–2198.

50 Reiner WG, Gearhart JP. Discordant sexual identity in some genetic males with cloacal exstrophy assigned to female sex at birth. *N Engl J Med* 2004;350(4):333–341.

Answers to multiple choice questions

1 b A sufficient bladder template is required for immediate closure. Small templates should be kept moist with saline and protected with nonadherent plastic wrap until large enough to close. Age <72 hours, a pubic diastasis that can be reduced without tension, and good bladder quality are also important considerations when deciding upon timing of closure and use of osteotomies. Creatinine in the immediate postoperative period reflects maternal creatinine and does not impact your decision in this case.

2 e Bladder capacity in a patient with a successful primary closure is a key determinant of eventual continence, with a suggested minimum capacity of 100 mL prior to reconstruction. Choice of osteotomy and immobilization method at closure are inconsequential in a successful closure. While she may take longer to develop continence, her age does not make it less likely. In general, females with exstrophy are thought to have better continence rates than males, with some achieving continence without BNR.

3 e In the absence of significant renal dysfunction or other mitigating medical/social/mental circumstance, the goal of reconstruction should be continence, rather than incontinent diversion.

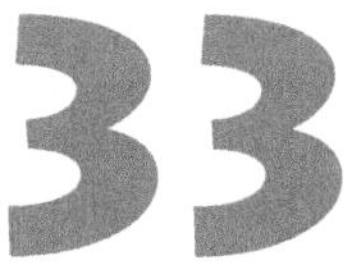

Bladder augmentation, bladder neck reconstruction, and continent diversions in children

Angela D. Gupta

The James Buchanan Brady Urological Institute and Department of Urology, The Johns Hopkins School of Medicine, Baltimore, MD, USA

KEY POINTS

- The aim of urinary reconstruction in the child is to emulate the storage and emptying patterns of the normal bladder: low pressure storage, a large capacity reservoir with a good compliance, and (when possible) spontaneous voiding.
- Patients best suited for a bladder neck reconstruction are those with an incompetent bladder neck.
- The goal of augmentation cystoplasty is to create a low pressure, large capacity, and compliant reservoir for adequate storage of urine while protecting the upper urinary tracts.
- The type of reconstruction offered to a patient and family needs to take into consideration the patient's intelligence and capability as well as the commitment and compliance with medical care to maintain the reconstruction.

CASE STUDY

A 16-year-old male presented with acute onset of abdominal pain, nausea, emesis, anorexia, and fever. He was born with bladder exstrophy–epispadias syndrome and had undergone neonatal closure of the bladder, followed at the age of 10 years by an ileocystoplasty with a Young–Dees bladder neck reconstruction (BNR) and catheterizable appendicovesicostomy. He occasionally voided spontaneously with a weak stream, and performed self-catheterization 2–3 times daily. The patient admitted that he had stopped catheterizing 2 weeks before his symptoms began and relied upon spontaneous voiding.

The patient was in mild distress, but alert and oriented. He was febrile, with generalized abdominal pain and guarding, but no distinct rebound tenderness. A catheter was placed in the Mitrofanoff, and CT with intravesical contrast revealed extravasation. He was taken to operating room urgently, and on exploration, was noted to have a large loculated collection of cloudy fluid in the left pelvic gutter. A 2 cm rupture was found in the posterolateral portion of the augmented bladder in the area of the apparent scar from the cystostomy of his original ileocystoplasty operation. The bladder was repaired with 3-0 vicryl suture in two layers; one catheter was left in the appendicovesicostomy, and another left in a separate cystostomy through a different opening. A Jackson–Pratt drain was placed in the left abdominal gutter.

The patient was continued on intravenous broad-spectrum antibiotics postoperatively. On the basis of culture sensitivities, the patient was switched to intravenous moxifloxacin for 48 hours on postoperative day 6. Nine days after surgery, the patient was discharged on oral moxifloxacin 400 mg twice daily for 14 days A cystogram on postoperative day 23 showed no extravasation, so the appendicovesicostomy catheter was removed, followed by the suprapubic catheter 5 days later. The patient was counseled to catheterize four times daily.

Handbook of Urology, First edition. J. Kellogg Parsons, John B. Eifler and Misop Han.
Published 2014 by John Wiley & Sons, Ltd.

Bladder neck reconstruction

The goal of BNR is to construct an outlet that provides enough resistance to achieve continence but does not obstruct the urinary tract. Many procedures including diversions will render the majority of patients continent, so it is important to properly select patients for a BNR. Patients best suited for a BNR are those with an incompetent bladder neck; pathologic diagnosis may include neurogenic dysfunction, exstrophy, and ureterocele [1].

Patient evaluation

First, the patient and family must be evaluated to ensure that they are compliant and willing to maintain the reconstruction. The commitment and ability to catheterize and to support the child through the learning process are essential for a successful postoperative procedure. The patient's long-term manual dexterity and intelligence are important to ascertain as intermittent self-catheterization (ISC) is required immediately after the procedure. There is always a chance that the patient may not spontaneously void after the procedure. Wheelchair-bound patients may benefit from a diversion for easier catheterization [2].

A thorough evaluation of the lower and upper urinary tracts should also be performed. A voiding cystourethrogram (VCUG) detects vesicoureteral reflux, and urodynamics reveal the bladder capacity, detrusor overactivity, and leak point pressure. These parameters will help in surgical options and planning; low capacity, compliance, or high storage pressure bladders may need concomitant augmentation cystoplasty. Bladder neck competence cannot always be diagnosed by any one modality, although the best visual image is given by videourodynamics.

Upper tract integrity should be assessed by renal ultrasound, CT urogram, or intravenous pyelogram (IVP) to determine the number of kidneys and whether they appear normal. Any congenital malformations should be known prior to surgical intervention, to allow for appropriate planning [2].

Techniques

The Young–Dees–Leadbetter repair tightens the bladder neck through the trigone over a silver probe and lengthens the urethra by displacing the ureters caudally. A fixed point of obstruction is constructed and to void the detrusor pressure must exceed that of the obstruction; otherwise, catheterization becomes necessary. The obstruction remedies the existing problem of the incompetent bladder neck. Continence success rates range from 57% to 79% with about 10% experiencing difficult catheterization postoperatively [2–4].

Bladder neck wrap procedures use a demucosalized bladder flap or a myofascial sling to wrap around the reconstructed urethra for added support. Success rates are slightly better. The Kropp procedure creates a one-way valve mechanism, similar to antirefluxing techniques used for ureteral reimplants, by tabularizing an anterior bladder flap and reimplanting it in the posterior trigonal area [2].

Augmentation cystoplasty

The goal of augmentation cystoplasty is to create a low pressure, large capacity, and compliant reservoir for adequate storage of urine without subjecting the upper urinary tracts to increased pressure. Patients experiencing incontinence are evaluated for urodynamic parameters to evaluate for capacity, compliance, and detrusor pressures. Cystoplasty involves bivalving of the bladder muscle and then insertion of the intestinal segment; therefore, patients require ISC postoperatively as the detrusor muscle can no longer produce coordinated contractions, although phasic contractions will occur and may be interpreted as overactivity on cystometry.

A proper evaluation consists of urodynamics, upper tract imaging, and voiding cystography if hydronephrosis is detected and routine bloodwork to reveal any level of renal insufficiency or metabolic derangement (i.e., acidosis) that may affect postoperative management. A mechanical bowel preparation to decrease bacterial exposure during surgery and parenteral antibiotics is preferred. Urine specimen should be taken to ensure sterile urine.

Techniques

In the pediatric patient, the native bladder does not routinely need to be resected; instead it is bivalved anteriorly a few centimeters from the bladder neck to the posterior trigonal area. The bowel segment is selected based on the mobility and adequate blood supply. Once the selected segment is detubularized it is sewn onto the bivalved bladder to emulate a sphere, such as to blunt contractions and to increase the storage of the reservoir as best as possible.

Ileum, the most commonly used section of the bowel, is the most compliant and has good mobility. The advantage of an ileocecocystoplasty is the reliable blood supply from the ileocolic artery. However, the loss of the distal portion of the ileum can result in a vitamin B12 deficiency and the loss of the ileocolic valve may cause the patient to experience clinically significant diarrhea.

The sigmoid cystoplasty is favored in patients with spinal dysraphisms that result in neuropathic bowels because the sigmoid in these patients tends to be dilated and redundant. The gastrocystoplasty uses the stomach as the intestinal segment, taking 10–15 cm of the greater curvature of the stomach and leaving the lesser curvature intact such as not to damage the vagus innervation.

Postoperative care includes continuous urinary reservoir drainage for 4 weeks, H2 blockers for gastrocystoplasty, daily bladder irrigation, and maintenance ISC for life. Long-term follow-up include annual renal ultrasounds, abdominal ultrasounds for stone disease, and electrolytes. At 5 years postoperatively, annual cystoscopy and urine cytologies should be initiated to screen for malignancy [1, 2].

Complications

Intestinal segments continue to produce mucus with the stomach producing the least and the colon making the most. Excess mucus can interfere in the patient's ability to empty the reservoir well, requiring the implementation of a lifelong regimen of bladder irrigation. Urinary stasis, abnormal urinary pH, and citrate levels, and foreign body exposure all contribute to the risk of urinary tract infection and stone formation. Bacteriuria occurs routinely in those who practice ISC and should only be treated if the patient has symptoms to suggest an infection. Metabolic complications are the most important to monitor for during both the perioperative period and long-term follow-up. The ileum and colonic segments continue to absorb ammonium, hydrogen ions, and chloride while secreting bicarbonate which can result in hyperchloremic acidosis. Incomplete bladder emptying increases the time of exposure of the urine to the bowel segment, and can worsen the metabolic derangement. The body may compensate for the acidosis by using inorganic salts from bones as a buffer, causing bone demineralization. Annual screening and appropriate bicarbonate repletion are essential for bone health. Gastric segments secret hydrogen ions and chloride, which increases bicarbonate levels resulting in a hypokalemic, hypochloremic alkalosis. Hematuria dysuria syndrome is seen in patients with gastrocystoplasties, consisting of bladder spasms, dysuria, suprapubic pain, gross hematuria, and perineal skin irritation from acidic urine [2].

Bladder perforation is a serious, relatively rare complication associated with lack of proper drainage, best diagnosed early and managed with definitive treatment. Patients typically present with acute abdominal pain. Diagnostic modalities include cystogram and CT cystogram.

The risk of malignancy in the augmented bladder with intestine has been debated and the data are conflicting [5, 6]. Nevertheless, for augmentations the recommendation is annual screening with cystoscopy and cytology beginning 5 years after surgery.

Continent diversions

A continent urinary diversion completely replaces the bladder and serves as a low pressure, compliant urinary reservoir with a catheterizable stoma for emptying. Indications include conditions for which the native bladder is completely dysfunctional or requires removal for malignancy. The patient evaluation is similar to that required of those undergoing augmentation as the same commitment to maintenance if the reconstruction applies.

Techniques

The Kock pouch is a reservoir made of about 80 cm of ileum (tailored to the size of the patient) with the continence mechanism made by a nipple valve fashioned with staplers. The distal 12–15 cm is used to make a stoma for catheterization. The gastroileal pouch uses both stomach and ileal segments, which makes the reconstruction more complicated, and offsets the metabolic derangements that occur with one or the other bowel segment. For patients who are at risk for short gut syndrome, this technique is the preferred continent diversion because less of the absorptive bowel is disconnected.

The Indiana pouch uses the distal ileum and the cecum. The cecum becomes the reservoir and the ureters are implanted into it, while the distal ileum becomes the catheterizable stoma. In this technique, the ileocecal valve is intact therefore assisting in the continence mechanism. Although this reconstruction is quite popular in adults, it is not used in children as much given the complications of vitamin B12 deficiency and diarrhea.

The MAINZ pouch is composed of ileum and cecum but uses two limbs of distal ileum. It has been applied to orthotopic diversions, augmentations, and continent diversions. The catheterizable stoma is made based on the Mitrofanoff principle. The channel must be implanted submucosally with adequate muscle backing so that it acts as a valve making the stoma continent. The channel should have a straight and direct route to the reservoir with a short intra-abdominal segment [1, 2].

Conclusion

The aim of urinary reconstruction in the child is to emulate the normal storage and emptying patterns that are afforded by the normal bladder; low pressure storage, large capacity reservoir with a good compliance, and if possible spontaneous voiding. There are numerous techniques available to reconstruct the native bladder or a neobladder, the most important factors in deciding which reconstruction to offer a patient are quality of life and commitment to long-term maintenance.

WHAT TO AVOID

- Evaluate upper tracts routinely throughout the patient's life.
- Monitor for vitamin B12 deficiency during long-term follow-up, especially if the reconstruction included the distal portion of the ileum.
- Children do NOT routinely need removal of diseased bladder unless there is a malignancy.

Multiple choice questions

1 Urinary tract reconstruction for continence requires:
  a Normal upper urinary tract
  b Compliant bladder
  c Acceptance and compliance with intermittent catheterization
  d VCUG

2 A good preoperative evaluation can avoid which complication associated with bladder neck repair?
  a Cystitis
  b Unmasking of detrusor hostility causing upper tract changes
  c Urolithiasis
  d Need for augmentation cystoplasty
  e Inability to void

3 To minimize uninhibited contractions during an enterocystoplasty and for the remainder of the reconstruction:
  a Use large bowel exclusively.
  b Create a stellate incision into the bladder to increase the circumference of the bowel anastomosis.
  c Reconfigure the bowel segment.
  d Excise the diseased bladder.
  e There is no way of minimizing the phasic contractions of the bowel.

References

1 Wein AJ, Kavoussi LR, Novick AC, Partin AW, Peters C, editors. *Campbell-Walsh Urology*. 10th ed. Philadelphia, PA: Saunders Elsevier; 2012.
2 Gearhart J, Rink R., Mouriquand P, *Pediatric Urology*. 2nd ed. Philadelphia, PA: Saunders Elsevier; 2010.
3 Purves T, Novak T, King J, Gearhart JP. Modified Young-Dees-Leadbetter bladder neck reconstruction after exstrophy repair. *J Urol* 2009;182(4 Suppl):1813–1817.
4 Donnahoo KK, Rink RC, Cain MP, Casale AJ. The Young-Dees-Leadbetter bladder neck repair for neurogenic incontinence. *J Urol* 1999;161(6):1946–1949.
5 Higuchi TT, Granberg CF, Fox JA, Husmann DA. Augmentation cystoplasty and risk of neoplasia: fact, fiction and controversy. *J Urol* 184(6):2492–2496.
6 Husmann DA. Malignancy after gastrointestinal augmentation in childhood. *Ther Adv Urol* 2009;1(1):5–11.

Answers to multiple choice questions

1 c
2 b
3 c

34 End-stage renal disease and transplantation

Angela D. Gupta

The James Buchanan Brady Urological Institute and Department of Urology, The Johns Hopkins School of Medicine, Baltimore, MD, USA

KEY POINTS

- Diabetes mellitus is the most common cause of end-stage renal disease (ESRD) in the adult population. Other causes include hypertension and glomerulonephritis.
- Renal donors and recipients should be screened for renal disease, malignancy, and active infection.
- The technical goals for the donor operation are to decrease ischemia time and preserve ureteral blood supply and renal vessel length.
- Major histocompatibility complex (MHC) is a protein that is expressed by all nucleated cells and allows for recognition of self and non-self by the immune system.
- Three classes of immunosuppressants are used most commonly to prevent rejection: calcineurin inhibitors, steroids, and antiproliferative agents.

CASE STUDY

A 45-year-old woman with a history of end-stage renal disease (ESRD) secondary to poorly controlled diabetes mellitus returns for a follow-up 4 months after undergoing autologous renal transplantation. She has been compliant with following up with her endocrinologist since surgery. She received a living donor transplant and has been maintained on tacrolimus, CellCept, and prednisone. On routine laboratory test, her serum creatinine is 2.5 mg/dL. Postoperatively her creatinine nadir was 0.9 mg/dL and at her last clinic visit 1 month prior to it was 1.1 mg/dL. Her tacrolimus level is found to be subtherapeutic. The patient admits to not filling her tacrolimus after a financial crisis in the family; she has been taking only half the dose of the tacrolimus in order to make it last longer. A renal biopsy demonstrates acute rejection.

End-stage renal disease

End-stage renal disease (ESRD) is defined as a glomerular filtration rate (GFR) <10 mL/min or serum creatinine >8 mg/dL [1]. At such a low GFR, the kidneys are no longer able to maintain electrolyte and water homeostasis in the body, requiring a form of renal replacement therapy. According to the US Renal Data System, in 2009, the US incidence and prevalence of ESRD were 115,705 and 2.2 million cases, respectively. Diabetes mellitus is the most common cause of ESRD followed closely by hypertension and glomerulonephritis [2].

The two types of renal replacement therapy are dialysis and renal transplantation. Half of the adult population with ESRD is treated with dialysis; children are

Handbook of Urology, First edition. J. Kellogg Parsons, John B. Eifler and Misop Han.
Published 2014 by John Wiley & Sons, Ltd.

more likely to receive transplantation. In the United States, renal transplantation is considered a standard of care for ESRD, and with expanded donor criteria, donated kidneys are matched to individuals who will be the most compatible recipients [1]. Cadaveric donor and living donor transplants have both been shown to improve quality of life and survival [1, 2].

Transplantation

Recipient evaluation

The diagnosis of ESRD makes a patient eligible for an evaluation for a renal transplant, but does not guarantee acceptance onto the waiting list to receive an organ. Factors taken into consideration include infection status, malignancy, obesity, compliance issues, substance abuse, and ability to withstand surgery [1]. Any active infection must be addressed prior to the transplantation. Pulmonary, dialysis access catheter, and urinary tract infections must be properly treated. CMV, HIV, HBV, HCV and, in children, EBV status should be investigated.

Patients with invasive malignancies can be considered for transplantation if they remain disease-free for 2–5 years following definitive treatment. Patients with low-grade and noninvasive disease can wait a shorter period of time, but this may need to be individualized to the type of malignancy and patient [3].

A number of factors increase perioperative morbidity and mortality, including cardiac disease, cerebrovascular disease, obesity, smoking, diabetes, and pulmonary disease. Patients with a history of any of the above and those older than 50 years should undergo a complete cardiac workup. Those who are smokers should be counseled to stop, especially in those with preexisting cardiovascular disease, as smoking increases the risk of posttransplant allograft loss [4].

Those with a history of substance abuse must undergo treatment and complete toxicology screening to be eligible for transplantation. For those with a history of alcohol dependency, alcohol should be discontinued for a period of at least 6 months prior to consideration. Financial and psychosocial consultations are usually provided to ensure that the patient has an intact support system and has a desire to be compliant with the postprocedural follow-up and maintenance.

Patients are screened for a few preexisting conditions that can decrease the likelihood of successful transplantation. Patients with known lower extremity vascular disease or abdominal or pelvic vascular surgery should have a diagnostic study to evaluate the vessels and determine the optimal location of renal revascularization. Doppler ultrasound is sufficient in most cases, but in complex cases, arteriography can be used to determine an alternate location as necessary. Renal thrombosis causes 2–7% of renal allograft loss in adults and 35% in children [5]. Predisposing causes include nephrotic syndrome, previous renal thrombosis, previous vascular access thrombosis, and antiphospholipid antibodies. Treatment for thrombophilias may involve intraoperative heparin and prophylactic subcutaneous heparin in the immediate postoperative period; longer-term management with warfarin may be required.

It is not uncommon for patients with ESRD to have anuria or oliguria and therefore a defunctionalized bladder prior to transplantation. A few weeks after transplantation, the majority of these bladders will regain a normal function and capacity [1]. In those that do not, techniques to create a low pressure, normal capacity bladder may be used without compromising the allograft [6]. Transplants have been successful in adults and children with urinary reservoirs or intestinal conduits [7, 8]. Men with bladder outlet obstruction secondary to benign prostatic hyperplasia may require medical or surgical treatment once the bladder begins to cycle again.

Pre-transplant nephrectomy is indicated in patients with grade IV or V hydronephrosis, large infected renal stones, solid renal tumors, symptomatic polycystic kidneys, recurrent pyelonephritis, persistent proteinuria, and persistent anti-glomerular basement membrane antibody levels. Nephrectomy should be done 6 weeks prior to transplant, and the open or laparoscopic technique can be used depending on the location and size of the kidneys [1].

Donor evaluation and selection

Renal donors should be screened for renal disease, any malignancy, and active infection. Deceased donors also have specimens collected for histocompatibility testing. Living donors go through a rigorous preoperative evaluation, the goal of which is to screen patients who would have the highest rate of normal renal function after nephrectomy and the lowest chance of developing future renal disease. Transmissible disease (i.e., malignancy or viral), renal disease, mental illness, and a high probability of perioperative morbidity or mortality disqualify a donor [1]. Diagnostic imaging to evaluate renal and vessel anatomy, serologic testing, and glucose tolerance test are all done to decrease the chance of allograft rejection and contamination and to maximize long-term outcomes for the donor. If there is a discrepancy in donor kidney function, the less functional kidney is donated. In women who wish to become pregnant in the future, typically the right kidney is donated since it is usually the right side that experiences hydronephrosis and pyelonephritis during pregnancy [1]. In all other cases, the left kidney is preferred for donation because of the longer renal vein, which facilitates the technical performance of the operation. Live renal donors need psychological support and long-term follow-up to ensure the best medical outcome of unilateral nephrectomy [9]. Hyperfiltration injury is commonly seen in donors after nephrectomy and these patients should be screened for long-term renal dysfunction for appropriate management.

Surgical technique

The technical goals for the donor operation are to decrease ischemia time, preserve ureteral blood supply, and maximize renal vessel length. Ischemia time should be minimized with hypothermia, which decreases the cellular energy requirement. If necessary, vascular reconstruction to ensure adequate vessel length for the anastomoses can be performed after donor nephrectomy and prior to transplantation.

In adults, the kidney is transplanted via a Gibson incision into the extraperitoneal space of the iliac fossa. During vascular occlusion, intravenous (IV) heparin is administered, and mannitol is given during the vascular anastomosis. If the recipient does not have aberrant vascular anatomy, spatial constrictions, or substantial arterial disease, the internal iliac artery and the external iliac vein are utilized for allograft anastomosis. First the renal artery and then the renal vein are anastomosed with nonabsorbable sutures. Mannitol and furosemide are administered to decrease reperfusion injury [1]. The ureteroneocystostomy is the last portion of the procedure and it can be either an antirefluxing or refluxing anastomosis. The majority of these are done in an extravesical fashion and a ureteral stent is inserted to bridge the suture line.

Immunology and immunosuppression

Once a renal transplant is performed, immunosuppressive medications are administered to prevent the host from rejecting the allograft. T and B cells are lymphocytes that drive the immune system to respond to antigens that are identified as foreign. T cells have a T-cell receptor, which recognizes these antigens with the help of an antigen-presenting cell, activating the production of cytokines and destruction of the infected cells via interactions of cell surface molecules. B cells detect antigens via IgM and IgD antibodies on the cell surface. Once activated via T-cell signaling, B cells produce antibodies that bind to the antigen and label it for destruction by the complement system. There is also a nonspecific immunity provided by the physical barriers, macrophages, natural killer cells, monocytes, and neutrophils. This immunity is not enhanced with repeated exposure and remains nonspecific, unlike that of T and B cells, which only initiate signaling pathways once presented with a very specific antigen.

Major histocompatibility complex (MHC) is a protein that is expressed by all nucleated cells and allows for recognition of self and nonself by the immune system. The MHC molecules are formed by a combination of many human leukocyte antigens (HLAs) to create genetic variability and improve the chances of survival against new pathogens. MHC class I antigens combining HLA A, B, and C are expressed by most nucleated cells and bind to the CD8 molecule on T lymphocytes to present intracellular peptides. These molecules allow the immune system to recognize cells that are self, preventing an immune response. MHC class II proteins combine HLA DR, DP, and DQ and are on the cell surface of antigen-presenting cells, dendritic cells, B lymphocytes, macrophages, and endothelial cells. ABO blood type is screened in those receiving organ transplants; however, HLA screening is also performed. The closer the donor organ matches the recipient's immune system, the better chance of avoiding graft rejection.

Types of immunosuppression

At the time of transplant, induction therapy in the form of antibodies may be utilized to decrease the chances of acute rejection. These antibodies block the antigens from being recognized by recipient T cells.

Three classes of immunosuppressants are used most commonly to prevent rejection: calcineurin inhibitors, steroids, and antiproliferative agents. Calcineurin activates T cells by increasing production of interleukin-2. Calcineurin inhibitors such as tacrolimus and cyclosporine blunt this response in a dose-dependent fashion and prevent rejection. Serum levels of these drugs must be monitored carefully to prevent toxicities, which include nephrotoxicity, diabetes, hypertension, and hyperlipidemia [10]. Steroids interfere with intracellular signaling and decrease the production of cytokine gene transcription [1]. Antiproliferative agents, such as azathioprine and mycophenolate mofetil, inhibit purine synthesis, downregulating the production of lymphocytes. Maintenance therapy traditionally involves one drug from all three categories.

mTOR inhibitors, such as sirolimus, inhibit the response of interleukin-2, blocking activation of T- and B-cell lymphocytes. There is no nephrotoxicity associated with sirolimus; however, myelosuppression and hyperlipidemia can occur. An mTOR inhibitor can be used in conjunction with calcineurin inhibitors or as a substitute [1, 10].

Rejection

There are three types of rejection. Hyperacute rejection occurs immediately after the graft is introduced into the body and is secondary to preformed antibodies in the bloodstream and may lead to graft loss. Acute rejection occurs within the first 6 months of transplantation and affects 30% of recipients. It presents with a rapid deterioration in graft function and the diagnosis is confirmed by renal biopsy. The Banff criteria are used to score its severity [10]. IV steroids are used as first-line treatment for acute rejection. Anti-CD3 monoclonal antibodies are used as second line, but require close monitoring for cytokine reactions. CD4 staining at biopsy indicates antibody-mediated rejection and anti-B-cell therapy or plasmapheresis should be utilized [10]. Chronic rejection is the gradual decline of graft function may be seen in conjunction with minimal mononuclear infiltrate, interstitial fibrosis, and vascular changes [1]. Prior occurrence of rejection is associated with chronic rejection [11].

WHAT TO AVOID

- Patients after diagnosis of malignancy can still be candidates for transplantation if they are malignancy-free for 2–5 years.
- Substance abuse does not exclude from wait list but patient must prove that he or she is drug free
- Vascular anatomy should be screened prior to the procedure to optimize surgical outcomes.
- Left kidneys are preferred when donating, because there is a longer renal vein which can be harvested for vascular anastomosis.

Multiple choice questions

1 The standard method of urinary tract reconstruction during renal transplantation is
  a Ureteroneocystostomy
  b Ureteroureterostomy
  c Vesicopyelostomy
  d Cutaneous ureterostomy

2 The donor renal vein is usually anastomosed to the recipient's
  a Internal iliac vein
  b Posterior gluteal
  c Common iliac
  d Inferior vena cava
  e External iliac vein

3 Which of the following are common causes of ESRD in the United States?
  a Hypertension
  b Diabetes
  c Nephrolithiasis
  d A and B
  e A, B, and C

References

1 Wein AJ, Kavoussi LR, Novick AC, Partin AW, Peters CA. *Campbell-Walsh Urology*. 10th ed. Philadelphia, PA: Saunders Elsevier; 2011.

2 US Renal Data System, USRDS 2009. *Annual Data Report: Atlas of End-Stage Renal Disease in the United States*. Bethesda, MD: National Institutes of Health, National Institute of Diabetes and Digestive and Kidney Diseases; 2009.
3 Kasiske BL, Cangro CB, Hariharan S, et al. The evaluation of renal transplantation candidates: clinical practice guidelines. *Am J Transplant* 2001;1(Suppl 2):3–95.
4 Sung RS, Althoen M, Howell TA, Ojo AO, Merion RM. Excess risk of renal allograft loss associated with cigarette smoking. *Transplantation* 2001;71(12): 1752–1757.
5 Ponticelli C, Moia M, Montagnino G. Renal allograft thrombosis. *Nephrol Dial Transplant* 2009;24(5): 1388–1393.
6 Barry JM. Kidney transplantation into patients with abnormal bladders. *Transplantation* 2004;77(7):1120–1123.
7 Hatch DA, Koyle MA, Baskin LS, et al. Kidney transplantation in children with urinary diversion or bladder augmentation. *J Urol* 2001;165(6 Pt 2):2265–2268.
8 Surange RS, et al. Kidney transplantation into an ileal conduit: a single center experience of 59 cases. *J Urol* 2003;170(5):1727–1730.
9 Hambro A. Narratives: an essential tool for evaluating living kidney donations. *Med Health Care Philos* 2012;15(2):181–194.
10 Hornick P, Rose M. *Transplantation Immunology: Methods and Protocols*. Totowa, NJ: Humana Press Inc.; 2006.
11 Humar A, Kerr S, Gillingham KJ, Matas AJ. Features of acute rejection that increase risk for chronic rejection. *Transplantation* 1999;68(8):1200–1203.

Answers to multiple choice questions

1 a Ureteroneocystostomy
2 e External iliac vein
3 d A and B

Uropharmacology

John B. Eifler

The James Buchanan Brady Urological Institute and Department of Urology, The Johns Hopkins School of Medicine, Baltimore, MD, USA

α-adrenergic receptor blockers (α-blockers)

Indications:

- Initial management of patients with BPH as well as combination therapy for BPH with 5α-reductase inhibitors, Phosphodiesterase-5 (PDE-5) inhibitors, or anticholinergic agents
- Off-label indications: medical expulsive therapy for ureteric stones (tamsulosin), neurogenic bladder, radiation-induced urethritis, nocturia (terazosin)

Mechanism of action:

- Block sympathetic nervous-system-mediated contraction of smooth muscle cells in the prostate and bladder neck

Side effects:

- Orthostatic hypotension
- Fatigue
- Dizziness
- Retrograde ejaculation
- Floppy iris syndrome

Note: The α_{1A}-adrenergic receptor is most prevalent in the prostate, and α_{1A}-specific inhibitors have been developed (tamsulosin, silodosin).

Approved agents:

- Nonselective
  - Terazosin (Hytrin)
  - Doxazosin (Cardura)
  - Alfuzosin (Uroxatral)
- Selective
  - Tamsulosin (Flomax)
  - Silodosin (Rapaflo)

5α-reductase inhibitors

Indications:

- BPH in men with enlarged gland (>30 cc or PSA > 1.5)
- Male pattern alopecia
- Off-label indications: hematuria related to BPH, prostate cancer chemoprevention, hirsutism

Mechanism:

- Inhibit the enzyme that converts testosterone to dihydrotestosterone
- Decreases prostate size

Side effects:

- Erectile dysfunction
- Decreased ejaculation
- Low libido
- Gynecomastia
- Increased risk of moderate- to high-grade prostate cancer

Approved agents:

- Finasteride (Proscar)
- Dutasteride (Avodart)

Handbook of Urology, First edition. J. Kellogg Parsons, John B. Eifler and Misop Han.
Published 2014 by John Wiley & Sons, Ltd.

Anticholinergics (muscarinic receptor antagonists)

Indications:
- Overactive bladder
- Hyperreflexic bladder
- Neurogenic bladder, to reduce the detrusor pressure during bladder filling in poorly compliant bladders and thereby protect the upper tracts
- Reduce frequency and severity of bladder spasms

Mechanism:
- The M_1, M_2, and M_3 muscarinic receptors are present in the smooth muscle of the bladder. Binding of acetylcholine to these sites stimulates smooth muscle contraction. The M_2 receptor is most common in the bladder but M_3 binding contributes most to detrusor contractions.
- CNS side effects of anticholinergic medications may be bothersome in elderly patients, with oxybutynin having particularly high CNS penetrance. Trospium (Sanctura) has low CNS penetrance.

Side effects:
- Constipation
- Xerostomia
- Headache
- Dizziness
- Somnolence
- Confusion (particularly in the elderly)
- Urinary retention

Approved agents:
- Oxybutynin (Ditropan)
- Solifenacin (Vesicare), bladder selective (less dry mouth than oxybutynin)
- Tolterodine (Detrol), bladder selective (less dry mouth than oxybutynin)
- Trospium (Sanctura), less risk of dizziness and confusion than oxybutynin
- Darifenacin (Enablex), M_3 receptor selective agent
- Fesoterodine (Toviaz)

Benzodiazepines

Indications:
- Severe bladder spasms

Mechanism:
- Potentiates the activity of GABA by binding A-type GABA receptors

Side effects:
- Contraindications:
  - Severe liver failure
  - Myasthenia gravis
  - Severe respiratory insufficiency
  - Sleep apnea syndrome
- Respiratory depression
- Muscle weakness
- Ataxia
- Somnolence
- Hypotension
- Risk of abuse

Commonly used agents:
- Diazepam
- Lorazepam

Botulinum Toxin

Indications:
- Hyperreflexic bladder (detrusor instability associated with neurologic condition)

Mechanism:
- Inhibits release of acetylcholine at the presynaptic nerve terminal, inhibiting smooth and skeletal muscle contractions. Botox is injected directly in the target tissue of interest. In the case of detrusor instability +/– urinary incontinence, botulinum toxin is injected directly into the detrusor muscle endoscopically.

Side effects:
- Urinary retention
- Respiratory depression (rare, but mentioned in black box warning)

Phenazopyridine (Pyridium)

Indications:
- Dysuria, symptomatic relief

Mechanism:
- The agent is excreted in the urine and provides direct topical analgesia through an unknown mechanism

Side effects:
- Contraindications: allergy to phenazopyridine, renal insufficiency (GFR < 50)
- Headache
- Nephrotoxicity (rare)
- Hemolytic anemia (rare)

Phosphodiesterase-5 inhibitors

Indications:
- Erectile dysfunction
- Off-label indications: premature ejaculation, lower urinary tract symptoms, penile rehabilitation following radical prostatectomy (which remains an experimental indication)

Mechanism:

Inhibit cGMP-specific PDE-5 in erectile tissue, which increases intracytoplasmic cGMP and leads to smooth muscle relaxation. During sexual arousal, nitric oxide (NO) is released from nerve endings as well as endothelial cells in the penis. This in turn leads to increased intracellular cGMP and relaxation of smooth muscle cells in the penis, which facilitates erection. Sildenafil does not induce erections but augments the erectile response.

Tadalafil (Cialis) has a longer half-life and may augment erectile function for 72 hours. Sildenafil and vardenafil cross-react slightly with PDE-6, which may cause visual disturbances. Tadalafil cross-reacts with PDE-11.

Side effects:
- *PDE-5 inhibitors are contraindicated in patients taking nitrates due to risk of hypotension.* Patients who discontinued nitrates for more than 2 weeks may safely take these medications.
- Other contraindications:
  - MI, stroke, or life-threatening arrhythmia within the previous 6 months
  - Severe resting hypotension or hypertension
  - History or retinitis pigmentosa
  - Severe liver failure
  - Renal failure (on dialysis)
  - Unstable angina or congestive heart failure (NYHA class II)
- Visual disturbances. This may manifest as blue-tinted vision, mediated by PDE-6 inhibition (sildenafil and vardenafil are most commonly associated with this side effect)
- Headache, facial flushing
- Back ache (particularly tadalafil)
- Nasal congestion
- Priapism
- Sudden loss of vision (nonarteritic anterior optic neuropathy (NAION)) may rarely occur

Approved agents:
- Sildenafil (Viagra)
- Vardenafil (Levitra)
- Tadalafil (Cialis)
- Avanafil (Stendra)

Intracavernous injection

Indications:
- Erectile dysfunction

Mechanism:
- Typically injections contain 1–3 different pharmacotherapies which synergistically relax smooth muscle in the corpora cavernosa. Typical components include papaverine (a benzylisoquinoline opium alkaloid with general vasodilatory properties), alprostadil (prostaglandin E1, a vasodilatory agent), and phentolamine (an α-adrenergic receptor inhibitor).

Side effects:
- Contraindications: history of priapism, psychologic instability, severe coagulopathy, reduced manual dexterity, concurrent use of MAOIs (which may cause hypertensive crisis if an α-adrenergic agonist is used to reverse priapism)
- Alprostadil: pain at injection site
- Papaverine: priapism, penile fibrosis
- Phentolamine: systemic hypotension, reflex tachycardia, nausea

Testosterone

Indications:
- Hypogonadism, often manifest in aging males by testosterone deficiency syndrome (loss of energy, decreased libido, lack of motivation, irritability) associated with decreased serum total testosterone levels
- Delayed puberty

Mechanism:
- Testosterone is the primary male androgen necessary for the development of male sexual organs (i.e., prostate, seminal vesicles, scrotum, and penis). Testosterone level is important for many processes in the male, including erectile function, libido, mood, energy level, muscle mass, and bone mass.

Side effects:
- Contraindication: prostate cancer or breast cancer
- Fluid retention
- Gynecomastia (due to aromatization to estrogens)
- Polycythemia
- It is unknown whether long-term testosterone therapy is associated with increased risk of prostate cancer or BPH

Index

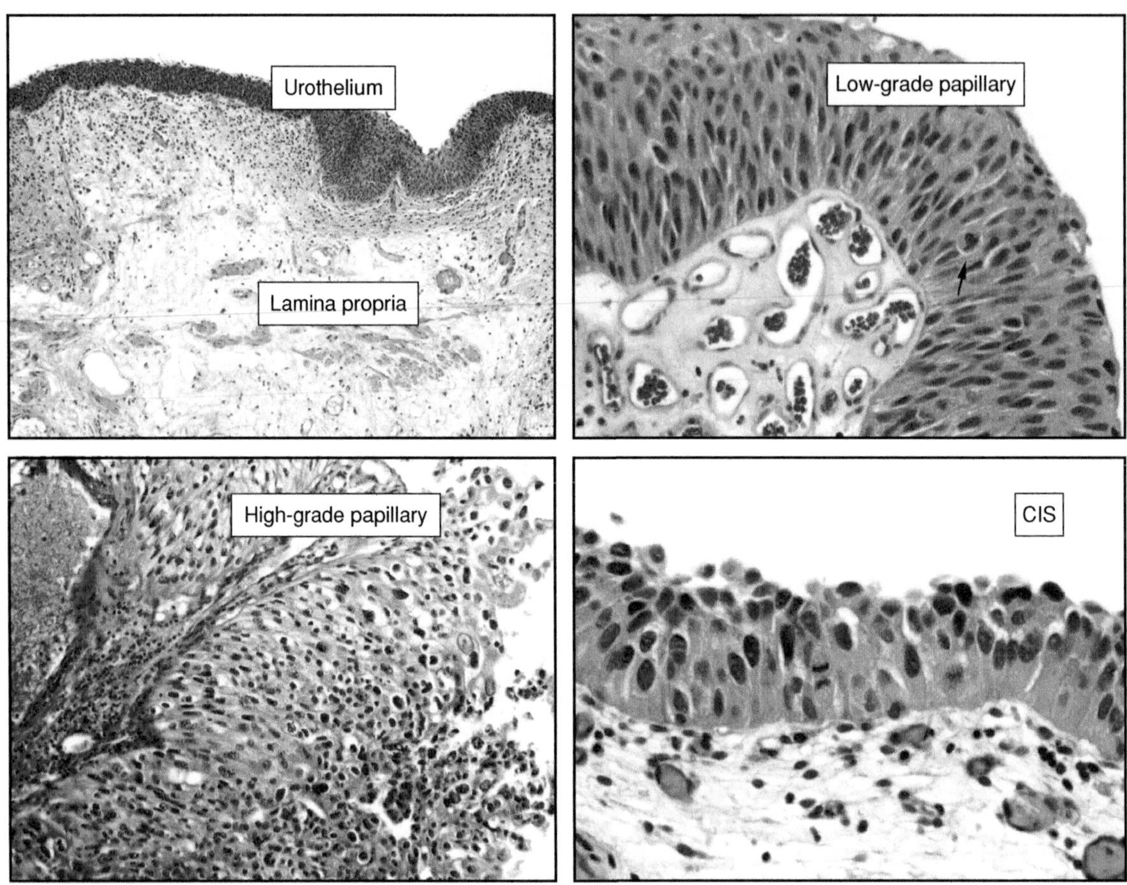

Plate 20.1 Micrographs demonstrating normal bladder (top left), low- and high-grade transitional cell carcinoma and carcinoma *in situ*.

Printed and bound by CPI Group (UK) Ltd, Croydon, CR0 4YY
27/10/2024
14580144-0005